Interpersonal Relationships and Health

INTERPERSONAL RELATIONSHIPS AND HEALTH

Social and Clinical Psychological Mechanisms

Edited by Christopher R. Agnew
  and
Susan C. South

3RD PURDUE SYMPOSIUM ON PSYCHOLOGICAL SCIENCES

OXFORD
UNIVERSITY PRESS

2081855

MAR 29 2016

OXFORD
UNIVERSITY PRESS

Oxford University Press is a department of the University of
Oxford. It furthers the University's objective of excellence in research,
scholarship, and education by publishing worldwide.

Oxford   New York
Auckland   Cape Town   Dar es Salaam   Hong Kong   Karachi
Kuala Lumpur   Madrid   Melbourne   Mexico City   Nairobi
New Delhi   Shanghai   Taipei   Toronto

With offices in
Argentina   Austria   Brazil   Chile   Czech Republic   France   Greece
Guatemala   Hungary   Italy   Japan   Poland   Portugal   Singapore
South Korea   Switzerland   Thailand   Turkey   Ukraine   Vietnam

Oxford is a registered trademark of Oxford University Press
in the UK and certain other countries.

Published in the United States of America by
Oxford University Press
198 Madison Avenue, New York, NY 10016

Library of Congress Cataloging-in-Publication Data
Interpersonal relationships and health: social and clinical psychological mechanisms / edited by
Christopher R. Agnew and Susan C. South.
    p. ; cm.
Includes bibliographical references and index.
ISBN 978–0–19–993663–2 (alk. paper)
I. Agnew, Christopher Rolfe, editor of compilation.   II. South, Susan C., editor of compilation.
[DNLM: 1. Psychoneuroimmunology.   2. Health.   3. Immune System Phenomena.
4. Interpersonal Relations. WL 103.7]
616.024
RC346.5—dc23
2014000743

9 8 7 6 5 4 3 2 1
Printed in the United States of America
on acid-free paper

CONTENTS

PREFACE

Relationships are ubiquitous in daily life. Not surprisingly, then, they have been the focus of intensive research, both with respect to their own underlying mechanisms but also regarding the extent to which they impact a number of consequential outcomes.

This project arises out of a recent explosion of interest, across multiple academic and research fields, in the ways that interpersonal relationships affect health and well-being. The current volume brings together leading scholars in social and clinical psychology, public health, medicine, and sociology to consider theoretical and empirical issues relevant to understanding the mechanisms linking close relationship processes with mental/physical health.

This book emerged as the result of the Third Purdue Symposium on Psychological Sciences (PSPS), held on the West Lafayette, Indiana, campus of Purdue University in May of 2012. PSPS would not have been possible without financial support from the estate of James V. Bradley. We are grateful for this support as we are of the support of Erica Wilson at Purdue and of Abby Gross at Oxford University Press.

Christopher R. Agnew
Susan C. South

CONTRIBUTORS

Christopher R. Agnew
Department of Psychological Sciences
Purdue University
West Lafayette, Indiana

Carolynne E. Baron
Department of Psychology
University of Utah
Salt Lake City, Utah

Steven R. H. Beach
Department of Psychology
University of Georgia
Athens, Georgia

Catherine M. Caska
Department of Psychology
University of Utah
Salt Lake City, Utah

Rebecca Y. M. Cheung
Department of Psychology
University of Notre Dame
South Bend, Indiana

M. Lynne Cooper
Department of Psychological Sciences
University of Missouri, Columbia
Columbia, Missouri

E. Mark Cummings
Department of Psychology
University of Notre Dame
South Bend, Indiana

J. Dennis Fortenberry
Section of Adolescent Medicine
Indiana University School of Medicine
Indianapolis, Indiana

Melissa M. Franks
Department of Human Development
    and Family Studies
Purdue University
West Lafayette, Indiana

Karen Hasselmo
Department of Psychology
University of Arizona
Tucson, Arizona

Rachel C. Hemphill
Department of Psychology
Kent State University
Kent, Ohio

Devon J. Hensel
Department of Sociology
Indiana University-Purdue University
    Indianapolis
Indianapolis, Indiana

James Iveniuk
Department of Sociology
The University of Chicago
Chicago, Illinois

Elizabeth Keneski
Department of Human Development
and Family Sciences
The University of Texas at Austin
Austin, Texas

Kalsea J. Koss
Department of Psychology
University of Notre Dame
South Bend, Indiana

Edward O. Laumann
Department of Sociology
The University of Chicago
Chicago, Illinois

Timothy J. Loving
Department of Human Development
and Family Sciences
The University of Texas at Austin
Austin, Texas

Christopher M. Murphy
Department of Psychology
University of Maryland,
Baltimore County
Baltimore, Maryland

Widyasita Nojopranoto
Department of Psychology
University of Arizona
Tucson, Arizona

Amber E. Q. Norwood
Department of Psychology
University of Maryland,
Baltimore County
Baltimore, Maryland

Gina M. Poole
Department of Psychology
University of Maryland,
Baltimore County
Baltimore, Maryland

Karen S. Rook
Department of Psychology and Social
Behavior
University of California at Irvine
Irvine, California

David A. Sbarra
Department of Psychology
University of Arizona
Tucson, Arizona

Richard B. Slatcher
Department of Psychology
Wayne State University
Detroit, Michigan

Timothy W. Smith
Department of Psychology
University of Utah
Salt Lake City, Utah

Susan C. South
Department of Psychological Sciences
Purdue University
West Lafayette, Indiana

Mary Ann Parris Stephens
Department of Psychology
Kent State University
Kent, Ohio

Linda J. Waite
Department of Sociology
The University of Chicago
Chicago, Illinois

Ruixue Zhaoyang
Department of Psychological Sciences
University of Missouri, Columbia
Columbia, Missouri

PART ONE
Introduction

Interpersonal Relationships and Health

Where the Social and Clinical Converge

CHRISTOPHER R. AGNEW AND SUSAN C. SOUTH

D o relationships between people influence physical and/or mental health? There is considerable evidence to suggest that the answer to this simple question is a resounding "yes." Recent years have witnessed burgeoning attention to the question and attempts at answers (e.g., Holt-Lunstad, Smith, & Layton, 2010; Newman & Roberts, 2013; Sbarra, Law, & Portley, 2011; Shor, Roelfs, Bugyi, & Schwartz, 2012). But, as is often the case with seemingly simple questions, it turns out the question is not so simple. There are numerous debated issues tucked within every aspect of the question. For instance, what is meant by relationships between people? Does any interpersonal relationship, of any degree of closeness, influence health? What constitutes influence on health, and can it truly be disentangled from mere association between health-related variables? Furthermore, given how many centuries have passed since Descartes, why are "physical and/or mental" health treated in the question as if they are separate entities? Moreover, why not flip the causation implied in the question—that relationships cause changes in health—and focus on the opposite ordering, as there would seem little doubt that health can also influence relationships?

The current volume attempts to dig deep into the seemingly simple question and its attendant offspring queries, focusing particular attention on the extensive and exciting research currently being conducted by social and clinical psychologists on the general topic of interpersonal relationships and health. As is evidenced throughout this book, social and clinical psychologists at times appear to be like the proverbial blind men trying to make sense of an elephant: working on parts of the question and, accordingly, being unable at times to discern the whole. The chapters collected here reflect what is known about the interplay between interpersonal relationships and health from two "camps" whose literature does not intermingle as much as one might suspect or hope. Although it may not restore sight to the blind, this volume attempts to bridge the awareness gap between the significant social and clinical psychological literatures on relationships and health, bringing them together here for consideration, to mutual advantage.

SOCIAL AND CLINICAL PSYCHOLOGICAL MECHANISMS AND HEALTH

Relationships are, by definition, social, as they involve more than one person. Social psychologists who are interested in interpersonal relationships have concentrated their research efforts on understanding decidedly relational topics, often guided by overarching theoretical frameworks developed to direct research in this realm, including evolutionary theory (e.g., Kenrick & Trost, 2000), attachment theory (e.g., Hazan & Shaver, 1994), and interdependence theory (e.g., Holmes, 2004). Irrespective of theoretical orientation, there is little question that health-relevant issues constitute an increasing focus of attention among social relationship researchers, albeit not generally the main focus. Those guided by evolutionary theory might, for example, generate and test hypotheses focused on gender differences in sexual behavior (Buss & Schmitt, 1993). Preference for particular contraceptive methods within heterosexual couples (including use of no method) is one such topic of interest and it has clear relevance to health, but more often than not the emphasis among relational scholars has been on theory-driven hypothesis testing as opposed to a principal concern with health outcomes per se.

Similarly, attachment theory proponents focus on the mental models of self and others that individuals develop beginning early in life and how these models influence a host of outcomes throughout life, including relational and health-oriented outcomes (Mikulincer & Shaver, 2007). Those who are characterized by a high level of attachment anxiety, for example, have been shown to have higher autonomic responses in interpersonal situations, a finding with obvious health implications (Fox & Hane, 2008). Yet the emphasis over the years has been more on understanding relational behavior (e.g., interaction patterns) and less so on connections with health outcomes. Similarly, interdependence theory adherents are concerned with how the structure of interpersonal situations influences cognition, affect, and behavior, including those related to health. Again, however, the emphasis has been centered on theory testing, with health used as a topic in which to advance theoretical arguments, and not to necessarily illuminate our understanding of health processes.

Attention among social psychologists has also focused on how interpersonal relationships initially form (e.g., Sprecher, Wenzel, & Harvey, 2008), are maintained (Canary & Dainton, 2003; Gaines & Agnew, 2003), and, often times, dissolve (e.g., Fine & Harvey, 2006; VanderDrift, Agnew, & Wilson, 2009). Those with interests at the intersection of relationships and health have ample opportunities to examine their interplay at each of these junctures, as each stage of a relationship may have implications for physical and mental health. For instance, relationship initiation involves some degree of personal risk. Some people are more likely to "put themselves out there" to make a new connection, while others find that attempting to establish a new relationship generates excessive anxiety, an emotional response that can have negative health implications (Watson & Pennebaker, 1989).

It is not particularly surprising to find that social psychologists who study interpersonal relationships and who delve into associated health issues have been more focused on developing and testing theoretical propositions concerning relationships. Part of this emphasis lies with their own academic interests and part may lie within their lack of systematic training on biological systems. As knowledge about the biology of relationships has flourished in recent years, however, an increasing number of social researchers are integrating biological components into their understanding (and models) of dyadic processes. The roles of genetics, epigenetics, and hormones, for example, have been of increasing interest among relationship researchers, both social (e.g., Slatcher & Robles, 2012) and clinical (e.g., South & Krueger, 2013).

Clinical psychologists with an interest in relationships often focus on problematic interactions between people (e.g., between members of a married couple, between a parent and his or her child). The emphasis has been on understanding relational processes with an orientation toward amelioration of problematic behavior patterns (e.g., Snyder, Heyman, & Haynes, 2005). Intervention implications and/or approaches are of interest. As in social psychology, theoretical developments are emphasized but often with an eye toward implications for treatment. For instance, the theoretical emphasis on acceptance and mindfulness that has found prominence in cognitive and behavioral therapies (Hayes, Follette, & Linehan, 2004) is now a key part of couple interventions (e.g., Christensen, Atkins, Baucom, & Yi, 2010).

There has been less emphasis in the clinical psychology tradition on the application of marital intervention to ameliorate physical health problems. But paralleling the rise in health psychology and the fact that many clinical psychologists find themselves working, at least in part, in medical settings, more and more clinical psychology research has turned to an examination of how partner and family relationships can impact physical health outcomes. As just one example, researchers from Iowa State found that relationship quality moderated the effect of hostility on self-reported physical health outcomes (Guyll, Cutrona, Burzette, & Russell, 2010).

The other main focus of clinical psychological research on relationships and health has been on the interplay between mental health and relationship functioning. As mentioned earlier, the direction of this effect is not as simple as to say that dysfunctional relationships lead to mental illness (e.g., Whisman & Bruce, 1999) or that mental illness leads to disrupted interpersonal relationships (e.g., Coyne, 1976); the truth is probably somewhere in the middle, that there is a bidirectional influence between the two. More work is needed to understand the ways in which stressful and dysfunctional interpersonal relationships can trigger mental illness and vice versa. In contrast to social psychological work, more theory may be useful here as a way to guide research in this area, in addition to examining the mediating and moderating role of explanatory variables at the individual (e.g., personality), couple (e.g., communication), and environmental (e.g., socioeconomic status) level.

OVERVIEW OF THIS VOLUME

Using interpersonal relationships as a venue for theoretical development or for ameliorating problematic individual behavior is what brings social and clinical psychology together. The authors whose work is presented in this volume share a common belief in the importance of relationships in accounting for myriad health outcomes. This volume is organized into overarching but interrelated sections. We begin with a focus on the biology of interpersonal relationships. The emergence of the study of relational factors in the realm of psychoneuroimmunology (PNI) is the focus of the opening chapter by Tim Loving and Elizabeth Kenecki. Loving and Kenecki describe early research efforts at the nexus of biology and relationships, including pioneering work by Ishigami, Solomon, Moos, Ader, and Cohen that set the stage for modern research efforts in PNI. Ingenious work by Kiecolt-Glaser, Glaser, and colleagues connecting social interaction with immune system activity provides compelling evidence of how relationships can influence physical outcomes. Loving and Kenecki point out that relationship researchers have much to contribute to the work of biologically oriented research psychologists. What is happening behaviorally and psychologically in a person deserves the same degree of focus as the physical. For example, understanding the human physiological stress response would be furthered by considering the social context and relational factors that may give rise to it. They also suggest that far too often undifferentiated "stress" is highlighted by psychoneuroimmunologists, to the exclusion of a comprehensive understanding of the psychological and relational: "despite the clear complexities and complex characteristics of social relationships, summaries of psychoneuroimmunology tend to overgeneralize the 'psycho' in the term as simply reflecting *stress*. . . while all too often portraying the neuroimmunological component of the field as far more complex and nuanced" (this volume, p. 21). They further note that a corresponding oversight among relationship researchers is also true: Relationship researchers, particularly those guided by attachment theory, could benefit enormously by integrating PNI approaches in their work.

Of all the physical systems that may be influenced by interpersonal factors, certainly the cardiovascular system has featured prominently in research efforts over the years. In Chapter 2, Tim Smith, Carolynne Baron, and Catherine Caska provide a comprehensive summary of research connecting social relationships and cardiovascular health, delineating various models, methods, and mechanisms connecting close relationships and diseases of the cardiovascular system. They detail in particular the cardiovascular benefits of marriage and consider how close pair relationships can influence heart health. Marital quality, whether assessed dimensionally or categorically, is a significant predictor of cardiovascular disease. Moreover, individual differences in dyadic behavior evidenced by couple members are known to have the ability to positively or negatively influence the cardiovascular system. The authors provide a useful review of efforts to understand the effects that relationships can have on neuroendocrine responses, metabolic syndrome, and parasympathetic responses.

Beyond the couple relationship, relationships among family members are also characterized by both strongly positive and strongly negative thoughts, emotions, and interactions. Perhaps more than any other people, family members have the ability to both induce and buffer personally felt stress. In Chapter 3, Richard Slatcher focuses on the role of the hormone cortisol in stressful daily family interactions. Cortisol, often referred to as the stress hormone, is produced by the body to help ready it to respond to perceived stressful situations. However, greater total cortisol output is taxing on the body and has been linked to a number of poor health outcomes, including reduced immune functioning, increased inflammation, greater probability of cardiovascular disease, and increased likelihood of mortality. Slatcher reviews the literature linking everyday family life to daily cortisol production and provides an overview of his exciting research on the role of family life in children's cortisol production and links to chronic conditions such as asthma.

Ongoing close interpersonal relationships are the context for both significant "ups" and "downs," with attendant impact on health processes and outcomes. The end of a relationship, however, can also have a marked influence on health. Relationship dissolution has been described as one of the most stressful of life events, with associated cognitive, affective, and conative consequences (e.g., Agnew, 2000). David Sbarra, Widyasita Nojopranoto, and Karen Hasselmo detail the associations between the end of a marriage and various health outcomes from multiple perspectives (see Chapter 4). Combining a review of work in social epidemiology with findings from social psychophysiology, they provide a rich overview of what is known about the effects of relationship termination on health. They also describe their own efforts to use extant epidemiological findings to guide more mechanistic lab studies rooted in psychological science. Such efforts are likely to provide critical insights going forward regarding how precisely relationship termination influences health outcomes.

The next section of this volume focuses less on biology and more on marital, family, and social processes and their influence on health and well-being. The initial chapter in this section (Chapter 5) looks at how a relatively healthy individual can influence a chronic physical illness faced by a partner. Mary Ann Parris Stephens, Rachel Hemphill, Karen Rook, and Melissa Franks describe how chronic illness may best be characterized as a couple problem rather than as a problem faced only by the person suffering the illness. They focus on diabetes and the significant lifestyle changes required to keep this chronic condition under control. Both self-regulatory and social-regulatory processes are at play in adopting the health practices necessitated by the condition. These authors describe their work on the Couples Coping With Diabetes project and the 2-Partner Diabetes Management project, exemplifying how relationships can influence health outcomes *and* vice versa.

Just as physical illness can be influenced by close partners, so, too, can mental illness. One mental illness with particularly pernicious effects is depression. In Chapter 6, Steve Beach describes how relationship partners and family members can influence the onset and course of depression. Building on his well-known marital discord model (Beach, Sandeen, & O'Leary, 1990), Beach presents a broadened version of this social-contextual model, named the couple and family discord model of depression, with application beyond the marital dyad to include nonmarital romantic pairs and parenting relationships. He also describes his recent efforts to include genetic and epigenetic research into the model. Beach notes how the new model both furthers theoretical understanding of depression and gives direction to new approaches to treatment: "Remaining open to diverse pathways and incorporating both behavioral processes (such as stress generation) and biological processes (such as gene methylation) has the potential to identify ways in which biological and behavioral pathways may reinforce each other or interact, thereby identifying new directions for both prevention of depression and stimulating the development of new interventions designed to help those already experiencing a depressive episode" (this volume, p. 150). Beach's work epitomizes how relationships and mental health are intertwined and mutually reinforcing.

Although relationships can be the venue for the most positive of interpersonal experiences, they can also feature some of the most disturbing (e.g., Cupach & Spitzberg, 2011). The negative health effects of physical violence are readily apparent, but both the frequency and severity of such violence among intimately involved partners are alarmingly high and at least somewhat surprising: It seems to defy logic that a person whom one most cherishes can serve as the target of blatantly harmful acts. In Chapter 7, Chris Murphy, Amber Norwood, and Gina Poole provide a biopsychosocial, social information processing (SIP) perspective on the topic, illuminating the multiple systems underpinning interpersonal violence. They lay out a variety of factors that have been shown to influence SIP in the context of interpersonal violence, including "hostile appraisals of the partner's behavior and intentions, arousal regulation in the context of interactional goals, generation and evaluation of response options, and behavioral enactment processes.. . . In developing prevention and intervention strategies, there may be considerable value in understanding how various contributing factors alter social cognition—that is, to determine the specific mediational processes involved using the SIP model" (this volume, p. 166). They review several recent studies of interpersonal violence risk predictors to illustrate the applicability of the SIP model as a mediational framework for understanding violence within close relationships.

Perpetrators and victims of violence are not the only ones who are impacted by it. Witnesses to conflict can also be affected. Within families, conflicts between parents are inevitable, but often the considerable impact on children in the household is underappreciated. Extending emotional security theory (EST), an attachment theory–derived model, Mark Cummings, Kalsea Koss, and Rebecca Cheung (Chapter 8) describe their process-oriented approach to understanding the causal mechanisms accounting for the association between marital conflict and child (mal)adjustment. These authors describe EST via a helpful analogy: ". . . think about emotional security as a bridge between the child and the world. When family and community relationships are functioning well, they serve as a secure base, supporting the child's exploration and relationships with others. When destructive family and community relations erode the bridge, children may become hesitant to move forward, lack confidence, or may move forward in an uncertain way, unable to find appropriate footing within themselves or in interaction with others" (this volume, p. 181). In addition to reviewing evidence from longitudinal investigations within the EST framework, they also review recent work focusing on children's security in the context of challenging geopolitical environments. Specifically, work with children born and raised in Northern Ireland reveals how group conflicts can influence felt security. Although reductions in prevailing tensions in recent years have been widely noted (e.g., Horgan, 2013), political and sectarian violence has plagued the region for decades and the authors assess its impact on family conflict and, ultimately, children's well-being.

On the other end of the age spectrum, research is also accumulating regarding the health implications of social connectedness among older people. As chronicled by Linda Waite, Jame Iveniuk, and Edward Laumann in Chapter 9, obtaining good data from an older sample has a number of challenges, including ensuring representativeness in sampling, the inclusion of both key psychological and biological measures, and detailed assessment of active social relations. They summarize findings from the National Social Life, Health and Aging Project (NSHAP), a national longitudinal study that successfully overcomes each of the noted data collection challenges. NSHAP also includes a detailed battery of questions related to sexual behavior, an understudied but important relational topic with health implications within this population. The authors are guided by their interactive biopsychosocial model (Lindau, Laumann, Levinson, & Waite, 2003), a model that includes consideration of an individual's (1) "orientation toward health rather than illness; (2) analytic capacity for outcomes of health or illness; (3) parity among the three domains of capital (biophysical, psychocognitive, and social) as factors in an individual's health endowment; (4) consideration of causality and feedback between various types of capital and health; (5) conceptualization of individual health or illness embedded in intimate dyads, the family, or other social networks; (6) interdependency of social and life course dynamics; and (7) the potential of capital inputs to act as assets or liabilities" (this volume, p. 203). Their findings underscore the critical importance of relational factors, at multiple levels, in accounting for a variety of health outcomes among the elderly.

Consensual sexual relations between people represent a true blending of relationship and health dynamics. This may be particularly so among adolescents, who are in the midst of significant developmental changes and are experiencing a number of important life events for the first time (e.g., first coitus). In Chapter 10, Dennis Fortenberry and Devon Hensel describe their research focused on the relational and sexual dynamics within the heterosexual relationships of young African American women. They set out to dispel the outmoded notion that early sexual relationships are casual, unstable, or inconsequential, while also highlighting the significant and enduring health consequences that such relationships can have, including pregnancy and sexually transmitted infections. Their longitudinal investigation focuses on trajectories of three related cognitive and emotional relationship assessments: relationship quality, relationship satisfaction, and sexual relationship satisfaction. Citing simultaneous declines in each of these assessments over time, the authors note that "even in young women with relatively little relational experience, these three dimensions declined in concert, supporting the idea that adolescents bring relational schema to their assessments of relationships.. . . These relational schema and self-schema may help explain how young adolescents assess somewhat ephemeral qualities such as satisfaction, especially with little actual experience in setting expectations for relationships" (this volume, p. 245). For the young women sampled in this study, the strong connections between relationship functioning and sexual satisfaction reinforce the notion that psychological evaluations of one's relationship are integrally connected to physical aspects of that relationship.

Risky sexual behavior (e.g., unprotected intercourse, concurrent sexual partnerships) is nested within relationships and can be considered a product of both individual personality traits and situational dynamics. As discussed in Chapter 11 by Lynne Cooper and Ruixue Zhaoyang, past research efforts have revealed the rather limited explanatory power of intraindividual factors in accounting for sexual behaviors. Although situational and relational factors have demonstrated larger effects, they still tend to be modest, for reasons summarized by the authors (e.g., considering single variables in isolation from others). This chapter focuses on the manner in which personality can indirectly influence sexual behavior via the tendency to seek out different kinds of relational and situational contexts. As the authors put it, "individuals by virtue of their personal preferences and needs selectively seek out certain types of relational and sexual niches, and that these niches in turn shape the individual's subsequent sexual experiences" (this volume, p. 260). Risky sexual behavior (and its attendant negative health consequences) can, thus, be viewed as an interaction between person, relationships, and situation.

We close the volume by attempting to synthesize some of the main points made across chapters. A number of threads serve to integrate the contents of this book, including an emphasis on the importance to health of both the quantity and quality of social relationships in people's lives, the changing demographics of those for whom we collect data concerning their relationships and health, the importance of developing and using appropriate research methods, and the continuing and overarching need for theory as a guide in the hunt for social and clinical mechanisms linking relationships to health. As can be seen throughout this book, much work has been done at the nexus of interpersonal relationships and health, but additional exciting developments are on the horizon.

REFERENCES

Agnew, C. R. (2000). Cognitive interdependence and the experience of relationship loss. In J. H. Harvey & E. D. Miller (Eds.), *Loss and trauma: General and close relationship perspectives* (pp. 385–398). Philadelphia, PA: Brunner-Routledge.

Beach, S. R. H., Sandeen, E. E., & O'Leary, K. D. (1990). *Depression in marriage: A model for etiology and treatment.* New York, NY: Guilford Press.

Buss, D. M., & Schmitt, D. P. (1993). Sexual strategies theory: An evolutionary perspective on human mating. *Psychological Review, 100,* 204–232.

Canary, D. J., & Dainton, M. (Eds.). (2003). *Maintaining relationships through communication: Relational, contextual, and cultural variations.* Mahwah, NJ: Erlbaum.

Christensen, A., Atkins, D. C., Baucom, B., & Yi, J. (2010). Marital status and satisfaction five years following a randomized clinical trial comparing traditional versus integrative behavioral couple therapy. *Journal of Consulting and Clinical Psychology, 78,* 225–235.

Coyne, J. C. (1976). Toward an interactional description of depression. *Psychiatry: Journal for the Study of Interpersonal Processes, 39,* 28–40.

Cupach, W. R., & Spitzberg, B. H. (Eds.). (2011). *The dark side of close relationships II.* New York, NY: Routledge.

Fine, M., & Harvey, J. (Eds.). (2006). *Handbook of divorce and relationship dissolution.* Mahwah, NJ: Lawrence Erlbaum Associates.

Fox, N. A., & Hane, A. A. (2008). Studying the biology of human attachment. In J. Cassidy & P. R. Shaver (Eds.), *Handbook of attachment: Theory, research and clinical applications* (pp. 811–829). New York, NY: Guilford Press.

Gaines, S. O., Jr., & Agnew, C. R. (2003). Relationship maintenance in intercultural couples: An interdependence analysis. In D. J. Canary & M. Dainton (Eds.), *Maintaining relationships through communication: Relational, contextual, and cultural variations* (pp. 231–253). Mahwah, NJ: Erlbaum.

Guyll, M., Cutrona, C., Burzette, R., & Russell, D. (2010). Hostility, relationship quality, and health among African American couples. *Journal of Consulting and Clinical Psychology, 78,* 646–654.

Hayes, S. C., Follette, V. M., & Linehan, M. M. (Eds.). (2004). *Mindfulness and acceptance: Expanding the cognitive-behavioral tradition.* New York, NY: Guilford Press.

Hazan, C., & Shaver, P. R. (1994). Attachment as an organizational framework for research on close relationships. *Psychological Inquiry, 5,* 1–22.

Holmes, J. G. (2004). The benefits of abstract functional analysis in theory construction: The case of interdependence theory. *Personality and Social Psychology Review, 8,* 146–155.

Holt-Lunstad, J., Smith, T., & Layton, J. (2010). Social relationships and mortality risk: A meta-analytic review. *PLoS Medicine, 7,* e1000316. *doi:10.1371/journal.pmed.1000316.*

Horgan, J. (2013). *Divided we stand: The strategy and psychology of Ireland's dissident terrorists.* New York, NY: Oxford University Press.

Kenrick, D. T., & Trost, M. R. (2000). An evolutionary perspective on human relationships. In W. Ickes & S. Duck (Eds.), *The social psychology of personal relationships* (pp. 9–35). New York, NY: Wiley.

Lindau, S. T., Laumann, E. O., Levinson, W., & Waite, L. J. (2003). Synthesis of scientific disciplines in pursuit of health: The Interactive Biopsychosocial Model. *Perspectives in Biology and Medicine, 46,* S74–S86.

Mikulincer, M., & Shaver, P. R. (2007). *Attachment in adulthood: Structure, dynamics, and change.* New York, NY: Guilford Press.

Newman, M. L., & Roberts, N. A. (Eds.). (2013). *Health and social relationships: The good, the bad, and the complicated.* Washington, DC: Amerian Psychological Association.

Sbarra, D. A., Law, R. W., & Portley, R. M. (2011). Divorce and death: A meta-analysis and research agenda for clinical, social, and health psychology. *Perspectives on Psychological Science, 6,* 454–474.

Shor, E., Roelfs, D. J., Bugyi, P., & Schwartz, J. E. (2012). Meta-analysis of marital dissolution and mortality: Reevaluating the intersection of gender and age. *Social Science and Medicine, 75,* 46–59.

Slatcher, R. B., & Robles, T. F. (2012). Preschoolers' everyday conflict at home and diurnal cortisol patterns. *Health Psychology, 31,* 834–838

Snyder, D. K., Heyman, R. E., & Haynes, S. N. (2005). Evidence based approaches to assessing couple distress. *Psychological Assessment, 17,* 288–307.

South, S. C., & Krueger, R. F. (2013). Marital satisfaction and physical health: Evidence for an orchid effect. *Psychological Science, 24,* 373–378

Sprecher, S., Wenzel, A., & Harvey, J. (Eds.). (2008). *Handbook of relationship initiation.* Mahwah, NJ: Erlbaum.

VanderDrift, L. E., Agnew, C. R., & Wilson, J. E. (2009). Non-marital romantic relationship commitment and leave behavior: The mediating role of dissolution consideration. *Personality and Social Psychology Bulletin, 35,* 1220–1232.

Watson, D., & Pennebaker, J. W. (1989). Health complaints, stress, and disease: Exploring the central role of negative affectivity. *Psychological Review, 96,* 234–254.

Whisman, M. A., & Bruce, M. L. (1999). Marital dissatisfaction and incidence of major depressive episode in a community sample. *Journal of Abnormal Psychology, 108,* 674–678.

PART TWO

Biology of Interpersonal Relationships

CHAPTER 1
Relationship Researchers Put the "Psycho" in Psychoneuroimmunology

TIMOTHY J. LOVING AND ELIZABETH KENESKI

The ability to connect with and form enduring intimate relationships with other humans is a defining feature of the human experience. Volumes of data support the conclusion that we are defined by a fundamental need to belong, and serious negative consequences result from an inability to fulfill that need (Baumeister & Leary, 1995; Loving & Sbarra, in press). Consider, for example, that social isolation is predictive of a host of morbidity outcomes and all-cause mortality (House, Landis, & Umberson, 1988); divorce is a risk factor for early death (Sbarra et al., 2011; Shor, Roelfs, Bugyi, & Schwartz, 2012); high-quality intimate relationships reduce risk for negative mental health outcomes (e.g., clinical depression); and frequency of sexual activity is predictive of overall life happiness (more so than is increased money/income; Blanchflower & Oswald, 2004). In fact, a recent qualitative benchmarking analysis revealed the statistical connection between social integration and mortality rivaled the effect observed for other, significant, public health risk factors (e.g., smoking, excessive alcohol intake, lack of physical exercise, and obesity; Holt-Lunstad, Smith, & Layton, 2010). Such findings underscore an important conclusion: Connecting with others and nurturing our dearest, most intimate relationships contributes to not only our psychological well-being but also our physical health.

Despite the clear importance of social relationships for health and health-relevant physiological outcomes, individuals who self-identify as close relationship researchers have generally not been recognized as key players in the study of mind–body interactions. In fact, as we outline in this chapter, within the burgeoning field of psychoneuroimmunology (i.e., the study of psychological, neuroendocrinological, and immunological interactions), the role of psychology has often taken a backseat to the biological components of the field (in terms of the lack of complexity in which psychological factors are conceptualized and measured within psychoneuroim-munological models). But there are some exceptions to this broad generalization. Specifically, in this chapter we suggest that the field of psychoneuroimmunol-ogy (PNI) has been greatly influenced by close relationship researchers or those who make use of the close relationship context to better understand mind–body connections.

We begin by providing a brief history of how the field of psychoneuroimmunol-ogy has evolved over the past 100 years, highlighting the developments we view as most relevant to close relationship research. Next, we review the manner in which psychology is often treated or referred to in PNI studies, and we note the limita-tions of such an approach. Using the extant work on adult attachment and psycho-neuroimmunology as an example, we draw attention to the contributions that can be made by close relationship researchers to PNI more broadly when researchers remain mindful of how their work fits within the broader PNI literature. Finally, we argue that close relationship researchers have a lot to gain by integrating more mainstream PNI ideas into their research projects.

PSYCHONEUROIMMUNOLOGY: A PRIMER AND BRIEF HISTORY

A number of histories of psychoneuroimmunology have been published, all with slightly different takes on the events leading up to the state of the field today (e.g., see Ader, 1995, 2000; Fleshner & Laudenslager, 2004; Kiecolt-Glaser, McGuire, Robles, & Glaser, 2002; Korneva, 1989; Masek, Petrovický, Sevcík, Zídek, & Franková, 2000). What we provide here is a brief primer of the field's history with a special focus on events that are particularly relevant to close relationship research-ers. We first provide our preferred definition of *psychoneuroimmunology* and outline the early beginnings of the field. We subsequently highlight the seminal studies that set the stage for modern conceptualizations of psychoneuroimmunology.

Early Seeds

Psychoneuroimmunology is the "study of interactions among behavior, neural and endocrine function, and immune system processes" (Ader, 2000, p. 167). There are variations on this definition (e.g., Irwin & Vedhara, 2005; Solomon, 1985), but we prefer Ader's because it emphasizes the role of behavior (more on that later). Although the idea that the mind and body have reciprocal influences on one another dates back hundreds of years (Loving & Campbell, 2011), phy-sician and clinical researcher Tohru Ishigami's paper on pulmonary tuberculosis (1919) is often identified as laying the early seeds for the field (Zachariae, 2009). Briefly, Ishigami observed that moods and other mental states could influence the disease course of tuberculosis (Taguchi, 2003a, 2003b as cited in Hashiramoto &

Katafuchi, 2009). For example, he noted that the psychological characteristic of optimism could essentially cure tuberculosis patients. His groundbreaking hypothesis was that "psychic acts" influence immune outcomes (i.e., phagocytic activity) via shifts in glucose and adrenaline. Yet, despite laying out a clear directional (or mediational) pathway between mental states and immune outcomes, his ideas generally lay dormant for the next 45 years.

Picking up where Ishigami left off, in 1964 George Solomon and Rudolf Moos published a paper entitled "Emotions, Immunity, and Disease: A Speculative Theoretical Integration" in the *Archives of General Psychiatry*. They opened their paper with the following:

> Recent advances in immunology, clarification and the psychophysiology of stress, continued progress in the discovery of emotional factors in relation to physical disease and the finding of apparent immunological disturbances in conjunction with mental illness lead to this attempt at a theoretical integration of the relationship of stress, emotions, immunological dysfunction (especially autoimmunity), and disease, both physical and mental. (p. 657)

It was in this publication that "psychoimmunology" was coined in print; however, the term itself had gone public several years prior when Solomon placed a sign on his laboratory door that read "Psychoimmunology Lab." Remarkably (by today's standards), his colleagues expressed concerns about the idea of studying psychological states as legitimate contributors to physical disease (and, thus, had reservations about the laboratory door sign). Luckily for the field, despite the skepticism of their peers, Solomon and Moos proceeded with their investigation of how emotions influence arthritic symptoms (Ader, 1995), which ultimately resulted in their "speculative theory." It is hard to overemphasize just how far ahead of their time Solomon and Moos were relative to the rest of the research and medical establishment. In fact, the publication of their *Archives of General Psychiatry* paper occurred 13 years before Engel formally proposed his (now widely accepted) biopsychosocial model of medicine in *Science* (1977). In other words, ideas regarding the interplay of social and psychological factors with health-relevant processes were certainly percolating at the time but nonetheless meeting widespread resistance. Indeed, it was another 10 years after Solomon and Moos's 1964 publication before the modern version of psychoneuroimmunology finally took root.

Modern Conceptualization

The current formulation of psychoneuroimmunology is credited to Robert Ader, a behavioral psychologist, and colleagues, who discovered a clear, experimentally induced link between the mind and immune function (Ader & Cohen, 1975), purely by what is now characterized as a "happy accident" (Wilson, 1997). Ader did not set out to pioneer a new field of psychoneuroimmunology; rather, he was simply interested in the behavioral conditioning that made people on chemotherapy develop aversions to certain foods. He designed a Pavlovian animal model experiment in which rats were given injections of cyclophosphamide—a stomach irritant (the unconditioned stimulus)—while being fed flavored water (the conditioned stimulus). As expected, rats that continually received the noxious drug often died. But here's the "happy accident": Ader observed that when trying to extinguish the physiological effects of the cyclophosphamide, the conditioned rats also died, even though they were now only receiving the conditioned stimulus (flavored water) without the stomach irritant. The discovery that immunosuppression could be conditioned by external stimuli was revolutionary. Ader somewhat joked later, "As a psychologist, I did not know there were no [known] connections between the brain and the immune system" (p. 168). Subsequently, his colleagues, including George Engel, persuaded him to submit a letter to *Psychosomatic Medicine* and detail his findings (Ader, 2000).

Despite the implications of his study, Ader received little reaction regarding the assertions in his letter. It was not until he teamed up with immunologist Nicholas Cohen (one of the few researchers to be struck by Ader's findings) to publish work on conditioning immune responses (Ader & Cohen, 1975) that the idea of psychologically conditioned immunosuppression received attention by peers. Specifically, Ader and Cohen injected rats with "foreign" cells (red blood cells from sheep) and found that not only did the rats being given cyclophosphamide produce fewer antibodies to the sheep cells but so did the rats who had been conditioned to associate the drug with the flavored water but were now only receiving water (sans cyclophosphamide). Ader and Cohen's work served as scientific evidence, thanks to the wonders of natural experiments, of a mind–body connection. In a classification of his work in this new scientific area of inquiry, Ader subsequently used the term "psychoneuroimmunology" in an address to the American Psychosomatic Society (Ader, 1980), which was followed shortly thereafter by the 1981 publication of the edited volume *Psychoneuroimmunology*. And thus a field was born.

CLOSE RELATIONSHIPS AND PSYCHONEUROIMMUNOLOGY

With respect to the intersection of close relationship processes and physical functioning, most attribute the widespread acceptance of the connection of these topics to the publication of House, Landis, and Umberson's (1988) seminal review linking the quantity and quality of social ties to mortality (e.g., Loving, Heffner, & Kiecolt-Glaser, 2006; Uchino, Uno, & Holt-Lunstad, 1999). This review was groundbreaking, and in many respects it laid out an agenda and justification for the subsequent decades of work linking social relationships and health (one that continues strongly to this day, as evidenced by the work showcased in this volume). Interestingly, in the abstract of their paper, House and colleagues wrote the following: "The mechanisms through which social relationships affect health and the factors that promote or inhibit the development and maintenance of social relationships remain to be explored" (p. 540). In other words, House and colleagues suggested, among other things, that the mediational mechanisms that lead from the quality (or quantity) of social relationships to physical health had not been the subject of systematic scientific scrutiny.

Interestingly, 4 years prior to the publication of House and colleagues' (1988) paper, a team of researchers at The Ohio State University was doing just what the paper's authors would soon suggest. In the early 1980s, Janice Kiecolt-Glaser (a clinical psychologist) and Ronald Glaser (an immunologist), along with their colleagues, began a line of work on the immunological and neuroendocrine mechanisms that link specific aspects of social relationships to health outcomes (or health-relevant physiological outcomes). The body of work that followed, and continues, from their labs sets the bar for how to systematically identify the multiple psychological, endocrinological, and immunological mechanisms that link close relationships to physical health.

One of their first papers on the topic, published in *Psychosomatic Medicine* in 1984 (Kiecolt-Glaser et al.), reported that medical students' self-reports of loneliness were inversely associated with natural killer cell activity (cells which defend against cancer and other viruses; Kiecolt-Glaser & Glaser, 1997), providing one biological mechanism through which quality and quantity of social relationships affect morbidity and mortality. Three years later (and still 1 year before the publication of House et al.'s 1988 article), Kiecolt-Glaser, Glaser, and colleagues' investigation of underlying mechanisms became more specific with their study of women who had separated from their husbands within the previous 6 years. Women who had separated more recently, and who were more attached to their former partners, demonstrated signs of immune downregulation as indicated by both qualitative and quantitative measures of immune function. Interestingly, in a sample of matched, married controls, poorer marital quality was also associated with poorer immune function, forecasting a line of work to be generated by their labs for the next several decades. These two papers are important as they provide some of the best examples of early work that connects features and processes of close, intimate relationships with specific biological outcomes implicated in morbidity and mortality.

Importantly, however, their work up to this point was appropriately characterized as psychoimmunological in that it did not address endocrine correlates of their findings nor did the studies provide an indication of what it was about marital quality, for example, that resulted in immune downregulation. Those additional pieces of the puzzle came into view in the early 1990s, shortly after William Malarkey, an endocrinologist, joined their interdisciplinary research team. They first published a paper on the link between negative marital conflict behavior and poorer immune function (Kiecolt-Glaser, Malarkey, Chee, & Newton, 1993), and they followed that paper with their 1994 (Malarkey, Kiecolt-Glaser, Pearl, & Glaser, 1994) and 1997 pieces (Kiecolt-Glaser, Glaser, Cacioppo, & MacCallum,

1997) linking marital conflict behaviors to endocrine function in newlyweds and older adults, respectively. Collectively, these studies clearly demonstrated that negative behaviors within the marital context, especially hostile behaviors, altered endocrine and immune parameters. What many would argue was still missing, however, was a clear demonstration that these alterations had *meaningful* health impacts. In other words, do the effects observed in the laboratory (or in a Petri dish, for that matter) really matter for real health outcomes?

To address this "limitation" (term used loosely), Kiecolt-Glaser and colleagues (2005) conducted an ingenious study in which spouses were given a series of eight standardized wounds on the volar surface of their nondominant forearms via gentle suction (i.e., suction blisters) prior to engaging in conflict and social support interactions across two separate visits to The Ohio State University's Clinical Research Center. Once again, hostility exhibited during laboratory-induced marital interactions proved culpable; the wounds of individuals in high-hostility relationships healed at 60% of the rate of those in low-hostility relationships (with the effects being more pronounced when comparing the rate of healing following the conflict versus the support interaction). Importantly, hostility was also related to levels of two important proinflammatory cytokines, IL-6 and IL1-β, providing additional insights into the micro-level factors responsible for wound healing and perhaps other morbidity outcomes.

In the meantime, several other labs across the country were exploring the link between social relationships and health via PNI models, albeit in different social contexts. A few of these lines of work have been particularly influential to close relationships scholars. First, Sheldon Cohen and his colleagues made use of a remarkable paradigm in which they exposed subjects to the common cold via rhinoviruses, which allowed them to determine what features of social relationships promote or hinder subsequent development of cold-like symptoms. For example, individuals with lower social network diversity (i.e., the number of types of individuals subjects speak to often, such as friends, family, coworkers, neighbors, etc.) were more susceptible to developing colds relative to those with greater social network diversity. Further emphasizing the effect of relationship quality versus quantity, the number of social ties was unrelated to susceptibility (Cohen, Doyle, Skoner, Rabin, & Gwaltney, 1997). Additionally, speaking to some of House and colleagues' (1988) conclusions and suggestions, Cohen and colleagues identified some partial mediators of this effect (including endocrine function and health behaviors) but also noted that no obvious third variable fully accounted for the social diversity–cold symptom connection. Consistent with the work reviewed earlier, this same paradigm has also implicated the critical effect interpersonal relationship functioning (including those with family and friends; Cohen et al., 1998) has on health outcomes and provided fairly nuanced ideas for specific psychological and social factors that influence those outcomes.

A series of studies by Dickerson and colleagues further highlight the relevance of social relationships, and the emotional or cognitive states linked to social relationships, for PNI-related outcomes (e.g., indicators of inflammation, cortisol).

For example, Dickerson and colleagues (2004) randomly assigned participants to either write about a distressing event for which they felt they deserved blame or write in response to a neutral prompt. Participants in the blame condition reported feeling more shame and guilt post writing and also experienced an increase in receptors for tumor necrosis factor-alpha (TNF-α; an indicator of proinflammatory cytokine activity). In another study, participants were assigned to give a speech in front of a panel of judges, in front of an inattentive confederate, or alone (Dickerson, Mycek, & Zaldivar, 2008). Only the participants in the socially threatening evaluated-speech condition demonstrated significant increases in the stress-related hormone cortisol. In fact, in a meta-analysis of 208 studies that examined laboratory stress and cortisol responses, Dickerson and Kemeny (2004) concluded that the stress-induction tasks in which participants perceive a potential social threat (i.e., a negative judgment by others) produce the most pronounced increases in cortisol (see Chapter 3, this volume). In addition to these studies, loneliness has also received a fair amount of scientific scrutiny. Specifically, feeling lonely has consistently been found to be associated with a variety of negative PNI outcomes (for a review, see Hawkley & Cacioppo, 2010). Thus, beyond the conventional conceptualization of "psycho" as simply "stress," emotions such as shame, guilt, and loneliness, and cognitive states such as social threat play an important role in how social relationships and social dynamics impact health-relevant biomarkers.

OVERGENERALIZING "STRESS"

What the lines of work reviewed above have in common is that they underscore the significance of the behaviors and emotions that occur within the close relationships context for neuroimmune outcomes. Negative behaviors, hostility, social network diversity, shame, guilt, loneliness, and other constructs have all been implicated as key upstream instigators (and, in some cases, downstream outcomes) of PNI processes. Yet, despite the clear complexities of social relationships, summaries of psychoneuroimmunology tend to overgeneralize the "psycho" in the term as simply reflecting *stress* (or, on occasion, depression; Irwin, 2008), while all too often portraying the neuroimmunological component of the field as far more complex and nuanced. Interestingly, as we noted at the outset, Robert Ader, who coined the term *psychoneuroimmunology*, was a behavioral *psychologist*. It should come as no surprise then that he had issues with an overreliance on the broad-based term "stress" in psychoneuroimmunological models and writings. For example, in a 1980 address, he noted:

> . . . there is little heuristic value in the concept of "stress." "Stress" has come to be used (implicitly, at least) as an explanation of altered psychophysiologic states. Since different experiential events have different behavioral and physiologic effects that depend upon the stimulation to which the individual is subsequently exposed and the responses the

experimenter chooses to measure, the inclusive label, "stress," contributes little to an analysis of the mechanisms that may underlie or determine the organism's response. In fact, such labeling, which is descriptive rather than explanatory, may actually impede conceptual and empirical advances by its implicit assumption of an equivalence of stimuli, fostering the reductionistic search for simple one-cause explanations. (Ader, 1980, p. 312)

Ader was concerned with the temptation researchers might have to overgeneralize the psychological component of the field to simply reflect stress. We suspect the root of this concern may have arisen from the widespread use of animal models in the field (which limit behavioral paradigms and more nuanced distinctions of psychological states). Yet, despite Ader's clear warning in 1980, he must have felt that much of the field was still not viewing "psycho" as appropriately complex, for he reiterated his concern 20 years later:

In animals and humans, a variety of psychosocial events that are perceived to be stressful to the organism are capable of influencing cell-mediated and humoral immune responses as well as nonspecific host defense reactions. However, the concept of "stress" permits few generalizations. The direction, magnitude and duration of the effects of "stress" depend on the qualitative and quantitative nature of and the temporal relationship between the immunogenic and stressful stimulation, the primary or secondary responses being measured and a variety of host factors. (Ader, 2000, p. 173)

In other words, it is complicated, and an overreliance on the term "stress" fails to capture that complexity (i.e., as Ader notes, it is overly reductionistic). Fortunately, others in the field have begun to push for more "plausible models" that do appreciate the complexity of human social relationships. This is perhaps best illustrated in a recent paper by Miller, Chen, and Cole (2009) in which they argue that the simple documentation of links between the various components of psychoneuroimmunology has little theoretical value unless those links are shown to matter for clear, objective health outcomes (e.g., similar to what was done in the Kiecolt-Glaser et al., 2005 wound healing paper). Miller and colleagues' paper is a must-read for those interested in the links between social relationships and health, but what matters most for the current review is a subtle aspect of their Figure 1. Specifically, they provide a series of top-down example models linking "psychological" factors to specific disease outcomes via shifts in endocrine and immune function. Importantly, their sample pathways do not all begin with "stress." Rather, they highlight the potential roles of variables such as social isolation, low socioeconomic status, attributional response uncertainty, and social threat perception. Moreover, they suggest that these different socially affected variables likely influence different types of health outcomes as a function of their theoretical relevance to the pathways being discussed (Miller et al., 2009).

This approach to PNI models is an important advancement and one we suspect would make Ader proud. The behavioral and psychological mediators (and moderators) that comprise "stress" deserve the same degree of scientific scrutiny currently received by the biological mediators (and moderators) of clinical health outcomes. It is here that we suggest close relationship researchers have an enormous amount to offer to the PNI field more broadly. Perhaps nowhere is this potential better illustrated than past and current work linking adult attachment to physiological and health outcomes. We now turn our attention briefly to this line of work, as we feel it highlights the opportunities available to close relationship researchers within the realm of biobehavioral research.

ADULT ATTACHMENT AND HEALTH

Adult attachment theory builds on the idea that early-life experiences and interactions with important others contribute to individuals' later levels of comfort with closeness (Bowlby, 1969; Simpson, Collins, & Salvatore, 2011). The varying levels of comfort affect how individuals perceive and respond to stressful contexts (Simpson & Rholes, 2012). Specifically, attachment anxiety (i.e., fearing abandonment) and attachment avoidance (i.e., discomfort with closeness) regulate individuals' stress responses to threatening situations. Given the link between attachment and stress responses, it should come as no surprise that research that has examined the links between adult attachment characteristics and correlates of physical health is, in many ways, one of the more comprehensive areas of close relationship-based psychoneuroimmunological-relevant work (with the exception of conflict paradigms mentioned earlier). Both relationship scholars and psychoneuroimmunologists have employed a wide range of measurement techniques to examine an array of hormonal, cardiovascular, immunological, and other physical health correlates of adult attachment styles.[1] This area of work, however, is limited in that it has generally not taken advantage of all that a PNI approach has to offer. In the following text, we provide a review of the advances in the area of adult attachment and psychophysiology and psychoneuroimmunology. We then argue that this area of work is an exemplar of the uncharted opportunities that await close relationship researchers who are willing to expand the scope of biological parameters utilized in their research.

The notion that attachment dynamics affect physical health originated with Bowlby's writings regarding the physiological regulation function of the attachment

1. We recognize that the field has generally rejected the notion that individuals fall into mutually exclusive adult attachment "styles" or "categories" (e.g., preoccupied, insecure) versus viewing adult attachment as reflecting overlapping dimensions (i.e., anxiety and avoidance). However, for the purposes of this literature review, in which some studies predate this shift in conceptualization and measurement, we will use the terms attachment "styles," "qualities," and "characteristics" interchangeably.

system (1969, 1980). Bowlby proposed that the physical distress caused by separation from an attachment figure motivates proximity-seeking and functions to foster close relationships. Following Hazan and Shaver's (1987) initial application of attachment theory to adult human relationships, it was not long before researchers began to test for potential connections between attachment characteristics and indicators of physical health. Several recent reviews lay out the theoretical developments in this line of work (see Diamond, 2001; Sbarra & Hazan, 2008). Below we highlight a few key empirical pieces that are central to the current state of this area of research in terms of actual (or possible) applications to PNI more broadly.

In many respects, the first mainstream study to link adult attachment to physiological processes was Feeney and Kirkpatrick's (1996) now-classic research demonstrating how adult attachment security and insecurity moderated individuals' cardiovascular reactivity to a stressful laboratory task when in the presence or absence of their romantic partners. Fraley and Shaver (1997) highlighted additional autonomic correlates of adult attachment; they demonstrated that certain insecure attachment styles were associated with increased electrodermal activity when participants attempted to suppress thoughts related to loss (which is closely linked to attachment formation; Bowlby, 1980). These studies are important because they tested theoretically derived predictions regarding the link between close relationship dynamics and physical outcomes, and they demonstrated the relative ease by which researchers can study physical correlates of relationship properties in the laboratory.

In recent years, a number of researchers, some of whom identify as close relationship scholars, have conducted additional research that further explores the link between adult attachment characteristics and health-relevant physiological outcomes, with much of that work focused on HPA-axis functioning as assessed by cortisol. For example, Diamond, Hicks, and Otter-Henderson (2008) expanded on the premise that attachment-oriented distress affects neuroendocrine processes by assessing daily cortisol rhythms in partners who were separated from one another due to business travel. Homebound partners with higher anxious attachment experienced significant increases in cortisol from preseparation to separation. Powers, Pietromonaco, Gunlicks, and Sayer (2006) highlighted "partner" effects of adult attachment as well. Specifically, they found that anxious attachment was associated not only with increased cortisol reactivity after conflict for highly anxious spouses (both men and women) but also for their partners (men with more anxious partners).

In addition to these studies, a search of the PsycINFO, Medline, and Academic Search Complete research databases produced 39 papers that have examined adult attachment characteristics and a health-related outcome (indicated with an asterisk in the References). Although certainly not an exhaustive list, these 39 papers generally represent the types of work and findings on this topic. Collectively, the papers, published in a range of interdisciplinary journals, represent research conducted by psychologists, neuroimmunologists, and the products of interdisciplinary collaborations. Of these studies, nine focus on the link between adult attachment and cortisol reactivity. We briefly present an overall summary of these studies next.

If we just consider those studies that tested associations between adult attachment (as assessed with the Experiences in Close Relationships Scale; Brennan, Clark, & Shaver, 1998) and cortisol, a fairly consistent pattern emerges: both non-relationship-centered stressors (e.g., Trier Social Stress Test) and relationship-centered stressors (e.g., conflict interactions) exacerbate acute cortisol reactivity, particularly for more anxious individuals. Such a finding is not surprising; social situations that are perceived as threatening routinely increase HPA-axis activity (Dickerson & Kemeny, 2004). However, a closer look at the results indicates a wide amount of variability in patterns of findings across studies. For example, several studies reported heightened cortisol reactivity in response to stress/conflict for more anxious men but not for more anxious women (Brooks, Robles, & Schetter, 2011; Powers et al., 2006); other studies reveal no gender differences in highly anxious individuals' cortisol reactivity to stress or conflict (Dewitte, De Houwer, Goubert, & Buysse, 2010; Quirin, Pruessner, & Kuhl, 2008), and at least one other study reported no effect of attachment anxiety on cortisol reactivity (Smeets, 2010). Additional variability is seen in studies that test for *partner* effects. For example, Brooks and colleagues (2011) found that women's attachment anxiety moderated their partners' cortisol reactivity during conflict, whereas several other studies found no evidence for partner effects (Laurent & Powers, 2007; Powers, Pietromonaco, Gunlicks, & Sayer, 2006). Still others have not examined partner effects, although their designs afford such analyses (Diamond, Hicks, & Otter-Henderson, 2011; Quirin et al., 2008; Smeets, 2010).

Collectively, these types of studies support the conclusion that adult attachment is implicated in physiological outcomes, but the divergent patterns of findings and analytical approaches pose challenges for researchers interested in building off prior work. We believe that this body of work lacks a consistent progression; researchers seldom attempt to reconcile how their (potentially divergent) patterns of findings relate to the extant work on the same topic. For example, what does it mean that attachment anxiety appears to moderate cortisol reactivity in some contexts and in some subjects but not in others? Are these simply statistical aberrations or are the findings indicative of something more central? Although each stand-alone study admirably assessed how one set of relationship cognitions and processes influence physiological outcomes in a novel way (e.g., measuring diurnal cortisol as opposed to acute reactivity, or examining baseline, anticipatory and recovery cortisol, etc.), it is typically very difficult to determine what the results mean in terms of the bigger picture (i.e., What psychological mechanisms account for the link between adult attachment and health-relevant physiology?).

At this point we suggest that it is fairly well established that adult attachment affects cortisol reactivity in a number of social and relationship contexts. This is important, as cortisol has known effects on immune function. In fact, many of the studies noted above focus on the health implications of cortisol dysregulation as a rationale for conducting the research, but very few take the next important step that would actually demonstrate those health effects. As the fields of relationship science and psychoneuroimmunology continue to engage in cross-talk, it becomes imperative that we move beyond simply demonstrating cortisol effects and begin demonstrating actual downstream health effects of attachment (or other relationship processes). Several very recent lines of work have done just this. For example, Jaremka and colleagues (2013) tested the biological mechanisms underlying the link between cortisol production and poorer health outcomes for individuals high on anxious attachment following conflict and support interactions. Salivary cortisol assays and blood cell counts revealed that spouses with higher attachment anxiety produced more cortisol and had lower T-cell counts (indicative of poorer immune function) relative to those with lower levels of attachment anxiety. Importantly, these two neuroimmune outcomes were associated with one another, supporting the plausible conclusion that increased cortisol in this social setting decreased specific immune cell counts, potentially undermining the body's ability to fight off disease. In an additional study from the same lab, Gouin and colleagues (2009) investigated the links between adult attachment avoidance, conflict behaviors, and production of interleukin-6 (IL-6, a proinflammatory cytokine linked to a number of age-related diseases). Their analysis revealed that more avoidantly attached spouses had larger increases in IL-6 following a conflict interaction, and these increases may be explained by increased negative behaviors on the part of the avoidantly attached individuals. These types of studies are critical as they provide the basis for the development of much-needed mediational models that incorporate all aspects of the psychoneuroimmunological process. Admittedly, such studies are costly, in terms of time, labor, and research costs. But the payout is substantial. Not only do these studies underscore the importance of key constructs close relationship researchers have spent decades studying, but they also demonstrate definitively that "stress" is indeed an overly broad term. We now offer a few humble suggestions regarding what close relationship researchers have to gain by shifting their research programs to focus more centrally on core psychoneuroimmunological outcomes.

A GOLDEN OPPORTUNITY

Knowledge regarding how close relationships affect health has grown considerably over the past 30 years due to advancements made in the field of psychoneuroimmunology. Interestingly, the vast majority of the PNI work has not been led by mainstream close relationship researchers despite the fact that the close relationship context has taken center stage in many of the human PNI studies to date. We suggest it is time for close relationship researchers, which we define here as those who identify with and spend most of their research hours focused on studying basic close relationship processes, to get into the game. Simply put, close relationship researchers have a lot to offer (Loving & Campbell, 2011). The chapters in this volume are evidence of this assertion. Importantly, in many respects current research addressing PNI processes in the close relationship context has only touched the tip of the iceberg, with conflict and conflict behaviors as well as adult attachment generally representing the majority of what is known about how close relationships "get under the skin." Close relationship researchers have the theoretical, methodological, and statistical tools to take this work to new levels if they remain open to collaborating with those who have more intimate knowledge of physiological processes (Loving & Campbell, 2011).

Promote Understanding of Psychoneuroimmunological Processes

Close relationships are central to who we are as human beings (Baumeister & Leary, 1995). As such, it is not surprising that the dynamics involved in the formation, maintenance, and dissolution of our relationships have profound influences on our overall health and well-being (Loving & Slatcher, 2013). In the decades to come, close relationship contexts will be incorporated more and more in PNI models. Close relationship researchers should be a part of this work because we have spent decades promoting understanding of the various dynamics at play in these relational processes and understand them far better than anybody else. Thus, we are in a prime position to provide a more nuanced understanding of the "psycho" in psychoneuroimmunology.

Promote Relationship Science

In addition to the potential to contribute more to psychoneuroimmunology, greater involvement with these types of studies can greatly benefit relationship science. For example, the research on adult attachment and physiology reviewed earlier has helped to test basic tenets and develop more refined models regarding the development and function of attachment security and insecurity in our day-to-day lives (perhaps not as much as it could for the reasons we note earlier, but it is a step in the right direction). Additionally, considering how close relationship phenomena affect neuroendocrine and immune outcomes (and vice versa) will further showcase the health relevance of close relationships. This is not a trivial contribution, because the more our topic of inquiry is shown to directly influence important biological outcomes, the more relevant relationship science becomes. For example, as close relationship researchers located within a College of Natural Sciences, the authors know all too well how some researchers in the "hard" (we prefer "physical") sciences view those of us in the "soft" (we prefer "social" or "behavioral") sciences. It is not until we start talking about how dynamics such as basic attraction, falling in love, feeling dependent, breaking up, and rumination (all constructs that have received attention in PNI studies) contribute to changes in hormone and/or immune parameters that a glimmer of respect for our discipline appears to develop. Put another way, by leading the charge when it comes to applying our theories, methods, and measures to basic PNI research, we are able to highlight the importance of our discipline to others.

Increased Funding Opportunities and Job Prospects

Finally, there is more to gain beyond the advancement of science and respect for our discipline. As most social and behavioral scientists are aware, public funding for basic research is dwindling. But, importantly, funding for health-related research continues to remain relatively abundant (and is increasing; Loving & Campbell, 2011). Thus, close relationship researchers can take advantage of these funding initiatives to study PNI-related outcomes, which will have the indirect effect of promoting basic relationship science as well. The merging of relationship science with mainstream psychoneuroimmunology also creates more job prospects for faculty and graduate students. Not only does an interdisciplinary background increase the types of jobs for which individuals are potentially qualified, but job search committees at many research institutions tend to be attracted to candidates whose research is highly fundable.

CONCLUSION

The field of psychoneuroimmunology is still, in many respects, in its infancy. Yet, over the 30 years subsequent to Robert Ader coining the term, close relationships have played a central role in providing a context through which to study basic mind–body connections. Specifically, most of the extant human PNI work that goes beyond standard laboratory stressors (e.g., speech tasks) makes use of some aspect of close relationships, although relationship scientists have generally not been the ones pioneering these studies. We suggest that the time is ripe for relationship scientists to adopt a more interdisciplinary approach to their work and to jump into the fray. Such an expanded focus will benefit the field as a whole via theory development, respect gained, and increased funding and job opportunities. In short, PNI researchers have been using close relationships to advance their field for the past three decades; it is time for us to return the favor.

REFERENCES

Ader, R. (1980). Psychosomatic and psychimmunologic research: Presidential address. *Psychosomatic Medicine, 42,* 307–321.

Ader, R. (1995). Historical perspectives on psychoneuroimmunology. In H. Friedman, T. W. Klein, & A. L. Friedman (Eds.), *Psychoneuroimmunology, stress, and infection* (pp. 1–24). Boca Raton, FL: CRS Press.

Ader, R. (2000). On the development of psychoneuroimmunology. *European Journal of Pharmacology, 405,* 167–176.

Ader, R., & Cohen, N. (1975). Behaviorally conditioned immunosuppression. *Psychosomatic Medicine, 37,* 333–340.

Baumeister, R., & Leary, M. (1995). The need to belong: Desire for interpersonal attachments as a fundamental human motivation. *Psychological Bulletin, 117,* 497–529.

Blanchflower, D. G., & Oswald, A. J. (2004). Money, sex and happiness: An empirical study. *Scandanavian Journal of Economics, 106,* 393–415.

Bowlby, J. (1969). *Attachment and loss, Vol. 1. Attachment.* New York, NY: Basic Books.

Bowlby, J. (1980). *Attachment and loss, Vol. 3. Loss.* London, UK: Pimlico.

Brennan, K. A., Clark, C. L., & Shaver, P. R. (1998). Self-report measurement of adult attachment: An integrative overview. In J. A. Simpson & W. S. Rholes (Eds.), *Attachment theory and close relationships* (pp. 46–76). New York, NY: Guilford Press.

*Brooks, K. P., Robles, T. F., & Schetter, C. (2011). Adult attachment and cortisol responses to discussions with a romantic partner. *Personal Relationships, 18,* 302–320.

*Carpenter, E. M., & Kirkpatrick, L. A. (1996). Attachment style and presence of a romantic partner as moderators of psychophysiological responses to a stressful laboratory situation. *Personal Relationships, 3,* 351–367.

*Ciechanowski, P., Walker, E., Katon, W., & Russo, J. (2002). Attachment theory: A model for health care utilization and somatization. *Psychosomatic Medicine, 64,* 660–667.

Cohen, S., Doyle, W. J., Skoner, D. P., Rabin, B. S., & Gwaltney, J. M. J. (1997). Social ties and susceptibility to the common cold. *Journal of the American Medical Association, 277,* 1940–1944.

Cohen, S., Frank, E., Doyle, W. J., Skoner, D. P., Rabin, B. S., & Gwaltney, J. M. J. (1998). Types of stressors that increase susceptibility to the common cold in healthy adults. *Health Psychology, 17,* 214–223.

*Dewitte, M., De Houwer, J., Goubert, L., & Buysse, A. (2010). A multi-modal approach to the study of attachment-related distress. *Biological Psychology, 85,* 149–162.

Diamond, L. M. (2001). Contributions of psychophysiology to research on adult attachment: Review and recommendations. *Personality and Social Psychology Review, 5,* 276–295.

*Diamond, L. M., & Hicks, A. M. (2005). Attachment style, current relationship security, and negative emotions: The mediating role of physiological regulation. *Journal of Social and Personal Relationships, 22,* 499–518.

*Diamond, L. M., Hicks, A. M., & Otter-Henderson, K. (2006). Physiological evidence for repressive coping among avoidantly attached adults. *Journal of Social and Personal Relationships, 23,* 205–229.

*Diamond, L. M., Hicks, A. M., & Otter-Henderson, K. D. (2008). Every time you go away: Changes in affect, behavior, and physiology associated with travel-related separations from romantic partners. *Journal of Personality and Social Psychology, 95,* 385–403.

Diamond, L. M., Hicks, A. M., & Otter-Henderson, K. D. (2011). Individual differences in vagal regulation moderate associations between daily affect and daily couple interactions. *Personality and Social Psychology Bulletin, 37,* 731–744.

*Dias, P., Soares, I., Klein, J., Cunha, J. S., & Roisman, G. I. (2011). Autonomic correlates of attachment insecurity in a sample of women with eating disorders. *Attachment and Human Development, 13,* 155–167.

Dickerson, S. S., & Kemeny, M. E. (2004). Acute stressors and cortisol responses: A theoretical integration and synthesis of laboratory research. *Psychological Bulletin, 130,* 355–391.

Dickerson, S. S., Kemeny, M. E., Aziz, N., Kim, K. H., & Fahey, J. L. (2004). Immunological effects of induced shame and guilt. *Psychosomatic Medicine, 66,* 124–131.

Dickerson, S. S., Mycek, P. J., & Zaldivar, F. (2008). Negative social evaluation, but not mere social presence, elicits cortisol responses to a laboratory stressor task. *Health Psychology, 27,* 116–121.

*Ditzen, B., Schmidt, S., Strauss, B., Nater, U., Ehlert, U., & Heinrichs, M. (2008). Adult attachment and social support interact to reduce psychological but not cortisol responses to stress. *Journal of Psychosomatic Research, 64,* 479–486.

*Ehrenthal, J. C., Friederich, H., & Schauenburg, H. (2011). Separation recall: Psychophysiological response-patterns in an attachment-related short-term stressor. *Stress and Health: Journal of the International Society for the Investigation of Stress, 27,* 251–255.

Engel, G. L. (1977). The need for a new medical model: a challenge for biomedicine. *Science, 196,* 129–136.

*Feeney, B. C., & Kirkpatrick, L. A. (1996). Effects of adult attachment and presence of romantic partners on physiological responses to stress. *Journal of Personality and Social Psychology, 70,* 255–270.

Fleshner, M., & Laudenslager, M. L. (2004). Psychoneuroimmunology: Then and now. *Behavioral and Cognitive Neuroscience Reviews, 3,* 114–130.

Fraley, R. C., & Shaver, P. R. (1997). Adult attachment and the suppression of unwanted thoughts. *Journal of Personality and Social Psychology, 73,* 1080–1091.

*Gouin, J., Glaser, R., Loving, T. J., Malarkey, W. B., Stowell, J., Houts, C., & Kiecolt-Glaser, J. K. (2009). Attachment avoidance predicts inflammatory responses to marital conflict. *Brain, Behavior and Immunity, 23,* 898–904.

Hashiramoto, A., & Katafuchi, T. (2009). Mental state and tuberculosis—Tohru Ishigami, 1918. *History and Opnion.* Retrieved January 22, 2014 from Mental state and tuberculosis—Tohru Ishigami, 1918.

Hawkley, L. C., & Cacioppo, J. T. (2010). Loneliness matters: A theoretical and empirical review of consequences and mechanisms. *Annals of Behavioral Medicine, 40,* 218–227.

Hazan, C., & Shaver, P. (1987). Romantic love conceptualized as an attachment process. *Journal of Personality and Social Psychology, 52,* 511–524.

*Hicks, A. M., & Diamond, L. M. (2011). Don't go to bed angry: Attachment, conflict, and affective and physiological reactivity. *Personal Relationships, 18,* 266–284.

Holt-Lunstad, J., Smith, T. B., & Layton, J. B. (2010). Social relationships and mortality risk: A meta-analytic review. *PLoS Medicine, 7,* 1–20.

House, J. S., Landis, K. R., & Umberson, D. (1988). Social relationships and health. *Science, 241,* 540–545.

Irwin, M. R. (2008). *Human psychoneuroimmunology*: 20 years of discovery. *Brain, Behavior, and Immunity, 22,* 129–139.

Irwin, M. R., & Vedhara, K. (2005). Human psychoneuroimmunology. Oxford, UK: Oxford University Press.

Ishigami, T. (1919). The influence of psychic acts on the progress of pulmonary tuberculosis. *American Review of Tuberculosis, 2,* 470–484.

Jaremka, L. M., Glaser, R., Loving, T. J., Malarkey, W. B., Stowell, J. R., & Kiecolt-Glaser, J. K. (2013). Attachment anxiety is linked to alterations in cortisol production and cellular immunity. *Psychological Science, 24,* 272–279.

*Kidd, T., Hamer, M., & Steptoe, A. (2011). Examining the association between adult attachment style and cortisol responses to acute stress. *Psychoneuroendocrinology, 36,* 771–779.

Kiecolt-Glaser, J. K., Garner, W., Speicher, C., Penn, G., Holliday, J., & Glaser, R. (1984). Psychosocial modifiers of immunocompetence in medical students. *Psychosomatic Medicine, 46,* 7–14.

Kiecolt-Glaser, J. K., & Glaser, R. (1997). Measurement of immune response. In S. Cohen, R. C. Kessler, & L. U. Gordon (Eds.), *Measuring stress: A guide for health and social scientists* (pp. 213–229). New York, NY: Oxford University Press.

Kiecolt-Glaser, J. K., Glaser, R., Cacioppo, J. T., & MacCallum, R. C. (1997). Marital conflict in older adults: Endocrinological and immunological correlates. *Psychosomatic Medicine, 59*, 339–349.

Kiecolt-Glaser, J. K., Loving, T. J., Stowell, J. R., Malarkey, W. B., Lemeshow, S., Dickinson, S. L., & Glaser, R. (2005). Hostile marital interactions, proinflammatory cytokine production, and wound healing. *Archives of General Psychiatry, 62*, 1377–1384.

Kiecolt-Glaser, J. K., Malarkey, W. B., Chee, M., & Newton, T. (1993). Negative behavior during marital conflict is associated with immunological down-regulation. *Psychosomatic Medicine, 55*, 395–409.

Kiecolt-Glaser, J. K., McGuire, L., Robles, T. F., & Glaser, R. (2002). Psychoneuroimmunology and psychosomatic medicine: back to the future. *Psychosomatic Medicine, 64*, 15–28.

*Kim, Y. (2006). Gender, attachment, and relationship duration on cardiovascular reactivity to stress in a laboratory study of dating couples. *Personal Relationships, 13*, 103–114.

*Kiss, I., Levy-Gigi, E., & Kéri, S. (2011). CD 38 expression, attachment style and habituation of arousal in relation to trust-related oxytocin release. *Biological Psychology, 88*, 223–226.

Korneva, E. A. (1989). Beginnings and main directions of psychoneuroimmunology. *International Journal of Psychophysiology, 7*, 1–18.

*Laurent, H., & Powers, S. (2007). Emotion regulation in emerging adult couples: Temperament, attachment, and HPA response to conflict. *Biological Psychology, 76*, 61–71.

*Lawler-Row, K. A., Younger, J. W., Piferi, R. L., & Jones, W. H. (2006). The role of adult attachment style in forgiveness following an interpersonal offense. *Journal of Counseling and Development, 84*, 493–502.

*Lee, L. A., Sbarra, D. A., Mason, A. E., & Law, R. W. (2011). Attachment anxiety, verbal immediacy, and blood pressure: Results from a laboratory analog study following marital separation. *Personal Relationships, 18*, 285–301.

Loving, T. J., & Campbell, L. (2011). Mind–body connections in personal relationships: What close relationships researchers have to offer. *Personal Relationships, 18*, 165–169.

Loving, T. J., Heffner, K. L., & Kiecolt-Glaser, J. K. (2006). Physiology and interpersonal relationships. In A. Vangelisti & D. Perlman (Eds.), *Cambridge handbook of personal relationships* (pp. 385–405). New York, NY: Cambridge University Press.

Loving, T. J., & Sbarra, D. A. (in press). Relationships and health. In J. A. Simpson & J. Dovidio (Eds.), *APA handbook of psychology: Interpersonal relations and group processes.* Washington, DC: American Psychological Association.

Loving, T. J., & Slatcher, R. B. (2013). Romantic relationships and health. In J. A. Simpson & L. Campbell (Eds.), *The Oxford handbook of close relationships,* (pp. 617–637). Oxford, UK: Oxford University Press.

Malarkey, W. B., Kiecolt-Glaser, J. K., Pearl, D., & Glaser, R. (1994). Hostile behavior during marital conflict alters pituitary and adrenal hormones. *Psychosomatic Medicine, 56*, 41–51.

*Marazziti, D., Dell'Osso, B., Baroni, S., Mungai, F., Catena, M., Rucci, P.,...Dell'Osso, L. (2006). A relationship between oxytocin and anxiety of romantic attachment. *Clinical Practice and Epidemiology In Mental Health, 2*, 28.

Masek, K., Petrovický, P., Sevcík, J., Zídek, Z., & Franková, D. (2000). Past, present and future of psychoneuroimmunology. *Toxicology, 142*, 179–188.

*Maunder, R. G., Hunter, J. J., & Lancee, W. J. (2011). The impact of attachment insecurity and sleep disturbance on symptoms and sick days in hospital-based health-care workers. *Journal of Psychosomatic Research, 70*, 11–17.

*Maunder, R., Lancee, W., Hunter, J., Greenberg, G., & Steinhart, A. (2005). Attachment insecurity moderates the relationship between disease activity and depressive symptoms in ulcerative colitis. *Inflammatory Bowel Diseases, 11*, 919–926.

*Maunder, R. G., Lancee, W. J., Nolan, R. P., Hunter, J. J., & Tannenbaum, D. W. (2006). The relationship of attachment insecurity to subjective stress and autonomic function during standardized acute stress in healthy adults. *Journal of Psychosomatic Research, 60*, 283–290.

*McNamara, P., Pace-Schott, E. F., Johnson, P., Harris, E., & Auerbach, S. (2011). Sleep architecture and sleep-related mentation in securely and insecurely attached people. *Attachment and Human Development, 13*, 141–154.

*McWilliams, L. A., Murphy, P. J., & Bailey, S. (2010). Associations between adult attachment dimensions and attitudes toward pain behaviour. *Pain Research and Management, 15*, 378–384.

Miller, G., Chen, E., & Cole, S. W. (2009). Health psychology: developing biologically plausible models linking the social world and physical health. *Annual Review of Psychology, 60*, 501–524.

*Picardi, A., Battisti, F., Tarsitani, L., Baldassari, M., Copertaro, A., Mocchegiani, E., & Biondi, M. (2007). Attachment security and immunity in healthy women. *Psychosomatic Medicine, 69*, 40–46.

*Pierrehumbert, B., Torrisi, R., Glatz, N., Dimitrova, N., Heinrichs, M., & Halfon, O. (2009). The influence of attachment on perceived stress and cortisol response to acute stress in women sexually abused in childhood or adolescence. *Psychoneuroendocrinology, 34*, 924–938.

*Powers, S. I., Pietromonaco, P. R., Gunlicks, M., & Sayer, A. (2006). Dating couples' attachment styles and patterns of cortisol reactivity and recovery in response to a relationship conflict. *Journal of Personality and Social Psychology, 90*, 613–628.

*Quirin, M., Pruessner, J. C., & Kuhl, J. (2008). HPA system regulation and adult attachment anxiety: Individual differences in reactive and awakening cortisol. *Psychoneuroendocrinology, 33*, 581–590.

*Raque-Bogdan, T. L., Ericson, S. K., Jackson, J., Martin, H. M., & Bryan, N. A. (2011). Attachment and mental and physical health: Self-compassion and mattering as mediators. *Journal of Counseling Psychology, 58*, 272–278.

*Rifkin-Graboi, A. (2008). Attachment status and salivary cortisol in a normal day and during simulated interpersonal stress in young men. *Stress: The International Journal on the Biology of Stress, 11*, 210–224.

*Roisman, G. I. (2007). The psychophysiology of adult attachment relationships: Autonomic reactivity in marital and premarital interactions. *Developmental Psychology, 43*, 39–53.

*Roisman, G. I., Tsai, J. L., & Chiang, K. (2004). The emotional integration of childhood experience: Physiological, facial expressive, and self-reported emotional response during the adult attachment interview. *Developmental Psychology, 40*, 776–789.

*Sadava, S. W., Busseri, M. A., Molnar, D. S., Perrier, C. K., & DeCourville, N. (2009). Investigating a four-pathway model of adult attachment orientation and health. *Journal of Social and Personal Relationships, 26*, 604–633.

*Sambo, C. F., Howard, M., Kopelman, M., Williams, S., & Fotopoulou, A. (2010). Knowing you care: Effects of perceived empathy and attachment style on pain perception. *Pain, 151*, 687–693.

Sbarra, D. A., & Hazan, C. (2008). Coregulation, dysregulation, self-regulation: An integrative analysis and empirical agenda for understanding adult attachment, separation, loss, and recovery. *Personality and Social Psychology Review, 12*, 141–167.

Sbarra, D. A., Law, R. W., & Portley, R. M. (2011). Divorce and death: A meta-analysis and research agenda for clinical, social, and health psychology. *Perspectives on Psychological Science, 6*, 454–474.

Shor, E., Roelfs, D. J., Bugyi, P., & Schwartz, J. E. (2012). Meta-analysis of marital dissolution and mortality: Reevaluating the intersection of gender and age. *Social Science and Medicine, 75*, 46–59.

Simpson, J. A., Collins, W. A., & Salvatore, J. E. (2011). The impact of early interpersonal experience on adult romantic relationship functioning. *Current Directions in Psychological Science, 20*, 355–359.

Simpson, J. A., & Rholes, W. S. (2012). Adult attachment orientations, stress, and romantic relationships. In P. Devine & A. Plant (Eds.), *Advances in experimental social psychology* (Vol. 45, pp. 279–328). San Diego, CA: Academic Press.

*Sloan, E. P., Maunder, R. G., Hunter, J. J., & Moldofsky, H. (2007). Insecure attachment is associated with the α-EEG anomaly during sleep. *Biopsychosocial Medicine, 1*, 1–20.

*Smeets, T. (2010). Autonomic and hypothalamic-pituitary-adrenal stress resilience: Impact of cardiac vagal tone. *Biological Psychology, 84*, 290–295.

Solomon, G. F. (1985). The emerging field of psychoneuroimmunology. *Advances: Journal of the Institute for the Advancement of Health, 2*, 6–19.

Solomon, G. F., & Moos, R. H. (1964). Emotions, immunity, and disease: A speculative theoretical integration. *Archives of General Psychology, 11*, 657–674.

Uchino, B. N., Uno, D., & Holt-Lunstad, J. (1999). Social support, physiological processes, and health. *Current Directions in Psychological Science, 8*, 145–148.

Wilson, W. (1997). A new vision for psychoneuroimmunology? *Positive Health, 19*. Retrieved September 5, 2012, from http://www.positivehealth.com/article/immune-functio n/a-new-vision-for-psychoneuroimmunology/

Zachariae, R. (2009). Psychoneuroimmunology: A bio-psycho-social approach to health and disease. *Scandinavian Journal of Psychology, 50*, 645–651.

CHAPTER 2

On Marriage and the Heart

Models, Methods, and Mechanisms in the Study
of Close Relationships and Cardiovascular Disease

TIMOTHY W. SMITH, CAROLYNNE E. BARON, AND
CATHERINE M. CASKA

A growing body of evidence indicates that the central intimate relationship for most adults can confer either risk for, or protection from, the greatest threat to their physical health. Marriage—or a similar close relationship—is a key element in the lives of most adults (Karney & Bradbury, 2005), and aspects of this relationship predict the development and course of cardiovascular disease (CVD) generally, and coronary heart disease (CHD) in particular (Robles, Slatcher, Trombello, & McGinn, 2014; Slatcher, 2010). CVD is the leading cause of death in the United States and other industrialized nations, and CHD is the most common form (American Heart Association, 2012).

The literature on marriage and CVD identifies several avenues for future research on the development and management of this major health challenge. Ultimately, such efforts may identify useful additions to health services that include roles for practitioners in the field of close relationships. In building the empirical base to justify and optimally inform such applications, however, there is a more immediate role for relationship scientists; the next generation of research on marriage and the heart will be more useful if it incorporates current conceptual and methodological approaches in relationship science.

In this chapter we review evidence regarding the association of marriage with CVD and the mechanisms that might contribute to such associations. We also discuss concepts and methods in current marital research that could advance this literature. We conclude by discussing additional directions in research and applications in the emerging science of marriage and the heart. Throughout our discussion, we illustrate the value of current concepts and methods of the interpersonal perspective (Horowitz & Strack, 2011; Kiesler, 1996; Pincus & Ansell, 2003) on personality, adjustment, and close relationships. This approach has the potential to facilitate the integration of research on marriage and the heart with the broader literature on psychosocial risk factors for CVD.

CARDIOVASCULAR DISEASE AND MODIFIABLE RISK FACTORS

The primary sources of morbidity and mortality in CVD involve atherosclerosis, a decades-long, progressive narrowing of major arteries, due to inflammation and fatty deposits in the artery wall (Fisher & Scheidt, 2012). Early stages of atherosclerosis appear in childhood and adolescence, and are common by young adulthood (Groner, Joshi, & Bauer, 2006; Urbina et al., 2009). Atherosclerosis in the coronary arteries advances to cause the clinical manifestations of coronary heart disease (CHD). Each manifestation results from ischemia of the heart muscle (i.e., myocardium), in which oxygen demands of this muscle exceed the supply that is limited by narrowing of the blood vessels. These manifestations include angina pectoris, or chest pain of cardiac origin; myocardial infarction, or death of heart muscle due to severe and prolonged ischemia (i.e., "heart attack"); and sudden cardiac death, which refers to death from CHD within minutes or hours of symptom onset. In the carotid arteries of the neck, progression of atherosclerotic lesions contributes to ischemic stroke. CHD is the more common condition, with nearly 800,000 new coronary events in the United States each year and over 400,000 deaths annually. In contrast, there are approximately 600,000 new occurrences of stroke and 140,000 stroke deaths each year (AHA, 2012).

Several modifiable biologic risk factors account for much of CVD (e.g., blood lipid and blood pressure levels), as do behavioral risk factors (e.g., smoking, physical activity level, diet), forming the main focus of prevention efforts. However, aspects of personality, emotional adjustment, environmental stressors, and social relationships also confer CVD risk. Some psychosocial characteristics (e.g., chronic anger, depression, job stress, social isolation) increase the risk for the initial development of CVD and a poor clinical course after diagnosis (e.g., reduced survival), whereas others decrease such risks (e.g., optimism, social support) (Everson-Rose & Lewis, 2005).

The presence and quality of personal relationships are particularly strong risk factors for premature death generally, and for CVD in particular (Barth, Schneider, & von Kanel, 2010; Holt-Lunstad, Smith, & Layton, 2010). A greater number of social connections or higher social integration, as opposed to social isolation, reduces risk for developing CVD. And among persons with established CVD, social isolation increases the risk of recurrent cardiovascular events and reduced survival. Beyond these structural indicators of social integration or support, the subjective experience of the availability of supportive social ties is similarly related to reduced risk and improved prognosis (Barth et al., 2010; Holt-Lunstad et al., 2010).

ASSOCIATION OF MARITAL STATUS AND QUALITY WITH CARDIOVASCULAR DISEASE

Given the central role of marriage and similar close relationships during adulthood, it is perhaps not surprising that the presence and quality of this particular social relationship are important influences at seemingly all stages in the natural history of CVD. Marital status is a commonly used indicator of social integration versus isolation, and the presence and quality of marital (or marriage-like) relationships is an important source of the subjective experience of social support (Cutrona, 1996).

Being married as opposed to single (i.e., never married, divorced, or widowed) is associated with increased longevity, a reduced risk of the initial development of CVD in general, and CHD in particular, although sometimes this marital benefit is more apparent for men than women (Eaker, Sullivan, Kelly-Hayes, D'Agostino, & Benjamin, 2007; Johnson, Backlund, Sorlie, & Loveless, 2000; Kiecolt-Glaser & Newton, 2001; Roelfs, Shor, Kalish, & Yogev, 2011). The negative health effects of marital disruption (i.e., separation, divorce) and widowhood are well established (Sbarra, Law, & Portley, 2011; Shor, Roelfs, Bugyi, & Schwartz, 2012; Shor, Roelfs, Curreli, Burg, & Schwartz, 2012), but the effects of marital status are not fully explained by these major life events. Compared to the never married, married persons have less risk of CVD and mortality from all causes, although these benefits might reflect factors that influence whether individuals marry, rather than the effects of marriage per se. The benefits of marriage are also evident among individuals who have already developed CHD, where being married is associated with a reduced risk of recurrent coronary events and with longer survival after diagnosis (Idler, Boulifard, & Contrada, 2012; King & Reis, 2012).

The negative consequences of separation and divorce for health in general (Sbarra et al., 2011; Shor et al., 2012) are also seen in the specific instance of CHD. Divorce is associated with increased levels of asymptomatic coronary atherosclerosis in otherwise healthy adults (Smith, Uchino, et al., 2011) and increased risk of clinical manifestations of CHD (Matthews & Gump, 2002). These findings suggest that beyond marital status the quality of marriage is a potentially important psychosocial risk factor. In studies that measure marital quality directly, low marital quality is associated with higher levels of ambulatory blood pressure (Holt-Lunstad, Birmingham, & Jones, 2008; Tobe et al., 2007), which is a strong predictor of later hypertension and other forms of CVD. For example, low marital quality predicts enlargement of the left ventricle of the heart, a change that often occurs in response to sustained high blood pressure and which is indicative of greater risk of serious cardiac events (Baker et al., 2000).

Regarding the association of marital quality with asymptomatic levels of athero-sclerosis before the clinical emergence of CHD, research has produced somewhat inconsistent findings. For example, for men low marital quality reduces otherwise beneficial effects of frequent contact with their spouse on progression of carotid atherosclerosis (Janicki, Kamarck, Shiffman, Stton-Tyrrell, & Gwaltney, 2005). In some studies low marital quality is associated with greater atherosclerosis at some sites (e.g., carotid arteries, aorta) but not in the coronary arteries (Gallo et al., 2003; Janicki et al., 2005), whereas other studies have found the expected association with coronary artery disease (Smith, Uchino, Berg, & Florsheim, 2012). These var-ied findings are somewhat surprising, given the systemic nature of the condition; atherosclerosis in one major location is typically associated with its presence else-where. However, as we discuss later, these varied findings may reflect the differing conceptualizations and approaches to measurement of marital quality.

Reports of greater conflict in marriage and similar close relationships (e.g., among unmarried but cohabiting partners) are associated with increased risk of incident CHD (e.g., fatal and nonfatal myocardial infarction) (De Vogli, Chandola, & Marmot, 2007), although in some studies these associations vary across mea-sures of specific marital difficulties (e.g., Eaker et al., 2007). In CHD patients, low marital quality predicts the progression of coronary atherosclerosis (Wang et al., 2007), greater risk of recurrent coronary events, and reduced survival (Idler et al., 2012; King & Reis, 2012; Orth-Gomer et al., 2000; Rohrbaugh, Shoham, & Coyne, 2006). Hence, inconsistencies in this literature notwithstanding, marital quality is associated with CVD across its decades-long natural history from asymp-tomatic atherosclerosis to the course of established disease.

CONCEPTUAL MODELS OF MARITAL QUALITY AND MARITAL PROCESSES

Most studies of marital quality and CVD utilize a single-dimension approach to the measurement of quality. In some cases, the measures are well validated (e.g., the Short Marital Adjustment Test, Locke & Wallace, 1959; Dyadic Adjustment Scale, Spanier, 1976). In other instances, scales are developed for a given study (cf., Eaker et al., 2007). But in most cases marital quality is assessed as a single broad dimension, ranging from good quality to bad (i.e., warmth, satisfaction vs. hostility, dissatisfaction).

Multidimensional Models of Marital Quality

This single-dimension model is inconsistent with developments in relationship science (Fincham & Rogge, 2010), where evidence suggests that positive (i.e., warmth, support) and negative (i.e., hostility, conflict, criticism) aspects of close relationships are independently related to overall quality (Henry, Berg, Smith & Florsheim, 2007; Herrington et al., 2008; Mattson, Paldino, & Johnson, 2007). Separate measurements of positive and negative relationship characteristics could refine our understanding of the association of marital quality with CVD. These features may be differentially related to disease, or their respective roles may differ for men and women or across the various stages of disease development and progression. Also, various combinations of positivity and negativity could have differing effects. For example, *ambivalence* (i.e., high negativity *and* high positivity) may be particularly stressful (Uchino et al., 2001).

Interpersonal theory (Horowitz & Strack, 2011; Kiesler, 1996; Pincus & Ansell, 2003) suggests that two broad dimensions describe social behavior: *affiliation* and *control*. Affiliation resembles closely the single-dimension model in most research on marital quality and CVD risk, and ranges from warmth, affection, and friendliness to hostility, coldness, and quarrelsomeness. Control describes social behavior as ranging from dominant and directive to submissive and yielding. Together, these two dimensions define the interpersonal circumplex, presented in Figure 2.1. Most psychosocial risk factors are strongly related to the affiliation axis, such that characteristics associated with low affiliation (i.e., high hostility, low warmth) confer increased risk and those associated with high affiliation confer protection (Smith et al., 2010). Further, this dimension of social behavior is consistently related to the psychophysiological mechanisms believed to link psychosocial risk factors to CVD (Smith et al., 2003; Smith & Cundiff, 2011). For example, social interactions that are low as opposed to high in affiliation evoke larger increases in heart rate and blood pressure (Gallo, Smith, & Kircher, 2000; Nealey-Moore, Smith, Uchino, Hawkins, & Olson-Cerny, 2007), and these cardiovascular responses predict CVD (Chida & Steptoe, 2010).

However, individual differences in control are also related to CVD (Smith & Cundiff, 2011). Individuals who characteristically display dominant social behavior have higher levels of coronary atherosclerosis (Smith et al., 2008), are at greater risk of CHD (Houston, Chesney, Black, Cates, & Hecker, 1992; Siegman et al., 2000), and have reduced life expectancy (Houston, Babyak, Chesney, Black, & Ragland, 1997). Further, social behavior (e.g., efforts to exert influence and control over others) and social situations or contexts (e.g., exposure to unwelcome control from others) related to the control dimension alter psychophysiological mechanisms implicated as a link between psychosocial risk factors and CVD (Smith, Cundiff, & Uchino, 2012). For example, effortful attempts to alter the opinions or behavior of interaction partners evoke heightened heart rate and blood pressure responses (Brown & Smith, 1992; Smith, Limon, Gallo, & Ngu, 1996).

This second interpersonal circumplex dimension has been neglected in research on marriage and CVD, even though the perception of excessive or unfair control by the spouse and related behaviors that involve control (e.g., criticism, blame) reduce marital quality (Ehrensaft, Langhinrichsen-Rohling, Heyman, O'Leary, & Lawrence, 1999; Sanford, 2010; Smith et al., 2010). Women and men may

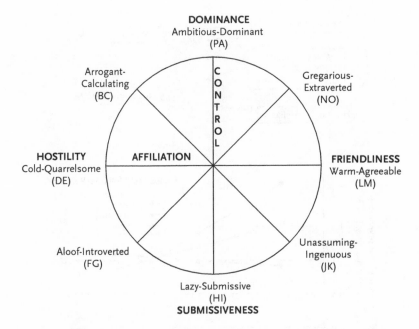

DOMINANCE
Ambitious-Dominant
(PA)

Arrogant-
Calculating
(BC)

CONTROL

Gregarious-
Extraverted
(NO)

HOSTILITY
Cold-Quarrelsome
(DE)

AFFILIATION

FRIENDLINESS
Warm-Agreeable
(LM)

Aloof-Introverted
(FG)

Unassuming-
Ingenuous
(JK)

Lazy-Submissive
(HI)
SUBMISSIVENESS

Figure 2.1: The interpersonal circumplex.

differ in the importance or salience of affiliation and control in close relationships (Helgeson, 2003); women may be more responsive to difficulties along the affiliation dimension, whereas men may be more responsive to threats to control (Brock & Lawrence, 2011; Smith, Gallo, Goble, Ngu, & Stark, 1998). Assessment of both dimensions of the interpersonal circumplex could provide a more detailed understanding of the association of marital processes with CVD.

To examine this possibility, Smith, Uchino, et al. (2011) rated affiliation and control evident in husbands' and wives' behavior during a discussion of a marital problem (c.f., Snyder, Heyman, & Haynes, 2005), generating composite scores for affiliation (i.e., warmth, hostility) and control (i.e., dominance, submissiveness) (Benjamin, Rothweiler, & Critchfield, 2006). In 150 outwardly healthy older couples with no prior evidence of CVD, the behavioral ratings were used to predict the severity of coronary artery calcification (CAC; Pletcher et al., 2004), a noninvasive index of coronary atherosclerosis.

As depicted in Figure 2.2 (top panel), behavioral ratings of affiliation accounted for approximately 6% of the variance in women's atherosclerosis, controlling for a wide variety of demographic, biomedical, and behavioral risk factors. Women who displayed low levels of affiliation during the discussion had more severe atherosclerosis. This first-order effect was qualified by an interaction of wives' and husbands' affiliation; wives' low levels of affiliation were related to greater atherosclerosis, especially if their husbands also displayed low affiliation (see Fig. 2.2, bottom panel). Suggesting a gender or marital role difference, levels of affiliation

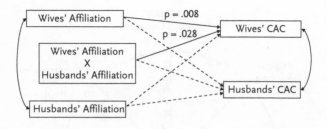

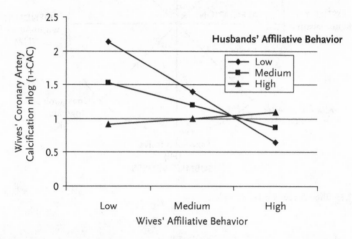

Figure 2.2: Association of husbands' and wives' affiliative behavior during marital disagreement discussion with coronary artery calcification (reprinted with permission from Smith, Uchino et al., 2011).

displayed by wives and husbands did not predict husbands' atherosclerosis—either as first-order or interactive effects.

The coding system permitted separate examination of hostile and warm aspects of affiliation. Wives' and husbands' levels of hostile behavior were unrelated to wives' atherosclerosis. Rather, low levels of warmth during the discussion predicted greater atherosclerosis among wives, underscoring the importance of separate measurements of positive and negative aspects of affiliation in studies of marital quality and CVD.

Ratings of control during the task accounted for about 6% of the variance in husbands' atherosclerosis, again controlling for traditional risk factors (Fig. 2.3, top panel). As depicted in Figure 2.3 (bottom panel), husbands who displayed high levels of control and husbands of wives who displayed high levels of control had more atherosclerosis. These first-order effects were qualified by an interaction of wives' and husbands' control; husbands in couples where the partners displayed very little control had the least atherosclerosis. When dominance and submissiveness were examined separately, submissive behavior was unrelated to disease; only dominance predicted husbands' atherosclerosis. Suggesting another gender or marital role difference, in first-order and interactive effects controlling behavior during the marital conflict discussions was unrelated to wives' atherosclerosis.

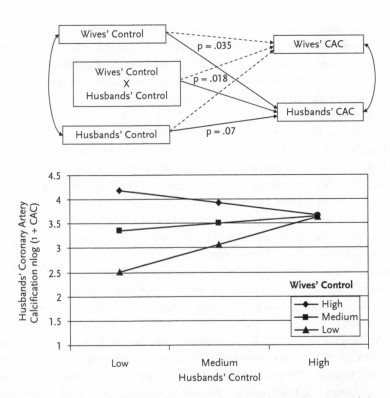

Figure 2.3: Association of husbands' and wives' controlling behavior during marital disagreement discussion with coronary artery calcification (reprinted with permission from Smith, Uchino et al., 2011).

These results suggest that more refined dimensional models of relationship quality may improve our understanding of marital processes in CVD. The interpersonal circumplex calls attention to the commonly studied dimension of affiliation but also control. The common practice of measuring only affiliation could lead to an underestimate of the association of marital processes with CVD in men. Further, measurement of both ends of these dimensions can provide further refinements. Low warmth predicted women's atherosclerosis, as opposed to the "usual suspect" of hostility. For men, the couple's expressions of dominance predicted disease; submissive behavior afforded no discernible protection. If replicated, these findings suggest refinements for future research and perhaps for interventions as well.

Categorical Models of Marital Adjustment

Recent studies suggest that marital quality may be best described as a category. Taxometric studies (Haslam, Holland, & Kuppens, 2012) have challenged traditional dimensional models by suggesting that marital discord may be more accurately represented as a discrete category, with an approximate prevalence of .2 among newlyweds (Beach, Fincham, Amir, & Leonard, 2005) and .3 among married couples generally (Whisman, Beach, & Snyder, 2008). Hence, the Smith, Uchino, et al. (2011) findings might be limited to artificial circumstances in which a dimensional structure is inaccurately imposed on the categorical reality of marital discord.

To address this issue, we reanalyzed the Smith, Uchino, et al. (2011) data, subjecting ratings of husbands' and wives' warmth, hostility, dominance, and submissiveness to a cluster analysis. Unlike taxometric methods, cluster analysis imposes rather than detects a categorical structure. However, our sample was too small to permit reliable taxometric analyses. Across multiple clustering methods, we obtained a two-cluster solution; a smaller (31%) discordant group was characterized by high levels of hostile and dominant behavior, and low levels of warmth (Smith, Uchino, Berg, & Florsheim, 2012). Compared to the nondiscordant group, husbands and wives in the discordant group also reported lower levels of overall marital adjustment and support from spouses, and higher marital conflict. They also reported larger increases in anger and anxiety during the conflict discussion.

As depicted in Figure 2.4, husbands and wives in the discordant couples had greater CAC than in nondiscordant couples, again controlling for traditional risk factors. Hence, in a behaviorally defined discordant group with other indications of marital distress (i.e., more reported distress, stronger negative affective responses to the discussion), husbands and wives had higher levels of asymptomatic atherosclerosis. These two sets of analyses suggest that whether defined as dimensions or categories, marital discord is associated with increased levels of asymptomatic disease. However, different aspects of discord may be important for men and women, and this possibility requires more refined approaches to the assessment of relationship quality in future studies of marriage and CVD.

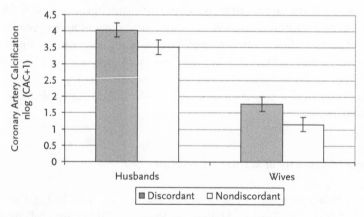

Figure 2.4: Levels of coronary artery calcification in cluster–analytically defined high and low discordant behavior couples (reprinted with permission from Smith, Uchino, Berg, & Florsheim, 2012).

As noted previously, a variety of negative affective characteristics are associated with increased risk for CHD, including depression, anger and hostility, and anxiety (Chida & Steptoe, 2009; Nicholson, Kuper, & Hemingway, 2006; Roy-Byrne et al., 2008; Suls & Bunde, 2005). Some positive traits (e.g., optimism) are associated with reduced risk (Boehm & Kubzansky, 2012; Rasmusen, Scheier, & Greenhouse, 2009).

Each of these individual-level risk and resilience factors is also associated with marital quality. Depression is a well-established correlate of close relationship difficulties and may function as a cause and consequence of marital problems (Chapter 6, this volume; Whisman & Schonbrun, 2010; Whisman & Uebelacker, 2009). Anxiety is similarly associated with marital difficulties (McCleod, 1994; Pankiewicz, Majkowicz, & Krzykowski, 2012; Zaider, Heimberg, & Masumi, 2010). Given the close association of depression and anxiety, it may be most accurate to consider marital distress as related to general internalizing disorder symptoms (i.e., negative affectivity), rather than depression and anxiety specifically (Brock & Lawrence, 2011; South, Kruger, & Iacono, 2011). Higher levels of trait anger and hostility are also associated with lower marital quality (Baron et al., 2007; Renshaw, Blais, & Smith, 2010), and optimism is associated with better marital quality both concurrently and over time (Assad, Donellen, & Conger, 2007; Smith, Ruiz, Cundiff, Baron, & Nealey-Moore, 2013).

Mechanisms underlying associations of individual differences in personality, social behavior, and emotional adjustment with marital quality are described in a second conceptual element in the interpersonal perspective: the transactional cycle (Kiesler, 1996). The transactional cycle describes the dynamic influences between individuals during social interaction. As depicted in Figure 2.5, the model can be adapted to describe reciprocal processes between members of a couple. One member's internal or covert experiences related to his or her partner (e.g., goals, affect, beliefs, attributions, expectations, appraisals, etc.) guide the member's overt behavior toward the partner. These actions constrain the range of the partner's likely overt responses, through effects on that partner's internal experience. Expressions of warmth by one couple member are appraised by the partner accordingly, with related effects on that partner's affect, attributions, expectations, and interaction goals. Typically, warmth has a positive emotional impact and activates affiliative goals and expectations of continued warmth. Those internal responses, in turn, increase the likelihood of warm partner responses and decrease the likelihood of cold or quarrelsome reactions. Expressions of hostility have the opposite effect on the partner's behavior, again through effects on that partner's internal experience.

As depicted in Figure 2.5, exposure to positive partner behavior (e.g., warmth, support) and the resulting internal experiences can prevent or dampen physiological responses that promote the development and progression of CVD, and they

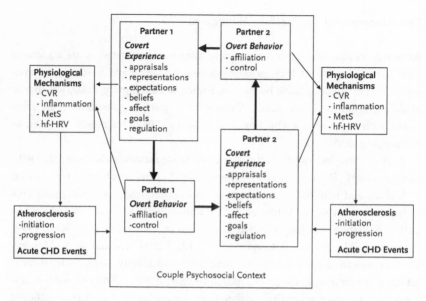

Figure 2.5: The dyadic transactional cycle: partners' covert processes and overt behavior are reciprocally related, creating and maintaining positive or negative dyadic interactions and patterns of relationship quality, with corresponding effects on physiology. CHD, coronary heart disease; CVR, cardiovascular reactivity.

may activate other physiological responses that inhibit disease development. We review these mechanisms later. In contrast, exposure to aversive partner behavior (e.g., neglect, hostility) and the very different internal experiences it encourages can heighten pathogenic physiological responses and inhibit salubrious ones. The individual's own overt behavior (e.g., anger expression, efforts to control the spouse) can also alter these physiological responses.

There are important contextual influences on these transactional processes. For example, low socioeconomic status and stressful work experiences make positive transactional patterns less likely and make negative cycles more so (Conger, Conger, & Martin, 2010; Karney & Bradbury, 2005; Neff, 2012; Story & Repetti, 2006). Once CVD is clinically apparent, the disease becomes an important contextual influence on couple transactions, as they cope with a serious chronic illness. For some couples, the chronic illness leads to positive and supportive interactions; for others the associated strain promotes negative interactions.

A variety of concepts in current research on marriage and other close relationships can be located within the various components of this expanded and dyadic version of the transactional cycle (e.g., adult attachment styles, regulatory processes, attributions for partner behavior, the role of affect, goals, relationship beliefs and standards, contextual factors, etc.). Hence, the model provides an integrative framework describing the range of marital processes that might influence cardiovascular health, as well as their ties to aspects of personality and emotional adjustment that have similar associations with CVD.

In interpersonal theory (Kiesler, 1996), an actor's behavior tends to "pull, invite, or evoke restricted classes of responses" from interaction partners (Pincus & Ansell, 2003, p. 215), in this case a romantic partner. In the interpersonal circumplex, "invited" or evoked behavior is similar to the initial actor's behavior in terms of affiliation and opposite in control. Warmth invites warmth in return, whereas cold or hostile actions invite hostility. Expressions of dominance or interpersonal control invite submissiveness or deference, in return; submissive actions invite dominant or controlling responses. This is known as the *complementarity principle*, but research suggests it is more apparent for affiliation than control (Sadler, Ethier, & Woody, 2011), because unfriendly dominance tends to evoke dominance in return, as opposed to the predicted unfriendly submissiveness. Complementarity in control is more common for interactions that are highly structured (i.e., where clear roles are defined) or high in warmth.

The transactional cycle and principle of complementarity provide an account of associations between individual-level difference risk factors and risk factors primarily seen as involving the quality of personal relationships. Rather than separate classes of influences on CVD, they may in fact represent two sides of a single psychosocial risk or protective process. Yet in most studies individual-level risk factors (e.g., personality, emotional adjustment) and social-environmental factors (e.g., social support, isolation, relationship quality) are examined separately. When studied together, their independent associations with CVD are the focus. Although important, the search for independent risk factors for CVD can obscure the actual influence of closely related psychosocial factors (Smith & Cundiff, 2014). Statistical separation of relationship quality and the emotional and personality factors closely associated with it could produce a less accurate and informative representation of the level of risk and the processes underlying it. In contrast, the interpersonal perspective encourages a more integrative and contextual approach.

METHODS IN THE ASSESSMENT OF MARITAL PROCESSES IN CARDIOVASCULAR DISEASE RISK

A variety of methodological approaches and specific instruments are available for the assessment of aspects of functioning in close relationships generally, and marriage in particular (Snyder et al., 2005). Multiple methods are available for assessing most of the central constructs in this domain, including structured clinical interviews, self-reports, partner reports, and structured behavioral observation procedures. These methods are used to assess specific relationship *behaviors* (e.g., rates and reciprocity of positive and negative responses during conflict discussions; frequency and severity of conflict; degree of warmth and support), *cognitions* (e.g., attributions for positive and negative couple events and partner behavior; beliefs, expectancies, and standards regarding spouse behavior), and *affect* (e.g., frequency, degree, and reciprocity of positive and negative affect during couple interaction; general positive and negative sentiments about the partner and relationship; emotion regulation in couple interactions). The close association of aspects of relationship functioning (e.g., marital satisfaction, marital conflict) with features of individual emotional distress (e.g., depression, anxiety, anger) and maladaptive behavior (e.g., aggressiveness) discussed earlier justifies measurement of these factors in overall assessment of couple functioning (Snyder et al., 2005). Thus, the transactional processes linking relationship processes and individual-level risk factors for CVD are readily acknowledged in current assessment approaches to couple distress.

Compared to the multifaceted and multimethod nature of current conceptual models and measurement approaches to relationship functioning and couple distress, research on relationship quality as a CVD risk factor has been limited. As noted earlier, most studies have utilized single-dimension approaches to overall relationship quality, measured through self-reports. Self-reports that capture only the single dimension of relationship sentiment or overall satisfaction/quality/distress may not capture adequately the variety dimensions and aspects of marital functioning that influence cardiovascular health. As described earlier, measures based on single-dimension models combine the separate positivity and negativity dimensions that could have distinct and varying associations with disease, and those that emphasize only affiliation fail to capture issues surrounding the degree of control in couple interactions.

Commonly used self-reports may have an additional limitation. In the Smith, Uchino, et al. (2011) study of affiliation and control, behavioral ratings of these processes predicted coronary artery disease but several commonly used self-report measures did not, even though behavioral and self-report measures were correlated as expected. This was also the case in the Smith, Uchino, Berg, and Florsheim (2012) reanalysis. The cluster–analytically derived grouping based on behavioral ratings was significantly associated with a cluster–analytically derived grouping based on self-reports of marital quality, but only the former was related to atherosclerosis. The behavioral "snapshot" of marital quality based on observations of couple interactions was a clearly superior predictor. If replicated, this suggests that the most widely used method in examining relationship quality (i.e., self-reports) may underestimate the magnitude of its association with CVD. Behavioral observations are time consuming and expensive, but some individuals are unwilling or unable to provide sufficiently accurate reports of the quality of their close relationships. More behavioral observation studies are needed to determine their predictive utility relative to self-reports.

Behavioral observations may have other limitations. Behavior observed during laboratory tasks predicts important relationship outcomes (Snyder et al., 2005), but they capture responses to analog enactments of relationship conflict discussions that may be less negative and briefer than those in natural environments (Margolin, Burnam, & John, 1989). Behavioral assessments of positive and negative behavior during positive couple interaction tasks (e.g., discussing affection and positive spouse attributes; providing support to the partner) may have independent associations with relationship outcomes over and above the much more commonly used conflict tasks (e.g., Graber, Laurenceau, Miga, Chango, & Coan, 2011). Greater attention to the potential separate influences of positivity and negativity could improve the predictive utility of behavioral assessments.

Measurement of couples' experiences in naturalistic daily activities is an emerging approach to understanding couple dynamics and the influence of couple processes on physical health. Methodological and quantitative methods for examining momentary experiences in the daily lives of couples are well developed (Laurenceau & Bolger, 2005), and these patterns of daily experience are related to the more traditional measures of couple relationship quality (Janicki, Kamarck, Shiffman, & Gwaltney, 2006; Margolin, Christensen, & John, 1996). Daily experience designs have been used to study disease and pathophysiologic mechanisms, both in the context of general daily experiences of stress (Kamarck et al., 2005; Kamarck, Shiffman, Sutton-Tyrrell, Muldoon, & Tepper, 2012) and in the context of couple and family processes (Janicki et al., 2005; Repetti, Wang, & Saxbe, 2011). These approaches can also be used to examine the transactional processes involved in dynamic associations of individual differences in personality and emotional adjustment with marital quality, as depicted in Figure 2.5 (Graber, Laurenceau, & Carver, 2011). Overall, more complete and sophisticated assessment of multiple aspects of couple functioning will be essential in the continuing development of research on close relationships and CVD. Such studies should not only include refined approaches that use the traditional self-report methodology but also make greater use of behavioral observation and daily experience approaches.

MECHANISMS LINKING MARITAL PROCESSES AND CARDIOVASCULAR DISEASE

One benefit of high marital quality is the promotion of a healthy lifestyle (e.g., avoiding smoking, greater physical activity, lower caloric and fat intake, maintenance of normal body weight, adherence to medical regimens). Couple partners clearly influence each other's health behavior (e.g., Hornish & Leonard, 2008), and warm or supportive efforts to influence a partner's behavior (e.g., praise, collaborative problem solving) are associated with better outcomes than are more direct and hostile forms of control (e.g., criticism, coercion) (Franks et al., 2006; Rosland, Heisler, & Piette, 2012). However, marital status and quality predict CVD even when behavioral risks are controlled.

Cardiovascular and Neuroendocrine Responses

Psychophysiological effects of close relationships are key mechanisms potentially contributing to the association of marital quality with CVD (Robles et al., 2014;

Slatcher, 2010), and cardiovascular reactivity (CVR) is perhaps the most widely studied to date. Unlike increases in blood pressure and heart rate during physical activity, CVR during psychological stressors exceeds the body's physiologic demands (Carroll, Phillips, & Bolanos, 2009). For example, during physical exertion increases in heart rate and blood pressure are closely coupled to the intensity of physical work and related momentary oxygen requirements of the muscles and other tissues involved in the activity. In psychological challenges, heart rate and blood pressure respond as if one is preparing for physically demanding action (i.e., fighting or fleeing), but no such strenuous activity is required. The physiological excessiveness of the resulting blood flow and oxygen supply figures prominently in models of psychological stress, CVR, and CVD, and considerable evidence supports this view (Carroll et al., 2012; Chida & Steptoe, 2010).

Compared to appropriate control conditions (e.g., neutral couple interactions), experimental manipulations of marital conflict evoke significantly larger increases in heart rate and blood pressure (e.g., Nealey-Moore et al., 2007; Smith et al., 2009), and measures of marital distress are associated with the magnitude of CVR during such stressors (for a review, see Robles et al., 2014). The effects of marital conflict on CVR are sometimes stronger for women than men (e.g., Smith, Uchino, MacKenzie, et al., 2013), and such effects have been interpreted as reflecting the greater importance women assign to relationship quality compared to men (Kiecolt-Glaser & Newton, 2001). However, other studies using similar procedures find no sex differences (e.g., Nealey-Morre et al., 2007; Smith, Uchino, et al., 2009).

The presence and direction of sex differences in CVR in response to marital stressors may depend on context. The common difference in which women respond with greater CVR than their male partners is negligible or even reversed when the origin of the marital problem discussed is controlled (Denton, Burleson, Hobbs, Von Stein, & Rodriguez, 2001; Newton & Sanford, 2003). Women show greater CVR than men during discussions of problems the women have identified, but not during discussion of problems nominated by their male partners. Also, couple tasks that threaten the affiliative tone of the interaction are more likely to evoke greater CVR among women, whereas interactions involving issues of control or status evoke more CVR among their male partners (Brown & Smith, 1992; Smith et al., 1998).

These sex differences may also depend on characteristics of the couple. Smith, Uchino, and colleagues (2009) asked middle-aged and older couples to participate in a discussion of an ongoing marital conflict issue and in a collaborative problem-solving task, where couples were given a map of a hypothetical town and a list of errands. They were asked to work together to find the most efficient route to accomplish the errands. As depicted in Figure 2.6, the conflict discussion evoked greater CVR than the collaborative task, and husbands and wives did not differ in their response to conflict. However, older men displayed greater CVR in response to the collaborative task than did their wives and as compared to middle-aged couples, a response as large as their CVR to marital conflict.

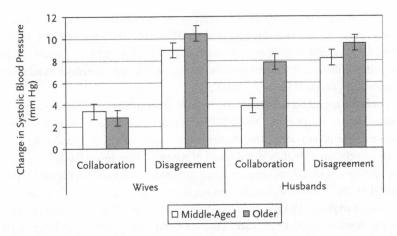

Figure 2.6: Systolic blood pressure reactivity during marital disagreement and collaborative problem-solving tasks among middle-aged and older married couples (reprinted with permission from Smith, Uchino, et al., 2009).

Overall, stressful marital interactions evoke substantial CVR, which could contribute to the association of marital strain with the development and course of CVD. A variety of factors, such as whether the stressor involves low affiliation or challenges to control, can moderate the presence and direction of sex differences in these responses, but stressful marital interactions evoke CVR for both genders. Importantly, low marital quality is associated with greater CVR outside the laboratory, such as those seen during ambulatory blood pressure monitoring (Holt-Lunstad, Birmingham, & Light, 2008; Tobe et al., 2007).

Marital stressors (e.g., conflict discussions) and levels of marital quality are related to other psychophysiological stress responses, such as elevations in cortisol and catecholamines (e.g., Ditzen et al., 2007; for a review, see Robles et al., 2014). Aspects of inflammation are an important set of physiological correlates and responses, given their role in the development and course of CVD (Fisher & Scheidt, 2012). Experimentally manipulated marital stressors evoke such responses and related consequences (e.g., delayed wound healing) (Kiecolt-Glaser, Loving, et al., 2005), and measured levels of marital difficulties are associated with systemic levels of inflammation (Kiecolt-Glaser, Gouin, & Hantsoo, 2010; Whisman & Sbarra, 2012). Depression is similarly associated with inflammation (Howren, Laubkin, & Suls, 2009); this mechanism could contribute to overlapping associations of depression and marital difficulties with CVD.

The neuropeptide *oxytocin* might link close relationships with CVD. In animal models, administration of oxytocin reduces inflammation and atherosclerosis, most likely by attenuating various physiological effects of stress (Nation et al., 2010). In both human and animal studies, oxytocin attenuates physiological stress responses (Carter et al., 2008; Uvnäs-Moberg, Arn, & Magnusson, 2005). There are two main models of this mechanism. In the "calm and connect" model, warm and supportive interactions evoke oxytocin release, which in turn reduces stress (Carter et al., 2008; Uvnäs-Moberg et al., 2005). In the "tend and befriend" model, strain and disruption in important relationships evokes oxytocin release, which motivates affiliation. If affiliative efforts are successful, stress is reduced and health is protected (Taylor et al., 2000, 2010).

Evidence regarding these differing hypotheses is mixed (cf. Gouin et al., 2010; Smith, Uchino, MacKenzie, et al., 2013), perhaps due to difficulties in oxytocin measurement (Campbell, 2010). In the largest study to date, we found only a very weak association of higher blood levels of oxytocin with lower levels of relationship quality in a sample of young married or cohabitating couples. Further, experimental manipulations of positive and negative couple interactions had no effect on plasma oxytocin (Smith, Uchino, MacKenzie, et al., 2013). However, in other studies administration of oxytocin (i.e., via intranasal spray to alter brain levels) increased positive behavior during stressful marital interactions and reduced cortisol responses to such stressors (Ditzen et al., 2009), and warm couple massage increased some indicators of oxytocin (i.e., salivary levels) but not the more commonly used measure of plasma levels (Holt-Lunstad, Birmingham, & Light, 2008).

Metabolic Syndrome

Elevated blood pressure, plasma lipids (i.e., high triglycerides, low-density lipoproteins), abdominal adiposity, and blood glucose (or insulin insensitivity) define the metabolic syndrome, a risk factor for diabetes and CVD (Eckel, Grundy, & Zimmet, 2005; Raikkonen et al., 2008). Chronic stress and high levels of negative affect increase the risk of metabolic syndrome (Goldbacher & Matthews, 2007), and depression is reciprocally related to components of the metabolic syndrome over time (Pan et al., 2012). Marital strain is also associated with greater risk of metabolic syndrome (Troxel et al., 2005; Whisman & Ubelacher, 2012).

Parasympathetic Processes and Emotion Regulation in Couples

The physiologic mechanisms described thus far emphasize sympathetic nervous system responses or hypothalamic-pituitary-adrenocortical activity (i.e., HPA axis). Recently, parasympathetic mechanisms have been described. The resting and reactive functioning of the parasympathetic nervous system can be measured noninvasively through heart rate variation known as respiratory sinus arrhythmia (RSA). At most times, heart rate is under parasympathetic inhibitory control, via the vagus nerve, holding heart rate below its intrinsic level. This inhibition changes across the respiratory cycle, decreasing during inhalation and returning with exhalation. Stretch receptors in the lungs respond during inhalation, reducing or "gating" parasympathetic inhibition, resulting in increased heart rate. Parasympathetic inhibition returns when stretch receptor activity decreases with exhalation, slowing heart rate. Hence, heart rate repeatedly rises and falls, within the range of respiration frequency. Variability in heart rate corresponding to this frequency is labeled "high-frequency" heart rate variability (hf-HRV), and it is quantified to provide measure of RSA (Thayer, Hansen, & Johnsen, 2008). Importantly, low tonic levels of resting RSA (i.e., "vagal tone") are associated with increased risk of CVD and other adverse health outcomes (Thayer & Lane, 2007; Thayer & Sternberg, 2006).

Neural circuits that regulate RSA are colocated in the prefrontal cortex with circuits and structures involved in the regulation of emotion and behavior. Evidence indicates that individual differences in resting hf-HRV reflect self-regulatory capacity, whereas momentary increases in hf-HRV reflect self-regulatory effort (cf. Segerstrom, Hardy, Evans, & Winters, 2012; Thayer, Hansen, Saus-Rose, & Johnsen, 2009).

We recently demonstrated that resting levels of hf-HRV are associated with higher levels of marital quality (Smith, Cribbet, et al., 2011), a finding consistent with other research (e.g., Diamond & Hicks, 2005; Diamond, Hicks, & Otter-Henderson, 2011; Kok & Fredrickson, 2010) and with the view that self-regulatory capacity facilitates the development and maintenance of close relationship quality. Further, in an experimental manipulation of the tone of marital interaction, we asked couples to engage in positive (i.e., discuss the spouses' positive characteristics), neutral (i.e., discuss the spouse's typical daily schedule), or negative interactions (i.e., discuss the spouses' negative characteristics), with a resting baseline assessment of hf-HRV before and after the task. As depicted in Figure 2.7, the positive marital interactions raised women's resting hf-HRV somewhat, whereas negative marital interactions reduced it (Smith, Cribbet, et al., 2011). In contrast, the tone of the interaction had no effects on men's resting hf-HRV.

These changes in women's resting hf-HRV were mediated by the magnitude of their husbands' negative affective response to the task and husbands' ratings of wives' behavior. Women whose husbands reported larger increases in negative

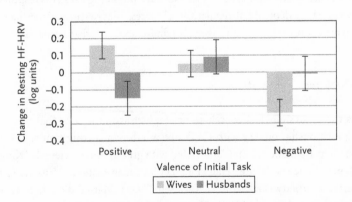

Figure 2.7: Change in husbands' and wives' high-frequency heart rate variability after positive, neutral, and negative marital interactions (reprinted with permission from Smith, Cribbet, et al., 2011).

affect during the task displayed a larger decrease in resting HF-HRV after the negative task. These women may have faced a greater challenge in regulating the tone of the interaction, posed by their husbands' negative affect. Importantly, the decrease in wives resting hf-HRV was not related to the magnitude of their own negative affect response to the task, and the initial negative task did not alter women's negative affect during the second resting baseline. Thus, it is unlikely that the decrease in women's hf-HRV simply reflected their own negative emotion. Women who displayed more directive or controlling behavior (as rated by their husbands) also had larger decreases in resting hf-HRV, perhaps reflecting greater efforts to manage the emotional tone of the interaction. Tests of both of these meditational paths were significant. Women whose husbands reported smaller increases in negative affect (or increases in warmth and calmness) during the positive interaction displayed larger increases in hf-HRV, in another significant mediated effect.

The lower levels of women's hf-HRV after negative interaction could indicate a temporary reduction in self-regulatory capacity, which if recurring could place them at greater risk of a variety of emotional, behavioral, and health difficulties (Thayer & Lane, 2007; Thayer et al., 2009). In terms of the impact of this depleted regulatory capacity on marital processes, it could leave women less able to resist negative complementarity during stressful marital interactions. The resulting higher levels of negative reciprocity could maintain and exacerbate stressful marital interactions. That is, when facing a continuing or new negative marital interaction, depleted women may be less able to "pause and plan" (Segerstrom et al., 2012); they may be less able to inhibit the automatic or "invited" hostile complementary response to their partner's hostile actions, and thereby fail to engage in more adaptive behavior, with the ultimate effect of continuing and perhaps escalating conflict and reduced relationship quality.

In contrast, the effects of positive marital interaction on women's hf-HRV suggest that such experiences can temporarily replenish this indicator of regulatory capacity (cf., Kok & Frederickson, 2010). Thus, difficulties in close relationships might threaten heart health not only through excessive physiological stress responses but also because they deplete self-regulatory resources. That is, stressful marital interactions may not only tax individuals but also drain them—perhaps especially women.

Sleep as Stress Restoration

Across these physiological processes, an implicit assumption is that mechanisms linking relationship quality with CVD operate during waking hours. Yet sleep is important as well. Poor sleep is associated with greater atherosclerosis (King et al., 2008), metabolic syndrome (Hall et al., 2008), inflammation (Mills et al., 2007), and earlier mortality (Gallachio & Kalsesen, 2009). Marital distress is associated with poor sleep (Troxel, 2010). This association appears bidirectional; marital strain contributes to poor sleep, and a poor night's sleep reduces the quality of marital interactions the next day (Hasler & Troxel, 2010). Marital difficulties also attenuate nighttime blood pressure "dipping," a normal physiological response that otherwise reduces CVD risk (Holt-Lunstad, Jones, & Birmingham, 2009).

Marriage as the Mechanism

The mechanisms discussed thus far are potential links between marital quality and CVD. For other psychosocial risk factors, marriage may be a mechanism. As described previously, marital difficulties are associated with individual difference characteristics that predict the development and course of CVD, such as depression, anxiety, anger, and optimism. Hence, efforts to understand mechanisms linking those characteristics with CVD might usefully consider marital processes as an additional link. These individual-level risk factors are associated with levels of stress exposure in the context of close relationships and with levels of stress-buffering social support, most likely through the sorts of transactional processes depicted in Figure 2.5. These affective risk factors also moderate the physiological reactivity to marital stressors described earlier. For example, individuals' levels of anger and hostility are positively associated with their own CVR during potential stressful marital interactions (i.e., actor effects) and with their partner's CVR (i.e., partner effects) (Smith & Brown, 1991; Smith & Gallo, 1999).

Marriage may be a mechanism for less frequently studied individual-level risk factors. For example, posttraumatic stress disorder (PTSD) is associated with increased risk of CVD (Boscarino, 2008; Kubzansky, Koenen, Spiro, Vokonas, & Sparrow, 2007; Kubzansky et al., 2009). As an anxiety disorder, more frequent, severe and prolonged anxiety could link PTSD with CVD (Roy-Byrne et al., 2008), as could high levels of depression and anger commonly associated with PTSD (Olatunji, Ciesielski, & Tolin, 2010; Orth & Wieland, 2006). PTSD is also associated with higher levels of marital distress, not only for the individuals with PTSD but for their partners as well (Lambert, Engh, Hasbun, & Holzer, 2012; Taft, Watkins, Stafford, Street, & Monson, 2011). PTSD is also associated with emotional distress among the partners, and the anger symptoms of PTSD may be a particularly important influence on partners' emotional adjustment and relationship quality (Monson, Taft, & Fredman, 2009). Thus, the effects of PTSD on CVD might occur not only within individuals but also between them. Consistent with this view, in a sample of US veterans returning from Iraq and Afghanistan, we recently found that those with PTSD demonstrated larger increases in anger and greater CVR during a discussion of an ongoing marital disagreement than did veterans without PTSD, and these effects of the veterans' PTSD were even stronger among their spouses (Caska, Smith et al., unpublished data).

Personality disorder symptoms have also been linked to CVD, where associations with borderline personality disorder (BPD) are particularly evident (El-Gabalawy, Katz, & Sareen, 2010; Lee et al., 2010; Moran et al., 2007). The negative emotionality, emotional instability, and highly variable but often quarrelsome interpersonal style prominent in BPD (Russell, Moskowitz, Zuroff, Sookman, & Paris, 2007; Trull & Brown, 2013) suggest that associations between BPD and CVD may parallel closely the associations of negative emotionality, trait anger, and hostility or antagonism with CVD described previously. The formal diagnosis of BPD may be most accurately seen as the extreme of a continuous dimension of related emotional and social behavioral symptoms, rather than a discrete natural category (Edens, Markus, & Ruiz, 2008; Haslam, Holland, & Kuppens, 2012). Further, continuous measures of personality pathology often are better predictors of a wide variety of outcomes than categorical representations (Markon, Chielewski, & Miller, 2011). Hence, variations in levels of continuously distributed BPD symptoms are a valid and potentially useful way to represent this personality construct. Importantly, BPD symptoms are associated with increased marital difficulties (South, Turkheimer, & Oltmanns, 2008; Stroud, Durbin, Saigal, & Knobloch-Fedders, 2010; Whisman & Schonbrun, 2009). Hence, the associations of BPD symptoms with CVD may involve disturbances in close relationships.

Stress-related mechanisms linking psychosocial risk factors with CVD can be conceptualized as involving four stress processes: *exposure* to stressors, physiological *reactivity* to stressors, physiological *recovery* after the stressor, and various aspects of *restoration* (e.g., sleep, positive social experiences) (Williams, Smith, Gunn, & Uchino, 2011). The presence and quality of marital and marriage-like relationships can influence CVD risk in each of these ways. Exposure to marital stressors evokes significant physiological stress responses of a nature and magnitude that can influence CVD. The degree of positivity or negativity evident in a particular interaction or in the relationship as a whole is also related to the magnitude of reactivity. Although there is less evidence regarding effects of specific marital interactions or levels of relationship quality on physiological recovery after stress exposure, it is reasonable to assume that good marriages and positive interactions would facilitate recovery, whereas strained marriages and negative interactions with the spouse would inhibit it (Smith, Uchino, et al., 2009). The recent research on close relationships and sleep suggests an important role for restoration as well. It may be that the robust effects of marriage and marital quality on CVD reflect the fact that these central aspects of our lives affect the full gamut of stress processes.

CONCLUSIONS AND FUTURE DIRECTIONS

The available evidence suggests that married individuals (and those involved in marriage-like relationships) are at reduced risk for the development of CVD, and among persons with established CVD these relationships are associated with a better clinical course (e.g., longer survival, reduced risk of recurrent events). However, the quality of this relationship is also important. Low marital quality is associated with asymptomatic atherosclerosis, the emergence of clinically apparent CVD, and reduced survival among CVD patients. Psychophysiological mechanisms underlying these associations have been identified, and marital processes may contribute to the effects of other individual-level psychosocial risk factors, such as depression, anxiety, anger and hostility, and optimism.

Relationship Science and the Interpersonal Perspective

The concepts and methods of current relationship science can be useful in advancing research on marriage and the heart. Multidimensional models of relationship quality can clarify which aspects of close relationships confer risk and resilience, and how those effects might vary across gender and age. Examination of specific couple processes involving interactional behavior, relationship cognition, and affective responses in close relationships can identify specific mechanisms that influence CVR risk and eventually guide the development of risk-reducing interventions. Multiple methods in current relationship science beyond the commonly used self-reports could also advance the field, such as behavioral assessment and daily experience approaches.

The concepts and methods of the interpersonal perspective (Horowitz & Strack, 2011; Kiesler, 1996; Pincus & Ansell, 2003) are a useful framework for the study of psychosocial risks for CVD in general (Smith & Cundiff, 2011), and for the study of marriage and the heart, in particular. The interpersonal circumplex identifies two broad dimensions of social behavior and more specific aspects of social interactions that could help clarify both the unhealthy and protective elements of close relationships. Further, the transactional cycle organizes research on elements of risky and protective marital processes, and it provides an important point of integration with research on individual-level psychosocial risk factors. The interpersonal tradition also includes a wide variety of well-validated approaches to the measurement of these processes (Horowitz & Strack, 2011).

A Central Role for Diversity

Future research must attend to the possibility that risks and mechanisms may differ for men and women. The development, course, and clinical presentation of CVD differ for men and women, as does the importance of various psychosocial risk factors (Low, Thurston, & Matthews, 2010). Early research focused on sex differences in the cardiovascular protection afforded by marriage and parallel sex differences in the degree of risk conferred by marital strain and disruption, but it now appears that men and women are both affected by these processes. Yet they may be differentially affected by specific marital processes, and through somewhat different mechanisms. Ethnicity must also be considered in future research. There are strong differences in CVD risk across ethnic groups (American Heart Association, 2012), and ethnic groups differ in a variety of aspects of marriage (Bryant et al., 2010; Cutrona, Russell, Burzette, Wesner, & Bryant, 2011).

Socioeconomic status (SES) is an important influence across all stages of CVD and, as depicted in Figure 2.5, SES is an important contextual influence on interaction patterns that determine marital quality and stability (Conger, Conger, & Martin, 2010; Matthews & Gallo, 2011). It is also important to examine these processes in the context of same-sex relationships, as similarities with heterosexual relationships must be tested rather than assumed (Peplau & Fingerhut, 2007). Given the long time course for the development, emergence, and course of CVD, it is important to note that levels of relationship quality, couple interaction patterns, and the physiological effects of stressful couple interactions often vary with age (e.g., Smith, Uchino, et al., 2009; Smith, Berg, et al., 2009).

Behavioral Genetics and Social Neuroscience of Close Relationships

Like many measures of the social environment (Kendler & Baker, 2007), marital status, marital quality, and marital disruption all display significant heritability. In genetically informative designs, associations of personality or emotional adjustment with marital quality reflect—at least in part—a common genetic factor (South & Kreuger, 2008; Spotts et al., 2005). Marital status and marital disruption may be associated with distinct genetic factors (Jersky et al., 2010), suggesting that genetic influences on relationship formation differ from those involved in staying together. Despite clear evidence of genetic influences on CVD, on virtually all of the psychosocial risk factors for CVD, and on the covariation of individual-level and social-environmental risk factors, little or no research on marriage and related psychosocial risk factors (e.g., personality, emotional adjustment) has utilized genetically informative designs.

Even if CVD risk factors reflecting marital processes and aspects of personality and emotional adjustment share genetic influences, transactional processes described in Figure 2.5 are probably the mechanisms by which heritable aspects of personality and emotionality become correlated with features of the social environment (Buss, 1987; Plomin, 2009; Scarr & McCartney, 1983). However, identification of such genetic factors could help elucidate endophenotypes underlying the risk processes reflected in recurring patterns of interpersonal transaction (Williams et al., 2011). The possible influence of common genetic factors also suggests a larger role for neuroscience approaches generally in future research on marriage and CVD. The brain bases of physiological mechanisms linking psychosocial risk factors with CVD have been initially identified (Gianaros & O'Connor, 2011), as have brain mechanisms in positive and negative aspects of relationships (Eisenberger, 2011; Tomlinson & Aron, 2012).

A Developmental Perspective

As noted previously, early indications of the vascular changes that progress to atherosclerosis and related CVD can be measured in childhood and adolescence (Charakida et al., 2009; Groner et al., 2006; Urbina et al., 2009). Further, exposure to adverse events in childhood (e.g., abuse, marital conflict and disruption) is associated with increased risk of CVD in adulthood (Dong et al., 2004; Miller, Chen, & Parker, 2011). Hence, although our focus has been on the effect of marital processes on the cardiovascular health of the married partners directly involved, these effects extend to their children as well. That is, the well-established effects of marital quality on child emotional and social adjustment (Cummings & Schatz, 2012) likely extend to physical health. Further, family experiences such as exposure to marital conflict influence the development of emotional and interpersonal characteristics that closely resemble psychosocial risk factors for CVD (e.g., negative affectivity, anger, antagonistic behavior, social isolation) and also influence the quality of the developing individual's own close relationships later in adulthood (Ehrensaft, Knous-Westfall, & Cohen, 2011). Thus, early experience apparently influences psychosocial risk for CVD across the life span.

In interpersonal theory and closely related models of attachment, early family experiences take the form of recurring patterns of parent–child transaction. Warm and responsive transactional cycles between parent and child promote secure attachment, and the related positive internal representations or working models of self, others, and relationships (i.e., schemas and scripts). In contrast, hostile, distant, or unresponsive parental behavior leads to maladaptive transactional patterns, and the development of negative internal representations or working models. From this perspective, individuals display continuities in the quality of important relationships across the life span, as early interactional patterns shape later interpersonal experiences (Shaver & Mikulincer, 2011).

As depicted in Figure 2.8, these continuities can be conceptualized as a series of adaptive or maladaptive transactional cycles, described previously (see Fig. 2.5). Strung together over time and across settings, these adaptive or maladaptive transactions form interpersonal trajectories, comprising recurring patterns in which positive or negative internal representations of the self, others, and relationships guide the individual's overt behavior toward important others. As described previously, that overt behavior has the effect of constraining the internal experiences and likely behavior of interaction partners across multiple contexts, with the result of recurrently evoking positive (e.g., warm, responsive) or negative (e.g., hostile, cold, rejecting, quarrelsome) behavior from others. Thus, these transactional trajectories create and sustain exposure to social environments that either heighten (top trajectory) or reduce (lower trajectory) the individual's level of psychosocial risk for CVD. Importantly, aspects of the individual's life context (e.g., low versus high early socioeconomic status, low versus high exposure to parental conflict,

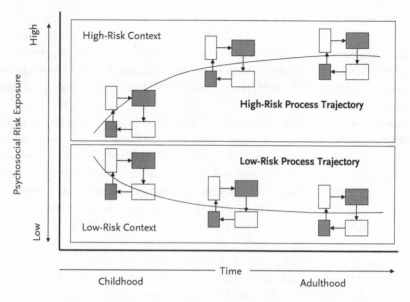

Figure 2.8: The transactional trajectory model: transactional cycles over time and across situations create high and low psychosocial risk exposure trajectories.

etc.) facilitate adaptive or maladaptive transactional patterns. Early in life, parent–child transactions are the key patterns, but over time there is a more important role for siblings and peers, and eventually the individual's own close relationship partner(s).

As noted previously, rather than the strictly social learning processes emphasized in interpersonal and attachment theory, it is possible that common genetic influences underlie these recurring transactions between the individual and the surrounding social context. Also, early experiences could shape later transactional patterns through epigenetic effects on the expression of genetic influences on emotion, self-regulation, social behavior, and physiological reactivity (Miller et al., 2011). However, even if genetic factors play a critical role, it is likely that the developmental, interpersonal, and transactional processes described here play a key role as well. Positive early experiences would facilitate the emergence of a lower risk "transactional phenotype" with recurring patterns involving high levels of social support and lower levels of interpersonal conflict. In contrast, early exposure to low warmth, neglect, high hostility, and hostile parental control would promote a high-risk trajectory involving social isolation, conflict, and contested control. From this perspective, marital quality as a cardiovascular risk or resilience factor reflects a central relationship context across a large span of the health-relevant trajectory, influencing the individual's own risk but also potentially the risk of offspring as well. Hence, facilitating positive trajectories that include sound marriages and preventing or altering negative trajectories involving strained relationships is an important element of risk reduction and prevention.

Intervention Implications

Although there is little controlled research evaluating the effects of marital interventions in the context of established CVD, such approaches have been described (Baucom, Porter, Kirby, & Hudepohl, 2012; Hilscher, Bartley, & Zarski, 2005; Rankin-Esquer, Deeter, Froelicher, & Taylor, 2000; Shields et al., 2012; Sperry, 2011). Further, there is evidence that couple-based interventions in chronic disease generally—and in a few small trials for CVD in particular—have beneficial effects on emotional adjustment and marital functioning (Martire, Schulz, Helgeson, Small, & Saghafi, 2010). If future research provides further evidence of the importance of marital processes in CVD, additional intervention research would be warranted. There is evidence that stress management interventions not only improve emotional adjustment among heart patients but can also reduce recurrent cardiovascular events and improve survival (Gullickson et al., 2011; Linden, Phillips, & Leclerc, 2007; Orth-Gomer et al., 2009). For distressed couples, several therapy approaches could reduce this psychosocial risk factor and related emotional risk factors, such as depression and anxiety (Lebow, Chambers, Christensen, & Johnson, 2012).

Given the decades long development of atherosclerosis before the clinical appearance of CVD, a variety of couple interventions could be used in CVD prevention efforts for clearly distressed but physically healthy couples. Further, empirically supported couple interventions for the prevention of couple distress among well-functioning couples (Markman & Rhoades, 2012) and for higher risk couples who are not yet distressed (Cordova et al., 2005) could be useful as well. There are important benefits of such interventions in terms of relationship quality and stability, emotional adjustment, and overall quality of life. It is possible that those benefits could extend to the prevention of cardiovascular disease as well. To explore that possibility effectively, researchers studying marriage and the heart should make greater use of current concepts and methods in the relationship science toolbox.

REFERENCES

American Heart Association. (2012). Heart disease and stroke statistics: 2012 update. *Circulation, 125,* e2–e220.

Assad, K. K., Donnellan, M. B., & Conger, R. D. (2007). Optimism: An enduring resource for romantic relationships. *Journal of Personality and Social Psychology, 93,* 285–297.

Baker, B., Paquette, M., Szalai, J. P., Driver, H., Perger, T., Helmers, K., ... Tobe, S. (2000). The influence of marital adjustment on 3-year left ventricular mass and ambulatory blood pressure in mild hypertension. *Archives of Internal Medicine, 160,* 3453–3458.

Baron, K. G., Smith, T. W., Butner, J., Nealey-Moore, J., Hawkins, M. W., & Uchino, B. N. (2007). Hostility, anger, and marital adjustment: concurrent and prospective associations with psychosocial vulnerability. *Journal of Behavioral Medicine, 30,* 1–10.

Barth, J., Schneider, S., & von Kanel, R. (2010). Lack of social support in the etiology and the prognosis of coronary heart disease: A systematic review and meta-analysis. *Psychosomatic Medicine, 72,* 229–238.

Baucom, D. H., Porter, L. S., Kirby, J. S., & Hudepohl, J. (2012). Couple-based interventions for medical problems. *Behavior Therapy, 43,* 61–76.

Beach, S. R. H., Fincham, F. D., Amir, N., & Leonard, K. E. (2005). The taxometrics of marriage: Is marital discord categorical? *Journal of Family Psychology, 19,* 276–285.

Benjamin, L. S., Rothweiler, J., & Critchfield, K. (2006). The use of structural analysis of social behavior (SASB) as an assessment tool. *Annual Review of Clinical Psychology, 2,* 83–109.

Boehm, J. K., & Kubzansky, L. D. (2012). The heart's content: The association between positive psychological well-being and cardiovascular health. *Psychological Bulletin, 138,* 655–691.

Boscarino, J. A. (2008). A prospective study of PTSD and early-age heart disease mortality among Vietnam veterans: implications for surveillance and prevention. *Psychosomatic Medicine, 70,* 668–676.

Brock, R. L., & Lawrence, E. (2011). Marriage as a risk factor for internalizing disorders: Clarifying scope and specificity. *Journal of Consulting and Clinical Psychology, 79,* 577–585.

Brown, P. C., & Smith, T. W. (1992). Social influence, marriage, and the heart: Cardiovascular consequences of interpersonal control in husbands and wives. *Health Psychology, 11,* 88–96.

Bryant, C. M., Wickerama, K. A. S., Bolland, J. B., Bryant, B. M., Cutrona, C. E., & Stanik, C. E. (2010). Race matters, even in marriage: Identifying factors linked to marital outcomes for African Americans. *Journal of Family, Theory and Review, 2,* 157–174.

Buss, D. M. (1987). Selection, evocation, and manipulation. *Journal of Personality and Social Psychology, 53,* 1214–1221.

Campbell, A. (2010). Oxytocin and human social behavior. *Personality and Social Psychology Review, 14,* 281–295.

Carroll, D., Ginty, A. T., Der, G., Hunt, K., Benzeval, M., & Phillips, A. C. (2012). Increased blood pressure reactions to acute mental stress are associated with 16-year cardiovascular disease mortality. *Psychophysiology, 49,* 1444–1448.

Carroll, D., Phillips, A. C., & Balanos, G. M. (2009). Metabolically exaggerated cardiac reactions to acute psychological stress revisited. *Psychophysiology, 46,* 270–275.

Carter, C. S., Grippo, A. J., Pournajafi-Nazarloo, H., Ruscio, M. G., & Porges, S. W. (2008). Oxytocin, vasopressin and sociality. *Progress in Brain Research, 170,* 331–336. doi: 10.1016/s0079-6123(08)00427-5.

Charakida, M., Deanfield, J. E., & Halcox, P. J. (2009). Childhood origins of arterial disease. *Current Opinion in Pediatrics, 19,* 538–545.

Chida, Y., & Steptoe, A. (2009). The association of anger and hostility with future coronary heart disease: A meta-analytic review of prospective evidence. *Journal of the American College of Cardiology, 53,* 774–778.

Chida, Y., & Steptoe, A. (2010). Greater cardiovascular responses to laboratory mental stress are associated with poor subsequent cardiovascular risk status: a meta-analysis of prospective evidence. *Hypertension, 55,* 1026–1032.

Conger, R. D., Conger, K. J., & Martin, M. J. (2010). Socioeconomic status, family processes, and individual development. *Journal of Marriage and Family, 72,* 685–704.

Cordova, J. V., Scott, R. L., Dorian, M., Mirgain, S., Yaeger, D., & Groot, A. (2005). The marriage check up: An indicated preventive intervention for treat-avoidant couples at risk for marital deterioration. *Behavior Therapy, 36,* 301–309.

Cummings, E. M., & Schatz, J. N. (2012). Family conflict, emotional security, and child development: Translating research findings into a prevention program for community families. *Clinical Child and Family Review, 15,* 14–27.

Cutrona, C. E. (1996). *Social support in couples: Marriage as a resource in times of stress.* Thousand Oaks, CA: Sage.

Cutrona, C. E., Russell, D. W., Burzette, R. G., Wesner, K. A., & Bryant, C. M. (2011). Predicting relationship stability among midlife African American couples. *Journal of Consulting and Clinical Psychology, 79*(6), 814–825. doi 10.1037/a0025874.

Denton, W. H., Burleson, B. R., Hobbs, B. V., Von Stein, M., & Rodriguez, C. P. (2001). Cardiovascular reactivity and initiate/avoid patterns of marital communication: A test of Gottman's psychophysiologic model of marital interaction. *Journal of Behavioral Medicine, 24,* 401–421.

De Vogli, R., Chandola, T., & Marmot, M. G. (2007). Negative aspects of close relationships and heart disease. *Archives of Internal Medicine, 167,* 1951–1957.

Diamond, L. M., & Hicks, A. M. (2005). Attachment style, current relationship security, and negative emotions: The mediating role physiological regulation. *Journal of Social and Personal Relationships, 22,* 499–518.

Diamond, L. M., Hicks, A. M., & Otter-Henderson, K. D. (2011). Individual differences in vagal regulation moderate associations between daily affect and daily couple interactions. *Personality and Social Psychology Bulletin, 37,* 731–744.

Ditzen, B., Neumann, I. D., Bodenmann, G., Von Dawans, B., Turner, R. A., Ehlert, U., ... von Dawans, B. (2007). Effects of different kinds of couple interaction on cortisol and heart rate responses to stress in women. *Psychoneuroendocrinology, 32,* 565–574.

Ditzen, B., Schaer, M., Gabriel, B., Bodenmann, G., Ehlert, U., & Heinrchs, M. (2009). Intranasal oxytocin increases positive communication and reduces cortisol levels during couple conflict. *Biological Psychiatry, 65,* 728–731.

Dong, M., Giles, W., Felitti, V., Dube, S., Williams, J., Chapman, D., & Anda, R. (2004). Insights into causal pathways for ischemic heart disease: Adverse childhood experiences study. *Circulation, 110,* 1761–1766.

Eaker, E. D., Sullivan, L. M., Kelly-Hayes, M., D'Agostino, R. B., & Benjamin, E. J. (2007). Marital status, marital strain, and risk of coronary heart disease or total mortality: The Framingham Offspring Study. *Psychosomatic Medicine, 69,* 509.

Eckel, R. H., Grundy, S. M., & Zimmet, P. Z. (2005). The metabolic syndrome. *Lancet, 365,* 1145–1128.

Edens, J. F., Marcus, D. K., & Ruiz, M. A. (2008). Taxonomic analyses of borderline personality features in a large-scale male and female offender sample. *Journal of Abnormal Psychology, 117,* 705–711.

Ehrensaft, M. K., Knous-Westfall, H. M., & Cohen, P. (2011). Direct and indirect transmission of relationship functioning across generations. *Journal of Family Psychology, 25,* 942–952.

Ehrensaft, M. K., Langhinrichsen-Rohling, J., Heyman, R. E., O'Leary, K. D., & Lawrence, E. (1999). Feeling controlled in marriage: A phenomenon specific to physically aggressive couples? *Journal of Family Psychology, 13,* 20–32. doi: 10.1037/0893-3200.13.1.20.

Eisenberger, N. I. (2011). The neural bases of social pain: Findings and implications. In G. MacDonald & L. A. Jensen-Campbell (Eds.), *Social pain: Neuropsychological and health implications of exclusion and loss* (pp. 53–78). Washington, DC: American Psychological Association.

El-Gabalawy, R., Katz, L. Y., & Sareen, J. (2010). Comorbidity and associated severity of borderline personality disorder and physical health conditions in a nationally representative sample. *Psychosomatic Medicine, 72,* 641–647.

Everson-Rose, S. A., & Lewis, T. T. (2005). Psychosocial factors and cardiovascular diseases. *Annual Review of Public Health, 26,* 469–500.

Fincham, F. D., & Rogge, R. (2010). Understanding relationship quality: Theoretical challenges and new tools for assessment. *Journal of Family Theory and Review, 2,* 227–242.

Fisher, J., & Scheidt, S. S. (2012). A whirlwind tour of cardiology. In R. Allan & J. Fisher (Eds.), *Heart and mind: The practice of cardiac psychology* (pp. 17–53). Washington, DC: American Psychological Association.

Franks, M. M., Stephens, M. A. P., Rook, K. S., Franklin, B., Keteyian, S., & Artinian, N. T. (2006). Spouses provision of health-related support and control to patients participating in cardiac rehabilitation. *Journal of Family Psychology, 20*, 311–318.

Gallicchio, L., & Kalesan, B. (2009). Sleep duration and mortality: A systematic review. *Journal of Sleep Research, 18*, 148–158.

Gallo, L. C., Smith, T. W., & Kircher, J. C. (2000). Cardiovascular and electrodermal responses to support and provocation: Interpersonal methods in the study of psychophysiological reactivity. *Psychophysiology, 37*, 289–301.

Gallo, L. C., Troxel, W. M., Kuller, L. H., Sutton-Tyrrell, K., Edmundowicz, D., & Matthews, K. A. (2003). Marital status, marital quality, and atherosclerotic burden in postmenopausal women. *Psychosomatic Medicine, 65*, 952.

Gianaros, P. J., & O'Connor, M. (2011). Neuroimaging methods in human stress science. In R. Contrada & A. Baum (Eds.), *Handbook of stress science: Biology, psychology, and health* (pp. 543–563). New York, NY: Springer.

Goldbacher, E. M., & Matthews, K. A. (2007). Are psychological characteristics related to risk of metabolic syndrome? A review of the literature. *Annals of Behavioral Medicine, 34*, 240–252.

Gouin, J-P., Carter, C. S., Pournajafi-Nazarloo, H., Glaser, R., Malarkey, W. B., Loving, T. J., ... Kiecolt-Glaser, J. K. (2010). Marital behavior, oxytocin, vasopressin, and wound healing. *Psychoneuroendocrinology, 35*, 1082–1090.

Graber, E. C., Laurenceau, J-P, & Carver, C. S. (2011). Integrating the dynamics of personality and close relationship processes: Methodological and data analytic implications. *Journal of Personality, 79*, 1403–1439.

Graber, E. C., Laurenceau, J-P., Miga, E., Chango, J., & Coan, J. A. (2011). Conflict and love: Predicting newlywed marital outcomes from two interaction contexts. *Journal of Family Psychology, 25*, 541–550.

Groner, J. A., Joshi, M., & Bauer, J. A. (2006). Pediatric precursors of adult cardiovascular disease: Noninvasive assessment of early vascular changes in children and adolescents. *Pediatrics, 118*, 1683–1691.

Gulliksson, M., Burrell, G., Vessby, B., Lundin, L., Toss, H., & Svardsudd, K. (2011). Randomized controlled trial of cognitive behavior therapy vs. standard treatment to prevent recurrent cardiovascular events in patients with coronary heart disease: Secondary prevention in Uppsala primary care project (SUPRIM). *Archives of Internal Medicine, 171*, 134–140.

Hall, M. H., Muldoon, M. F., Jennings, R., Buysee, D. J., Flory, J. D., & Manuck, S. B. (2008). Self-reported sleep duration is associated with the metabolic syndrome in midlife adults. *Sleep, 31*, 635–643.

Haslam, N., Holland, E., & Kuppens, P. (2012). Categories versus dimensions in personality and psychopathology: A quantitative review of taxometric research. *Psychological Medicine, 42*, 903–920.

Hasler, B. P., & Troxel, W. M. (2010). Couples' nighttime sleep efficiency and concordance: Evidence for bidirectional associations with daytime relationship functioning. *Psychosomatic Medicine, 72*, 794–801.

Helgeson, V. S. (2003). Gender-related traits and health. In J. Suls & K. Wallston (Eds.), *Social psychological foundations of health and illness* (pp. 367–394). Chichester, UK: Blackwell.

Henry, N. J. M., Berg, C. A., Smith, T. W., & Florsheim, P. (2007). Positive and negative characteristics of marital interaction and their association with marital satisfaction in middle-aged and older couples. *Psychology and Aging, 22*, 428–441.

Herrington, R. L., Mitchell, A. E., Castellani, A. M., Joseph, J. I., Snyder, D. K., & Gleaves, D. H. (2008). Assessing disharmony and disaffection in intimate relationships: Revision of the Marital Satisfaction Inventory factor scales. *Psychological Assessment, 20*, 341–350.

Hilscher, R. L., Bartley, A. G., & Zarski, J. (2005). A heart does not beat alone: Coronary heart disease through a family systems lens. *Family, Systems, and Health, 23,* 220–235.

Holt-Lunstad, J., Birmingham, W., & Jones, B. Q. (2008). Is there something unique about marriage? The relative impact of marital status, relationship quality, and network social support on ambulatory blood pressure and mental health. *Annals of Behavioral Medicine, 35,* 239–244.

Holt-Lunstad, J., Birmingham, W. A., & Light, K. C., 2008). Influence of a "warm touch" support enhancement intervention among married couples on ambulatory blood pressure, oxytocin, alpha amylase, and cortisol. *Psychosomatic Medicine, 70,* 976–985.

Holt-Lunstad, J., Jones, B., & Brimingham, W. (2009). The influence of close relationships on nocturnal blood pressure dipping. *International Journal of Psychophysiology, 71,* 211–217.

Holt-Lunstad, J., Smith, T. B., & Layton, J. B. (2010). Social relationships and mortality risk: A meta-analytic review. *PLoS Medicine, 7,* e1000316.

Hornish, G., & Leonard, K. E. (2008). Spousal influence on general health behaviors in a community sample. *American Journal of Health Behavior, 32,* 754–763.

Horowitz, L. M., & Strack, S. (Eds.). (2011). *Handbook of interpersonal psychology.* Hoboken, NJ: Wiley.

Houston, B. K., Babyak, M. A., Chesney, M. A., Black, G., & Ragland, D. R. (1997). Social dominance and 22-year all-cause mortality in men. *Psychosomatic Medicine, 59,* 5–12.

Houston, B. K., Chesney, M. A., Black, G. W., Cates, D. S., & Hecker, M. L. (1992). Behavioral clusters and coronary heart disease risk. *Psychosomatic Medicine, 54,* 447–461.

Howren, M. B., Lamkin, D. M., & Suls, J. (2009). Associations of depression with C-reactive protein, IL-1, and IL-6: A meta-analysis. *Psychosomatic Medicine, 71,* 171–186.

Idler, E. L., Boulifard, D. A., & Contrada, R. J. (2012). Mending broken hearts: Marriage and survival following cardiac surgery. *Journal of Health and Social Behavior, 53,* 33–49.

Janicki, D. L., Kamarck, T. W., Shiffman, S., & Gwaltney, C. J. (2006). Application of ecological momentary assessment to the study of marital adjustment and social interactions during daily life. *Journal of Family Psychology, 20,* 168–172.

Janicki, D. L., Kamarck, T. W., Shiffman, S., Stton-Tyrrell, K., & Gwaltney, C. J. (2005). Frequency of spousal interaction and 3-year progression of carotid artery intima medial thickness: The Pittsburgh Healthy Heart Project. *Psychosomatic Medicine, 67,* 889–896.

Jersky, B. A., Panizzon, M. S., Jacobson, K. C., Neale, M. C., Grant, M., … & Lyons, M. (2010). Marriage and divorce: A genetic perspective. *Personality and Individual Differences, 49,* 473–478.

Johnson, N., Backlund, E., Sorlie, P., & Loveless, C. (2000). Marital status and mortality: The National Longitudinal Mortality Study. *Annals of Epidemiology, 10,* 224–238.

Kamarck, T. W., Schwartz, J. E., Shiffman, S., Muldoon, M. F., Sutton-Tyrrell, K., & Janicki, D. L. (2005). Psychosocial stress and cardiovascular risk: What is the role of daily experience? *Journal of Personality, 73,* 1749–1774.

Kamarck, T. W., Shiffman, S., Sutton-Tyrrell, K., Muldoon, M. F., & Tepper, P. (2012). Daily psychological demands are associated with 6-year progression of carotid artery atherosclerosis: The Pittsburgh Healthy Heart Project. *Psychosomatic Medicine, 74,* 432–439.

Karney, B. R., & Bradbury, T. N. (2005). Contextual influences in marriage: Implications for policy and intervention. *Current Directions in Psychological Science, 14,* 171–174.

Kendler, K. S., & Baker, J. H. (2007). Genetic influences on measures of the environment: A systematic review. *Psychological Medicine, 37,* 615–626.

Kiecolt-Glaser, J. K., Gouin, J. P., & Hantsoo, L. (2010). Close relationships, inflammation, and health. *Neuroscience and Biobehavioral Reviews, 35,* 33–38.

Kiecolt-Glaser, J. K., Loving, T. J., Stowell, J. R., Malarkey, W. B., Lemeshow, S., Dickinson, S. L., & Glaser, R. (2005). Hostile marital interactions, proinflammatory cytokine production, and wound healing. *Archives of General Psychiatry, 62,* 1377–1384.

Kiecolt-Glaser, J. K., & Newton, T. L. (2001). Marriage and health: His and hers. *Psychological Bulletin, 127,* 472–503.

Kiesler, D. J. (1996). *Contemporary interpersonal theory and research: Personality, psychopathology, and psychotherapy.* New York, NY: Wiley.

King, C. R., Knutson, K. L., Rathouz, P. J., Sidney, S., Liu, K., & Lauderdale, D. S. (2008). Short sleep duration and incident coronary artery calcification. *Journal of the American Medical Association, 300,* 2859–2866.

King, K. B., & Reis, H. T. (2012). Marriage and long-term survival after coronary artery bypass grafting. *Health Psychology, 31,* 55–62.

Kok, B. E., & Fredrickson, B. L. (2010). Upward spirals of the heart: Autonomic flexibility, as indexed by vagal tone, reciprocally and prospectively predicts positive emotions and social connectedness. *Biological Psychology, 85,* 432–436.

Kubzansky, L. D., Koenen, K. C., Jones, C., & Eaton, W. W. (2009). A prospective study of posttraumatic stress disorder symptoms and coronary heart disease in women. *Health Psychology, 28,* 125–130.

Kubzansky, L. D., Koenen, K. C., Spiro, A., III, Vokonas, P. S., & Sparrow, D. (2007). Prospective study of posttraumatic stress disorder symptoms and coronary heart disease in the Normative Aging Study. *Archives of General Psychiatry, 64,* 109–116.

Lambert, J. E., Engh, R., Hasbun, A., & Holzer, J. (2012). Impact of posttraumatic stress disorder on the relationship quality and psychological distress of intimate partners: A meta-analytic review. *Journal of Family Psychology, 26*(5), 729–737. doi: 10.1037/a0029341.

Laurenceau, J-P., & Bolger, N. (2005). Using diary methods to study marital and family processes. *Journal of Family Psychology, 19,* 86–97.

Lebow, J. L., Chambers, A. L., Christensen, A., & Johnson, S. M. (2012). Research on the treatment of couple distress. *Journal of Marital and Family Therapy, 38,* 145–168.

Lee, H. B., Bienvenu, J., Cho, S., Ramsey, C., Bandeen-Roche, K., Eaton, W., & Nestadt, G. (2010). Personality disorders and traits as predictors of incident cardiovascular disease: Findings from the 23-year follow-up of the Baltimore ECA Study. *Psychosomatics, 51,* 289–296.

Linden, W., Phillips, M. J., & Leclerc, J. (2007). Psychological treatment of cardiac patients: A meta-analysis. *European Heart Journal, 28,* 2972–2984.

Locke, H., & Wallace, K. (1959). Short marital adjustment and prediction tests: Their reliability and validity. *Marriage and Family Living, 21,* 251–255.

Low, C. A., Thurston, R. C., & Matthews, K. A.(2010). Psychosocial factors in the development of heart disease in women: Current research and future directions. *Psychosomatic Medicine, 72,* 842–854.

Margolin, G., Burnam, B., & John, R. (1989). Home observation of married couples reenacting naturalistic conflicts. *Behavioral Assessment, 11,* 101–118.

Margolin, G., Christensen, A., & John, R. S. (1996). The continuance and spillover of everyday tensions in distressed and nondistressed families. *Journal of Family Psychology, 10,* 304–321.

Markman, H. J., & Rhoades, G. K. (2012). Relationship education research: current status and future directions. *Journal of Marital and Family Therapy, 38,* 169–200.

Markon, K. E., Chmielewski, M., & Miller, C. J. (2011). The reliability and validity of discrete and continuous measures of psychopathology: A quantitative review. *Psychological Bulletin, 137,* 856–879.

Martire, L. M., Schulz, R., Helgeson, V. H., Small, B. J., & Saghafi, E. M. (2010). Review and meta-analysis of couple-oriented interventions for chronic illness. *Annals of Behavioral Medicine, 40,* 325–342.

Matthews, K. A., & Gallo, L. C. (2011). Psychological perspectives on pathways linking socioeconomic status and physical health. *Annual Review of Psychology, 62,* 501–530.

Matthews, K. A., & Gump, B. B. (2002). Chronic work stress and marital dissolution increase risk of posttrial mortality in men from the Multiple Risk Factor Intervention Trial. *Archives of Internal Medicine, 162*, 309–315.

Mattson, R. E., Paldino, D., & Johnson, M. D. (2007). The increased construct validity and clinical utility of assessing relationship quality using separate positive and negative dimensions. *Psychological Assessment, 19*, 146–151.

McLeod, J. D. (1994). Anxiety disorders and marital quality. *Journal of Abnormal Psychology, 103*, 767–776.

Miller, G. E., Chen, E., & Parker, K. J. (2011). Psychological stress in childhood and susceptibility to the chronic diseases of aging: Moving toward a model of behavioral and biological mechanisms. *Psychological Bulletin, 137*, 959–997.

Mills, P. J., von Känel, R., Norman, D., Natarajan, L., Ziegler, M. G., & Dimsdale, J. E. (2007). Inflammation and sleep in healthy individuals. *Sleep, 30*, 729–735.

Monson, C. M., Taft, C. T., & Fredman, S. J. (2009). Military-related PTSD and intimate relationships: From description to theory-driven research and intervention development. *Clinical Psychology Review, 29*, 707–714.

Moran, P., Stewart, R., Coid, J. W., Bebbington, P., Bhugra, D., Jenkins, R., & Coid, J. W. (2007). Personality disorder and cardiovascular disease: Results from a national household survey. *Journal of Clinical Psychiatry, 68*, 69–74.

Nation, D. A., Szeto, A., Mendez, A. J., Brooks, L. G., Zaias, J., Herderick, E. E., … McCabe, P. M. (2010). Oxytocin attenuates atherosclerosis and adipose tissue inflammation in socially isolated ApoE-/- mice. *Psychosomatic Medicine, 72*, 376–382.

Nealey-Moore, J. B., Smith, T. W., Uchino, B. N., Hawkins, M. W., & Olson-Cerny, C. (2007). Cardiovascular reactivity during positive and negative marital interactions. *Journal of Behavioral Medicine, 30*, 505–519.

Neff, L. A. (2012). Putting marriage in its context: The influence of external stress on early marital development. In L. Campbell & T. J. Loving (Eds.), *Interdisciplinary research on close relationships* (pp. 179–203). Washington, DC: American Psychological Association.

Newton, T. L., & Sanford, J. M. (2003). Conflict structure moderates associations between cardiovascular reactivity and negative marital interaction. *Health Psychology, 22*, 270–278.

Nicholson, A., Kuper, H., & Hemingway, H. (2006). Depression as an aetiologic and prognostic factor in coronary heart disease: a meta-analysis of 6362 events among 146,538 participants in 54 observational studies. *European Heart Journal, 27*, 2763–2774.

Olatunji, B. O., Ciesielski, B. G., & Tolin, D. F. (2010). Fear and loathing: A meta-analytic review of the specificity of anger in PTSD. *Behavior Therapy, 41*, 93–105.

Orth, U., & Wieland, E. (2006). Anger, hostility, and posttraumatic stress disorder in trauma-exposed adults: A meta-analysis. *Journal of Consulting and Clinical Psychology, 74*, 698–706.

Orth-Gomér, K., Schneiderman, N., Wang, H. X., Walldin, C., Blom, M., & Jernberg, T. (2009). Stress reduction prolongs life in women with coronary disease: The Stockholm Women's Intervention Trial for Coronary Heart Disease (SWITCHD). *Circulation: Cardiovascular Quality and Outcomes, 2*, 25–32.

Orth-Gomér, K., Wamala, S. P., Horsten, M., Schenck-Gustafsson, K., Schneiderman, N., & Mittleman, M. A. (2000). Marital stress worsens prognosis in women with coronary heart disease: The Stockholm Female Coronary Risk Study. *Journal of the American Medical Association, 284*, 3008–3014.

Pan, A., Keum, N., Okereke, O., Sun, Q., Kivimaki, M., Rubin, R. & Hu, F. (2012). Bidirectional association between depression and metabolic syndrome: A systematic review and meta-analysis of epidemiologic studies. *Diabetes Care, 35*, 1171–1180.

Pankiewicz, P., Majkowicz, M., & Krzykowski, G. (2012). Anxiety disorders in intimate partners and the quality of their relationship. *Journal of Affective Disorders, 140*, 176–180.

Peplau, L. A., & Fingerhut, A. W. (2007). The close relationships of lesbians and gay men. *Annual Review of Psychology, 58,* 405–424.

Pincus, A. L., & Ansell, E. B. (2003). Interpersonal theory of personality. In T. Millon & M. J. Lerner (Eds.), *Handbook of psychology, Vol. 5. Personality and social psychology* (pp. 209–229). New York, NY: John Wiley.

Pletcher, M. J., Tice, J. A., Pignone, M., & Browner, W. S. (2004). Using the coronary artery calcium score to predict coronary heart disease events: A systematic review and meta-analysis. *Archives of Internal Medicine, 64,* 1285–1292.

Plomin, R. (2009). Nature of nurture. In K. McCartney & R. Weinberg (Eds.), *Experience and development* (pp. 61–80). New York, NY: Psychology Press.

Raikkonen, K., Kajantie, E., Rautanen, A., & Eriksson, J. G. (2008). Metabolic syndrome. In L. J. Luecken & L. C. Gallo (Eds.), *Handbook of physiological research methods in health psychology* (pp. 299–322). Thousand Oaks, CA: Sage.

Rankin-Esquer, L. A., Deeter, A., Froelicher, E., & Taylor, C. B. (2000). Coronary heart disease: Intervention for intimate relationship issues. *Cognitive and Behavioral Practice, 7,* 212–220.

Rasmussen, H. N., Scheier, M. F., & Greenhouse, J. B. (2009). Optimism and physical health: A meta-analytic review. *Annals of Behavioral Medicine, 37,* 239–256.

Renshaw, K. D., Blais, R. K., & Smith, T. W. (2010). Components of negative affectivity and marital satisfaction: The importance of actor and partner anger. *Journal of Research in Personality, 44,* 328–334.

Repetti, R. L., Wang, S., & Saxbe, D. E. (2011). Adult health in the context of everyday family life. *Annals of Behavioral Medicine, 42,* 285–293.

Robles, T. F., Slatcher, R. B., Trombello, J. M., & McGinn, M. M. (2014). Marital quality and health: A meta-analytic review. *Psychological Bulletin, 140,* 140–187.

Roelfs, D. J., Shor, E., Kalish, R., & Yogev, T. (2011). The rising relative risk of mortality for singles: Meta-analysis and meta-regression. *American Journal of Epidemiology, 174,* 379–389.

Rohrbaugh, M. J., Shoham, V., & Coyne, J. C. (2006). Effect of marital quality on eight-year survival of patients with heart failure. *American Journal of Cardiology, 98,* 1069–1072.

Rosland, A., Heisler, M., & Piette, J. (2012). The impact of family behaviors and communication patterns on chronic illness outcomes: A systematic review. *Journal of Behavioral Medicine, 35,* 221–239.

Roy-Byrne, P. P., Davidson, K. W., Kessler, R. C., Asmundson, G. J. G., Psych, R. D., Goodwin, R. D.,...Stein, M. B. (2008). Anxiety disorders and comorbid mental illness, *General Hospital Psychiatry, 30,* 208–225.

Russell, J. J., Moskowitz, D. S., Zuroff, D. C., Sookman, D., & Paris, J. (2007). Stability and variability in affective experience and interpersonal behavior in borderline personality dosorder. *Journal of Abnormal Psychology, 116,* 578–588.

Saldler, P., Ethier, N., & Woody, E. (2011). Interpersonal complementarity. In L. M. Horowitz & S. Strack (Eds.), *Handbook of interpersonal psychology: Theory, research, assessment, and therapeutic interventions* (pp. 123–142). Hoboken, NJ: Wiley.

Sanford, K. (2010). Perceived threat and perceived neglect: Couples' underlying concerns during conflict. *Psychological Assessment, 22,* 288–297.

Sbarra, D. A., Law, R. W., & Portley, R. M. (2011). Divorce and death: A meta-analysis and research agenda for clinical, social, and health psychology. *Perspectives in Psychological Science, 6,* 454–474.

Scarr, S., & McCartney, K. (1983). How people make their own environments: A theory of genotype-environmental effects. *Child Development, 54,* 424–435.

Segerstrom, S. C., Hardy, J. K., Evans, D. R., & Winters, N. F. (2012). Pause and plan: Self-regulation and the heart. In R. A. Wright & G. H. E. Gendolla (Eds.), *How motivation affects cardiovascular response: Mechanisms and applications* (pp. 181–198). Washington, DC: American Psychological Association.

Shaver, P. R., & Milulincer, M. (2011). An attachment-theory framework for conceptualizing interpersonal behavior. In L. M. Horowitz & S. Strack (Eds.), *Handbook of interpersonal psychology: Theory, research, assessment, and therapeutic interventions* (pp. 15–35). Hoboken, NJ: Wiley.

Shields, C. G., Finley, M. A., Chawla, N., & Meadors, P. (2012). Couple and family interventions for health problems. *Journal of Marital and Family Therapy, 38,* 265–280.

Shor, E., Roelfs, D. J., Burgyi, P., & Schwartz, J. E. (2012). Meta-analysis of marital dissolution and mortality: Reevaluating the intersection of gender and age. *Social Science and Medicine, 75,* 46–59.

Shor, E., Roelfs, D. J., Curreli, M., Clemow, L., Burg, M. M., & Schwartz, J. E. (2012). Widowhood and mortality: A meta-analysis and meta-regression. *Demography, 49,* 575–606.

Siegman, A. W., Kubzansky, L. D., Kawachi, I., Boyle, S., Vokonas, P. S., & Sparrow, D. (2000). A prospective study of dominance and coronary heart disease in the normative aging study. *American Journal of Cardiology, 86,* 145–149.

Slatcher, R. B. (2010). Marital functioning and physical health: Implications for social and personality psychology. *Social and Personality Psychology Compass, 3,* 1–15.

Smith, T. W., Berg, C. A., Florsheim, P., Uchino, B. N., Pearce, G., Hawkins, M., . . . Olson-Cerny, C. (2009). Conflict and collaboration in middle-aged and older couples: I. Age differences in agency and communion during marital interaction. *Psychology and Aging, 24,* 259–273.

Smith, T. W., & Brown, P. C. (1991). Cynical hostility, attempts to exert social control, and cardiovascular reactivity in married couples. *Journal of Behavioral Medicine, 14,* 579–590.

Smith, T. W., Cribbet, M. R., Nealey-Moore, J. B., Uchino, B. N., Williams, P. G., Mackenzie, J., & Thayer, J. F. (2011). Matters of the variable heart: Respiratory sinus arrhythmia response to marital interaction and associations with marital quality. *Journal of Personality and Social Psychology, 100,* 103–119.

Smith, T. W., & Cundiff, J. (2011). An interpersonal perspective on risk for coronary heart disease. In L. M. Horowitz & S. Strack (Eds.), *Handbook of interpersonal psychology: Theory, research, assessment, and therapeutic interventions* (pp. 471–490). Hoboken, NJ: Wiley.

Smith, T. W., & Cundiff, J. M. (in press). Aggregation of psychosocial risk factors: Models and methods. In S. R. Waldstein, W. J. Kop, & L. I. Katzel (Eds.), *Handbook of cardiovascular behavioral medicine.* New York, NY: Springer.

Smith, T. W., Cundiff, J., & Uchino, B. N. (2012). Interpersonal motives and cardiovascular response: Mechanisms linking dominance and social status with cardiovascular disease. In R. A. Wright & G. H. E. Gendolla (Eds.), *How motivation affects cardiovascular response: Mechanisms and applications* (pp. 287–305). Washington, DC: American Psychological Association.

Smith, T. W., & Gallo, L. C. (1999). Hostility and cardiovascular reactivity during marital interaction. *Psychosomatic Medicine, 61,* 436–445.

Smith, T. W., Gallo, L. C., Goble, L., Ngu, L. Q., & Stark, K. A. (1998). Agency, communion, and cardiovascular reactivity during marital interaction. *Health Psychology, 17,* 537–545.

Smith, T. W., Limon, J. P., Gallo, L. C., & Ngu, L. Q. (1996). Interpersonal control and cardiovascular reactivity: Goals, behavioral expression, and the moderating effects of sex. *Journal of Personality and Social Psychology, 70,* 1012–1024.

Smith, T. W., Ruiz, J. M., Cundiff, J. M., Baron, K. G., & Nealey-Moore, J. B. (2013). Optimism and pessimism in social context: An interpersonal perspective on resilience and risk. *Journal of Research in Personality, 47,* 553–562.

Smith, T. W., Traupman, E. K., Uchino, B. N., & Berg, C. A. (2010). Interpersonal circumplex descriptions of psychosocial risk factors for physical illness: Application to hostility, neuroticism, and marital adjustment. *Journal of Personality, 78,* 1011–1036.

Smith, T. W., Uchino, B. N., Berg, C. A., & Florsheim, P. (2012). Marital discord and coronary artery disease: A comparison of behaviorally defined discrete groups. *Journal of Consuling andt Clinical Psychology, 80,* 87–92.

Smith, T. W., Uchino, B. N., Berg, C. A., Florsheim, P., Pearce, G., Hawkins, M., … Yoon, H.-C. (2008). Associations of self-reports versus spouse ratings of negative affectivity, dominance, and affiliation with coronary artery disease: Where should we look and who should we ask when studying personality and health? *Health Psychology, 27,* 676–684.

Smith, T. W., Uchino, B. N., Berg, C. A., Florsheim, P., Pearce, G., Hawkins, M., … Olsen-Cerny, C. (2009). Conflict and collaboration in middle-aged and older couples: II. Cardiovascular reactivity during marital interaction. *Psychology and Aging, 24,* 274–286. doi: 10.1037/a0016067.

Smith, T. W., Uchino, B. N., Florsheim, P., Berg, C. A., Butner, J., Hawkins, M., … Yoon, H-C. (2011). Affiliation and control during marital disagreement, history of divorce, and asymptomatic coronary artery calcification in older couples. *Psychosomatic Medicine, 73,* 350–357. doi: 10.1097/PSY.0b013e31821188ca.

Smith, T. W., Uchino, B. N., MacKenzie, J., Hicks, A., Campo, R. A., Reblin, M., … Light, K. C. (2013). Effects of couple interactions and relationship quality on plasma oxytocin and cardiovascular reactivity: Empirical findings and methodological considerations. *International Journal of Pschophysiology, 88,* 271–281.

Snyder, D. K., Heyman, R. E., & Haynes, S. N. (2005). Evidence-based approaches to assessing couple distress. *Psychological Assessment, 17,* 288–307.

South, S. C., & Kruger, R. F. (2008). Marital quality moderates the genetic and environmental influnces on the internalizing disorders. *Journal of Abnormal Psychology, 117,* 826–837.

South, S. C., Kruger, R. F., & Iacono, W. G. (2011). Understanding the general and specific connections between psychopathology and marital distress: A model-based approach. *Journal of Abnormal Psychology, 120,* 935–947.

South, S. C., Turkheimer, E., & Oltmanns, T. F. (2008). Personality disorder symptoms and marital functioning. *Journal of Consulting and Clinical Psychology, 76,* 769–780.

Spanier, G. B. (1976). Measuring dyadic adjustment: New scales for assessing the quality of marriage and similar dyads. *Journal of Marriage and Family, 36,* 15–28.

Sperry, L. (2011). Treating patients with heart disease: The impact of individual and family dynamics. *The Family Journal, 19,* 96–100.

Spotts, E. L., Lichtenstein, P., Pedersen, N., Neiderhiser, J. M., Hansson, K., Cederblad, M., & Reiss, D. (2005). Personality and marital satisfaction: A behavioral genetic analysis. *European Journal of Personality, 19,* 205–227.

Story, L. B., & Repetti, R. (2006). Daily occupational stressors and marital behavior. *Journal of Family Psychology, 20,* 690–700.

Stroud, C. D., Durbin, C. E., Saigal, S. D., & Knobloch-Fedders, L. M. (2010). Normal and abnormal personality traits are associated with marital satisfaction for both men and women: A actor-partner interdependence model analysis. *Journal of Research in Personality, 44,* 466–477.

Suls, J., & Bunde, J. (2005). Anger, anxiety, and depression as risk factors for cardiovascular disease: The problems and implications of overlapping affective dispositions. *Psychological Bulletin, 131,* 260–300.

Taft, C. T., Watkins, L. E., Stafford, J., Street, A. E., & Monson, C. M. (2011). Posttraumatic stress disorder and intimate relationship problems: A meta-analysis. *Journal of Consulting and Clinical Psychology, 79,* 22–33.

Taylor, S. E., Klein, L. C., Lewis, B. P., Gruenewald, T. L., Gurung, R. A. R., & Updegraff, J. A. (2000). Biobehavioral responses to stress in females: Tend-and-befriend, not fight-or-flight. *Psychological Review, 107*, 411–429. doi: 10.1037/0033-295x.107.3.411.

Taylor, S. E., Saphire-Bernstein, S., Seeman, T. E., & Saphire-Bernstein, S. (2010). Are plasma oxytocin in women and plasma vasopressin in men biomarkers of distressed pair-bond relationships? *Psychological Science, 21*, 3–7.

Thayer, J. F., Hansen, A. L., & Johnson, B. D. (2008). Non-invasive assessment of autonomic influences on the heart: Impedance cardiography and heart rate variability. In L. Leuken & L. Gallo (Eds.), *Handbook of physiological research methods in health psychology* (pp. 183–209). Thousand Oaks, CA: Sage.

Thayer, J. F., Hansen, A., Saus-Rose, E., & Johnsen, B. (2009). Heart rate variability, prefrontal neural function, and cognitive performance: The neurovisceral intergration perspective on self-regulation, adaptation, and health. *Annals of Behavioral Medicine, 37*, 141–153.

Thayer, J. F., & Lane, R. D. (2007). The role of vagal function in the risk for cardiovascular disease and mortality. *Biological Psychology, 74*, 224–242.

Thayer, J. F., & Sternberg, E. (2006). Beyond heart rate variability: Vagal regulation of allostatic systems. *Annals of the New York Academy of Science, 1088*, 361–372.

Tobe, S. W., Kiss, A., Sainsbury, S., Jesin, M., Geerts, R., & Baker, B. (2007). The impact of job strain and marital cohesion on ambulatory blood pressure during 1 year: The double exposure study. *American Journal of Hypertension, 20*, 148–153.

Tomlinson, J. M., & Aron, A. (2012). Relationship neuroscience: Where we are and where we might be going. In O. Gillath, G. Adams, & A. Kunkel (Eds.), *Relationship science: Integrating evolutionary, neuroscience, and sociocultural approaches* (pp. 13–26). Washington, DC: American Psychological Association.

Troxel, W. M. (2010). It's more than sex: Exploring the dyadic nature of sleep and implications for health. *Psychosomatic Medicine, 72*, 578–586.

Troxel, W., M., Matthews, K. A., Gallo, L. C., & Kuller, L. H. (2005). Marital quality and the occurrence of the metabolic syndrome in women. *Archives of Internal Medicine, 165*, 1022–1027.

Trull, T. J., & Brown, W. C. (2013). Borderline personality disorder: A five-factor model perspective. In T. A. Widiger & P. T. Costa, Jr. (Eds.), *Personality disorders and the five-factor model of personality* (3rd ed., pp. 119–132). Washington, DC: American Psychological Association.

Uchino, B. N., Holt-Lunstad, J., Uno, D., & Flinders, J. B. (2001). Heterogeneity in social networks of young and older adults: Prediction of mental health and cardiovascular reactivity during acute stress. *Journal of Behavioral Medicine, 24*, 361–382.

Urbina, E. M., Williams, R. V., Alpert, B. S., Collins, R. T., Daniels, S. R., Hyaman, L… & McCrindle, B. (2009). Noninvasive assessment of subclinical atherosclerosis in children and adolescents: Recommendations for standard assessment for clinical research: A scientific statement of the American Heart Association. *Hypertension, 54*, 919–950.

Uvnäs-Moberg, K., Arn, I., & Magnusson, D. (2005). The psychobiology of emotion: The role of the oxytocinergic system. *International Journal of Behavioral Medicine, 12*, 59–65.

Wang, H., Leineweber, C., Kirkeeide, R., Svane, B., Schenck-Gustafsson, K., Theorell, T., & Orth-Gomer, K. (2007). Psychosocial stress and atherosclerosis: Family and work stress accelerate progression of coronary artery disease in women. *Journal of Internal Medicine, 261*, 245–254.

Whisman, M. A., Beach, S. R. H., & Snyder, D. K. (2008). Is marital discord taxonic and can taxonic status be assessed reliably? Results from a national, representative sample of married couples. *Journal of Consulting and Clinical Psychology, 76*, 745–755.

Whisman, M. A., & Sbarra, D. A. (2012). Marital adjustment and interleukin-6 (IL-6). *Journal of Family Psychology, 26*, 290–295.

Whisman, M. A., & Schonbrun, Y. C. (2009). Social consequences of borderline personality disorder symptoms in a population-based survey: Marital distress, marital violence, and marital disruption. *Journal of Personality Disorders, 23,* 410–415.

Whisman, M. A., & Schonbrun, Y. C. (2010). Marital distress and relapse prevention for depression. In C. S. Richards & M. G. Perri (Eds.), *Relapse prevention for depression* (pp. 251–269). Washington, DC: American Psychological Association.

Whisman, M. A., & Uebelacker, L. A. (2009). Prospective associations between marital discord and depressive symptoms in middle-aged and older adults. *Psychology and Aging, 24,* 184–189.

Whisman, M. A., & Uebelacker, L. A. (2012). A longitudinal investigation of marital adjustment as a risk factor for metabolic syndrome. *Health Psychology, 31,* 80–86.

Williams, P. G., Smith, T. W., Gunn, H. E., & Uchino, B. N. (2011). Personality and stress: Individual differences in exposure, reactivity, recovery, and restoration. In R. Contrada & A. Baum (Eds.), *Handbook of stress science: Biology, psychology, and health* (pp. 231–245). New York, NY: Springer.

Zaider, T. I., Heimberg, R. G., & Masumi, I. (2010). Anxiety disorders and intimate relationships: A study of daily processes in couples. *Journal of Abnormal Psychology, 119,* 163–173.

CHAPTER 3

Family Relationships and Cortisol in Everyday Life

RICHARD B. SLATCHER

When asked to describe what comes to mind when hearing the word *family*, it is not uncommon for people to conjure up images of happy experiences, relaxing times, and a place of refuge. But in reality, time with family is not always so harmonious. Even in generally happy and well-adjusted families there can be arguments, yelling, crying, and other negative emotions. Everyday lives of families can be stressful for both parents and children. There are also outside forces that exert a daily push and pull on the family environment, including work, peer relationships, financial difficulties, and even traffic hassles. When these outside forces are brought home by family members in the form of bad moods, emotional withdrawal, impatience, and/or less time spent with family, the ways in which other family members react to these outside forces—and how the person bringing them home reacts to them—is critically important for the mental and physical health of family members. In the best of cases, relationships in the home can provide a restorative place that buffers or diffuses the effects of outside stressors. In other cases, relationships at home—between spouses, children, siblings, and parents—can be stressors themselves.

Research has shown that the type of social environment that family members come home to has important consequences for the body's stress physiology and, ultimately, physical health. In this chapter, I present an overview of the links between family relationships in everyday life and the production of cortisol, the primary stress hormone produced by the body. The chapter begins with a description of cortisol—what it is, how it can be measured in naturalistic settings, and its implications for physical health. I then review key findings linking marital relationships to cortisol production before turning to a discussion of how family relationships impact children's cortisol production. Throughout the chapter, I will emphasize key findings from the past 5 years relating to associations between family relationships and cortisol that have not yet been reviewed elsewhere (to the author's knowledge). The final section of the chapter will cover cutting-edge work that is attempting to answer critical mechanistic questions of how family relationships "get under the skin" to affect cortisol, and, ultimately, physical health. The chapter will conclude with a preview of some of the work that our research group is conducting to tie together various aspects of links between family relationships, stress physiology, and health outcomes in order to clarify stress-health links.

CORTISOL RESPONSES TO STRESS

How might the relationships that we have at home translate into between-person differences in how our immune systems operate, how often we get sick, and how long we live? In the 50 years since Selye's (1956) pioneering rat studies on the physiological affects of stress, scientists across a variety of disciplines have sought to understand the biological mechanisms through which stress adversely impacts physical health. The allostatic load model suggests that chronic strain leads to alterations in the body's regulatory "set points," speeding up eventual wear and tear (McEwen, 1998b). Frequent activation of the body's stress response that accompanies chronic stress can lead to greater "load" on a variety of organs and tissues, including the cardiovascular system. It is this overload on the body's various biological systems that is thought to lead to serious health problems if chronic stress is not reduced. Extending this model to everyday family life, it is believed that biological systems involved in the stress response are chronically activated in families in which there are consistently high stress levels (due to a variety of factors described later in this chapter). This chronic activation, in turn, results in greater allostatic load and poorer health outcomes among family members within and across generations (Kiecolt-Glaser & Newton, 2001; Miller, Chen, & Parker, 2011; Repetti, Robles, & Reynolds, 2011; Repetti, Wang, & Saxbe, 2011; Slatcher, 2010).

A key biological system implicated in allostatic load is the HPA (hypothalamic-pituitary-adrenal) axis, a complex cascade network in which the hypothalamus, pituitary gland, and adrenal glands work in concert to produce the stress hormone cortisol (ultimately secreted by the adrenal cortex). The HPA axis has attracted particular attention from researchers due to its sensitivity to psychological stress and its effects on multiple biological systems throughout the body. This system is present in organisms ranging from birds to humans and can be engaged by an array of psychological and physical stressors (McEwen, 1998a; McEwen & Stellar, 1993; Miller, Chen, & Zhou, 2007; Sapolsky, Romero, & Munck, 2000). Activation of the HPA occurs when neurons in the paraventricular nucleus of the hypothalamus secrete corticotropin-releasing hormone (CRH). CRH then travels to the anterior pituitary gland, which responds to its presence by secreting a burst of adrenocorticotropin hormone (ACTH). ACTH then is carried through peripheral circulation to the adrenal glands, which proceed to synthesize and release cortisol. It is hard to overstate the biological reach of cortisol, for which receptors exist in virtually every cell of the human body. Cortisol is a regulatory hormone, involved in learning, memory, and emotion in the central nervous system; regulation of glucose storage and utilization in the metabolic system, particularly in times of threat (the fight-or-flight response); and regulation of the magnitude and of the inflammatory response and maturation of lymphocytes in the immune system (Miller et al., 2007; Sapolsky et al., 2000).

Cortisol production has a diurnal rhythm, with levels peaking approximately 30 minutes after a person wakes, declining sharply in the morning hours, then slowly decreasing over the afternoon and evening to its nadir shortly before bedtime. Flattened diurnal cortisol slope (less decline in cortisol throughout the day) is thought to be a marker of a dysregulated stress response system because it indicates that people's stress hormones are remaining unusually high as the day progresses, thus contributing to greater allostatic load (McEwen, 1998a). Dysregulation of the HPA axis—including flatter cortisol slopes but also greater total cortisol output (assessed through area under the curve analysis, or AUC)—is associated with a number of poor health outcomes, including compromised immune functioning (Cohen et al., 2012), inflammation (DeSantis et al., 2012; Rueggeberg, Wrosch, Miller, & McDade, 2012), diabetes (Schoorlemmer, Peeters, van Schoor, & Lips, 2009), lung disease (Schoorlemmer et al., 2009), hippocampal atrophy (Sapolsky, 2000), and cardiovascular disease (Matthews, Schwartz, Cohen, & Seeman, 2006). Recent evidence suggests that flatter diurnal cortisol slopes especially are indicative of poorer future health, with links to mortality in two studies (Kumari, Shipley, Stafford, & Kivimaki, 2011; Sephton, Sapolsky, Kraemer, & Spiegel, 2000). In one study, flatter cortisol slopes were associated with lowered cell counts and activity of circulating natural killer cells and greater mortality among patients with metastatic breast cancer (Sephton et al., 2000). Further, in a prospective cohort analysis of 4,047 civil servants from the Whitehall II study (Kumari et al., 2011), flatter cortisol slopes predicted greater all-cause mortality and were especially predictive of an increased risk of cardiovascular death.

Given the association between HPA dysregulation and physical health problems, links between family relationships—which can be both stress inducing and stress buffering—and cortisol production have begun to receive increased attention from researchers. Although most cortisol researchers have investigated the effects of acute stressors on cortisol in lab settings (for a review, see Dickerson & Kemeny, 2004; Halpern, Campbell, Agnew, Thompson, & Udry, 2002), it is currently believed that chronic, naturalistic stressors have a more profound impact on physical health via the HPA than do acute stressors (Miller et al., 2007). Cortisol studies conducted in daily life are beginning to provide a picture of how everyday stressors impact cortisol production in situ and, unlike laboratory studies, allow for examination of how real-life stressors impact diurnal cortisol patterns. Field studies of links between everyday life and HPA axis functioning have become more common since the introduction of salivary cortisol assays in the late 1980s. In these studies, participants generally provide between three and seven saliva samples per day (either by passively drooling into a tube for approximately 2 minutes or by chewing on a cotton swab, which then becomes soaked with saliva), usually over 1 to 7 days. The samples then either can be analyzed with commercially purchased assay kits or sent to a laboratory for analysis, which generally charges between $5 and $10 per sample. Although there is a learning curve for those who have not conducted salivary cortisol studies, the expense is quite low by biological research standards and collecting assays is relatively straightforward (for an excellent review and field guide to conducting salivary cortisol studies in everyday life, see Saxbe, 2008).

Understanding the specific psychological processes and events in everyday family life that lead to HPA axis dysregulation is key to clarifying how stress impacts physical health. Such an understanding adds to the allostatic load literature by defining the emotional, cognitive, and behavioral responses that family members have around one another when coping with the daily hassles and chronic stressors of daily life. While the allostatic load model takes into account the repeated "hits" on biological systems, the psychological literature has begun to outline what constitutes those hits (Repetti, Robles, et al., 2011). Next, I review the literature linking everyday family life to daily cortisol production, first focusing on how adults' cortisol levels are impacted by daily experiences in the home and then turning to how everyday family experiences impact children's production of cortisol.

EVERYDAY FAMILY ENVIRONMENTS AND ADULT CORTISOL

Social and emotional experiences in the family—particularly within the couple relationship—impact adults' daily cortisol production. For instance, couples' daily physical intimacy (including holding hands, touching, hugging, kissing, and sexual intercourse) is associated with lower cortisol production, and this link is mediated by greater levels of daily positive affect (Ditzen, Hoppmann, & Klumb, 2008). In a recent naturalistic study of 31 dual-earner married couples with children in the United States, wives who were more satisfied in their marriages had steeper (more "healthy") cortisol slopes throughout the day (Saxbe, Repetti, & Nishina, 2008). Further, marital satisfaction moderated the links between cortisol during the day (while women were at work) and cortisol at night; among wives high in marital satisfaction, the links between daily cortisol and nighttime cortisol were attenuated. These findings are in line with cross-sectional work demonstrating associations between aspects of marriage and daily cortisol patterns. Those studies have shown that less positive marital relationships and greater marital role concerns are linked to flatter diurnal cortisol slopes (Adam & Gunnar, 2001; Barnett, Steptoe, & Gareis, 2005), whereas greater marital satisfaction is linked to steeper cortisol slopes (Vedhara, Stra, Miles, Sanderman, & Ranchor, 2006).

The influence that family dynamics have on adult family members' HPA axis activity is not limited to the marital relationship. Stress related to household chores, for instance, has been shown to impact cortisol levels at home. In a recent study of dual-earner German couples, time devoted to housework was linked to greater cortisol production over the course of the day (Klumb, Hoppmann, & Staats, 2006). Housework, not surprisingly, also appears to be detrimental to unwinding after work: Husbands and wives who spend a higher percentage of their time at home on housework have higher evening cortisol levels and weaker declines in cortisol from afternoon to evening (Saxbe, Repetti, & Graesch, 2011). Interestingly, how people describe their homes—as either restorative or stressful—is linked to HPA axis functioning. In a recent study, spouses gave home tours to interviewers that were videotaped and then linguistically analyzed for words like "clutter," "unfinished," and "restful" (Saxbe & Repetti, 2010a). Over the 3 days following the home tours, wives with higher stressful home scores showed flatter cortisol slopes, whereas wives with higher restorative home scores had steeper cortisol slopes.

The effect of parenthood on cortisol functioning has received only limited attention, but studies suggest that from child delivery onward, having children impacts HPA functioning. In a study of women who recently gave birth, there were significant differences in postnatally depressed and postnatally nondepressed mothers: Those who were depressed showed a smaller morning rise in cortisol (CAR) than those not depressed (Taylor, Glover, Marks, & Kammerer, 2009), an effect similar to that seen in people reporting posttraumatic stress disorder. The mere presence of children in the home appears to attenuate recovery from daily stressors; among mothers of 2-year-olds, the greater the number of children in the home, the flatter the mother's cortisol slope (Adam & Gunnar, 2001). Similarly, working mothers have been shown to secrete greater cortisol over a 24-hour period than working women without children (Luecken et al., 1997).

Stress biology also is affected by the worries that people bring home with them from work. For instance, negative mood when people are at work is associated with day-to-day increases in angry marital behavior (Schulz, Cowan, Pape Cowan, & Brennan, 2004), and greater work-related stress is associated with less responsiveness to spouses and increased distraction after the work day ends (Story & Repetti, 2006). It is also the case that work stress impacts cortisol levels at home and that being in a highly satisfying marriage attenuates this effect (Saxbe et al., 2008). Further, increased work hours are linked to greater cortisol output over the course of the day—impacting both one's own and spouses' cortisol levels (Klumb et al., 2006).

When one comes home from work, it can be difficult to unwind. Even on the weekends, when we are spending time with family engaging in leisure pursuits, worries about work can sometimes stay with us. We recently investigated the physiological impact of work worries at home in a sample of dual-earner couples with young children (Slatcher, Robles, Repetti, & Fellows, 2010). Men's increases in work worries at home not only led to greater increases in their own cortisol levels (an actor effect) but also were linked to increases in their wives' cortisol levels (a partner effect). Interestingly, wives' work worries impacted their own cortisol levels but had no affect on their husbands' cortisol levels. Why might husbands' work worries impact their wives' stress biology, but not vice versa? Previous laboratory findings suggest that wives are more biologically sensitive to changes in marital behaviors than husbands are (Robles & Kiecolt-Glaser, 2003; Smith, Gallo, Goble, Ngu, & Stark, 1998). This also is in line with more recent work showing that couples' cortisol levels covary (Saxbe & Repetti, 2010b).

In addition to studying how outside stressors impact spouses at home, we are investigating the aspects of marriage that may help buffer the effects of those stressors. One relationship process that we believe may be especially important is self-disclosure—the opening up to another person about one's thoughts, feelings, and emotions. It is now well known that self-disclosure has positive benefits for romantic relationships (Laurenceau, Barrett, & Rovine, 2005; Reis & Shaver, 1988; Slatcher & Pennebaker, 2006). Although there are a large number of experimental studies showing that self-disclosure through expressive writing is associated with better physical health (Frattaroli, 2006; Slatcher & Pennebaker, 2005) and stress biology (Smyth, Hockemeyer, & Tulloch, 2008), surprisingly few studies have investigated the effect of self-disclosure in one's close relationships—the context in which most self-disclosure naturally occurs—on health-related outcomes. Our research has shown that wives who report low levels of self-disclosure to their husbands show a much stronger association between the worries about work that they carry home with them and cortisol levels at home than those who are highly disclosing (Slatcher et al., 2010). Wives low in self-disclosure who also reported low levels of marital satisfaction showed especially strong links between work worries and cortisol levels. These findings suggest that self-disclosure may be a way in which women "inoculate" themselves against the physiological effects of work stress.

Having shown that family relationships impact adults' cortisol levels, researchers are now beginning to test the effectiveness of couples interventions on HPA axis activity. The results of these studies so far are mixed. In one study, married couples were randomly assigned to either a behavioral monitoring control group or participated in a 4-week "warm touch" support enhancement intervention (Holt-Lunstad, Birmingham, & Light, 2008). The intervention led to increases in salivary oxytocin (a hormone that promotes pair bonding) and reductions in salivary alpha amylase (an index of sympathetic nervous system activity), but no changes in cortisol. More recently, the effects of couples relationship education (CRE) on cortisol have been tested. CRE, which is geared toward improving positive communication and conflict management (Markman, Rhoades, Delaney, & White, 2010), is effective in boosting relationship quality and stability in married couples (Carroll & Doherty, 2003). Couples who go through a CRE intervention show significantly reduced cortisol responses during couple conflict discussions compared to preintervention levels (Ditzen, Hahlweg, Fehm-Wolfsdorf, & Baucom, 2011). These data suggest that improving relationship functioning through interventions may buffer the harmful effects of repeated conflict on stress physiology.

Although more research is still needed, the past decade has seen a growing number of studies investigating how family relationships impact adults' cortisol production in daily life. This work has shown that the quality of family relationships—especially couple relationships—impacts HPA functioning and can buffer the effects of outside stressors such as the worries about work that people bring home with them. However, the effects of family relationships on cortisol are not limited to adult family members. Next, I review findings suggesting that family relationships can have potent effects on children's cortisol levels as well.

EVERYDAY FAMILY ENVIRONMENTS AND CHILD CORTISOL

Alterations of the HPA axis are considered a primary mechanism through which early-life experiences impact adult health (McEwen, 1998a; Repetti, Taylor, & Seeman, 2002). There have been a great number of studies examining the effects of stress on cortisol production in childhood, which have been exhaustively reviewed elsewhere (e.g., Gunnar & Quevedo, 2007). This review focuses specifically on family experiences and naturalistic assessments of cortisol in daily life throughout child development.

Prenatal Development

The impact of stress on human stress physiology begins in the earliest stages of life. The effects of stress on mothers' cortisol levels in pregnancy appear to have important implications for the long-term health of the child. Low birth weight remains one of the greatest concerns of perinatal health, and maternal stress is linked to clinically meaningful reductions in birth weight (Maina et al., 2008). Glucocorticoids may be a common link between prenatal stressors, intrauterine growth, and birth weight (Seckl & Meaney, 2004), but the evidence so far is mixed. In one study, mothers' higher CARs were associated with lower birth weight, but mothers' distress was unrelated to cortisol or birth weight (Bolten et al., 2011). In another study, higher cortisol concentrations at awakening and throughout the day and flatter CARs were associated with shorter length of gestation; negative affect was associated with higher cortisol throughout the day, but not to gestational length. Although this type of work in humans is only just starting, a recent review provides suggestive evidence that prenatal stress or anxiety in the mother is associated with raised basal cortisol or raised cortisol reactivity in offspring, from infancy through adolescence (Glover, O'Connor, & O'Donnell, 2010).

Infancy and Early Childhood

In the first year of life, external regulation of infants' arousal by primary caregivers is needed to protect infants from excessive stress. Caregivers who respond sensitively to the infant help to regulate this arousal, providing the infant with a secure base (Bowlby, 1969). Insensitive or intrusive parenting behaviors are believed to be stressful for newborns because of their uncontrollable nature (Ainsworth, Blehar, Waters, & Wall, 1978). Among 3-month-olds, maternal sensitivity is associated with faster cortisol recovery from the mild everyday stress of being bathed (Albers, Riksen-Walraven, Sweep, & de Weerth, 2008). Additionally, infants of mothers experiencing parenting stress show higher daily cortisol output (Saridjan et al., 2010).

This pattern continues into the preschool years. Although relatively few studies have examined how everyday family behaviors impact young children's diurnal cortisol, research has shown that mothers who report higher maternal parenting quality have kindergarteners who show steeper ("healthier") cortisol slopes in daily life (Pendry & Adam, 2007). In a recent study, we investigated the links between everyday conflict at home—assessed with a naturalistic observation tool called the Electronically Activated Recorder (EAR)—and preschoolers' diurnal cortisol patterns (Slatcher & Robles, 2012). Typically, participants carry the EAR (in a pocket, purse, etc.) for 1–4 days, unobtrusively capturing 30- to 50-second audio snippets every 9–12 minutes (Mehl, Robbins, & Deters, 2012). Essentially, the EAR provides an acoustic window into people's daily behaviors. Preschoolers in our study wore a child EAR inside a "special magic shirt" with a pocket to hold the EAR that had different cartoon characters sewn onto it; this helped to build children's enthusiasm for wearing the EAR, while at the same time helping to protect the EAR and make it more unobtrusive. Greater EAR-assessed conflict at home with parents and siblings was linked to children having higher initial morning cortisol levels and flatter cortisol slopes across the day (e.g., less "healthy" diurnal cortisol rhythms). Although it is now commonplace for studies of adolescents to include momentary self-reports of daily behaviors (Conner, Tennen, Fleeson, & Barrett, 2009), the inability of young children to complete these type of reports (and the inherent biases of parent reports) make everyday studies of family life and early childhood health less common. Studying actual behaviors at home offers a potential way of getting around some of these stubborn methodological difficulties. Emerging technologies such as the EAR offer a fairly low-cost way of studying the effects of early family environments on HPA axis functioning (the most current version of the EAR is now iPod touch based). Toward the end of this chapter I describe a new study being conducted at Wayne State University that is using the EAR to examine how everyday family behaviors are linked to diurnal cortisol patterns and health outcomes in youth with asthma.

Middle Childhood

The time of middle childhood is a period of relative calm in terms of HPA axis development (Gunnar & Quevedo, 2007), but the family continues to exert an influence on daily cortisol production. The pattern of findings generally is consistent with what we see in earlier childhood, with recent stressful events and parents' lower marital satisfaction being associated with greater overall cortisol output and flatter diurnal slopes (Bevans, Cerbone, & Overstreet, 2008; Pendry & Adam, 2007; Wolf, Nicholls, & Chen, 2008). Much of the work with this age group has looked at the extreme end of adverse family environments, investigating the effects of maltreatment and neglect. Cicchetti and Rogosch (2001a, 2001b), for example, have reported that children who experienced multiple, severe, prolonged abuse had greater daily cortisol output. A major challenge in interpreting the existing literature is that it remains unclear whether altered cortisol levels are due to ongoing adversity or prior-experienced adversity. In well-known studies of children in Romanian orphanages characterized by extreme neglect, children still in the orphanages showed a lack of diurnal rhythm in cortisol production during the daytime hours (Carlson & Earls, 1997), whereas after an average of 6.5 years post adoption, children exhibited the normal expected decrease in cortisol from wakeup to bedtime (Gunnar, Morison, Chisholm, & Schuder, 2001). More recently, it was shown that preadoption deprivation among internationally adopted children—as reported by adoptive parents—was associated with higher morning cortisol levels and larger diurnal cortisol decreases, but only among those children who had physical growth delays (e.g., shorter than expected height).

Current negative experiences at home also affect daily cortisol production at this age. These effects appear to be strongest during the evening, when cortisol levels are typically at their lowest and when children are at home with their families. Living with chronic stress at home (Bevans et al., 2008; Schreier & Evans, 2003; Wolf et al., 2008), marital dysfunction (Pendry & Adam, 2007), and family strife, crowding, and noise (Evans, 2003; Evans & Kim, 2007) all are associated with higher evening cortisol. A few recent studies have investigated the long-term effects of home-life adversity, showing that maltreatment in childhood is associated with greater daily cortisol output among adult women with chronic pain (Nicolson, Davis, Kruszewski, & Zautra, 2010), while low parental care is associated with increased CAR and increased afternoon/evening cortisol levels in healthy men and women (Engert, Efanov, Dedovic, Dagher, & Pruessner, 2011). Recent intervention research is encouraging, showing, for example, that atypical diurnal cortisol patterns of children in foster care can be altered—becoming comparable to nonfoster children—following a family-based treatment intervention (Fisher, Stoolmiller, Gunnar, & Burraston, 2007), and a poverty-alleviation intervention has led to reductions in daily cortisol production among low-income children with depressed mothers in Mexico (Fernald & Gunnar, 2009).

Adolescence

Adolescence is a critical time to study links between family environment and HPA axis activity, as transitions into early, middle, and late adolescence are each characterized by significant changes in family contexts (Graber, Brooks-Gunn, & Petersen, 1996; Lerner, 2002). The quality of youths' family environment both shapes and is shaped by these transitions, with important implications for the HPA axis and, more broadly, for physical health (Holmbeck et al., 2010; Poulin & Heckhausen, 2007). For example, transitions from elementary to middle school and from middle to high school are each associated with greater family conflict, particularly among high-stress families (Gutman & Eccles, 2007; Herrenkohl et al., 2010; Obradović & Hipwell, 2010; Seidman, Lambert, Allen, & Aber, 2003). Within families, parental monitoring shifts as youth assert greater behavioral autonomy (Barber, Stolz, & Olsen, 2005; Darling, Cumsille, & Martinez, 2008). Links between low family support, decreased monitoring, and precocious behavioral autonomy suggest that family environments may be crucial to supporting youths' behavioral autonomy in ways that influence health-related outcomes (Dishion, Poulin, & Skaggs, 2000; Laird, Criss, Pettit, Dodge, & Bates, 2008; Ryan, Deci, Grolnick, & La Guardia, 2006).

HPA axis activity increases substantially during adolescence (Gunnar & Quevedo, 2007; Oskis, Loveday, Hucklebridge, Thorn, & Clow, 2009). Although fewer studies of family effects on daily cortisol have been conducted in adolescence than in earlier developmental periods, the current evidence suggests that parental warmth has an inverse, linear association with basal cortisol levels (Marsman et al., 2012). Further, adolescents living in homes where mothers and their partners report poorer marital functioning have significantly higher average cortisol levels than adolescents in homes where parents report higher marital functioning (Pendry & Adam, 2007). There also appears to be significant synchrony between parent and child cortisol at this age. In a recent study (Papp, Pendry, & Adam, 2009), family members' cortisol levels were measured seven times a day on 2 typical weekdays. After accounting for the effects of time of day and relevant demographic and health control variables on cortisol levels, multilevel modeling indicated the presence of significant covariation over time in mother–adolescent cortisol. Importantly, mother–adolescent cortisol synchrony was strengthened among dyads characterized by mothers and adolescents spending more time together, and in families rated higher on levels of parent–youth shared activities and parental monitoring or supervision.

In a new study funded by the National Institutes of Health (NIH), we are using the EAR (described previously) to gain a fly-on-the wall perspective on how everyday family interactions impact youth health via their effects on the HPA axis. This project, Asthma in the Lives of Families Today (ALOFT), takes a multimethod biopsychosocial approach by investigating the links between everyday family behaviors and asthma morbidity in a sample of 180 youth aged 10–15 years in Detroit, Michigan. With the ALOFT study, we are collecting longitudinal data over three waves in a 2-year period, having participants in the study wear EAR, and collecting parent and child daily diaries of family functioning, biological measures (including diurnal cortisol, gene expression, and epigenetic markers), and clinical asthma evaluations. Asthma is a chronic inflammatory disease of the respiratory tract that stems from a complex interaction of environmental, psychological, and genetic factors (Howard, Meyers, & Bleecker, 2003). Because asthma symptoms are modulated by cortisol—not only cortisol produced by the body but also synthetic cortisol administered via oral steroids (e.g., prednisone) to control asthma—scientists are beginning to look to asthma as a target disease for understanding how stress "gets under the skin" to affect health. Next, I conclude this chapter with a discussion of the biological mechanisms through which cortisol dysregulation stemming from family-related stressors may ultimately impact physical health and how these are being tested with the ALOFT study.

HOW DO THE EFFECTS OF FAMILY ENVIRONMENTS ON CORTISOL ULTIMATELY IMPACT HEALTH?

The biological mechanisms through which families exert their influence on physical health via cortisol remain poorly understood. Among cortisol's physiological functions is modulation of the immune system—its primary role in this regard is to suppress inflammation. Based on this role, one would predict that the high levels of cortisol that accompany stress would lead to a dampening of inflammation in inflammatory diseases such as asthma, similar to what occurs when corticosteroids are exogenously administered (e.g., when one applies hydrocortisone to an itchy bug bite or takes prednisone for more serious inflammation). In reality, empirical evidence suggests just the opposite: Stress *exacerbates* inflammation (Miller, Rohleder, & Cole, 2009; Pervanidou, Margeli, Lazaropoulou, Papassotiriou, & Chrousos, 2008).

Over the past decade, Miller and colleagues (Miller, Cohen, & Ritchey, 2002) have proposed a theory of glucocorticoid resistance (immune system resistance to the regulatory effects of cortisol) that offers a plausible explanation for why chronic stress is linked to both high levels of circulating cortisol and high levels of inflammation. The basic idea behind the glucocorticoid resistance model is that chronic stress interferes with the immune system's responsiveness to cortisol, which normally should dampen the body's inflammatory immune response. In support of this idea, new evidence shows that the persistent secretion of cortisol associated with chronic stress leads to a downregulation of glucocorticoid receptor expression and functioning (Cohen et al., 2012; Miller & Chen, 2006; Miller et al., 2002; Miller, Gaudin, Zysk, & Chen, 2009). Among those with chronic inflammatory diseases (which include diseases such as asthma, arthritis, and cardiovascular disease), this downregulation can lead to increased inflammation and, in the case of asthma, reduced efficacy of glucocorticoid therapy (including both inhaled and oral steroids)—a mainstay of asthma treatment (Lee, Brattsand, & Leung, 1996). For example, among children with asthma, high levels of chronic family stress are associated with a 5.5-fold reduction in leukocyte (white blood cell) glucocorticoid receptor mRNA. This indicates that immune cells' receptors—which normally respond to cortisol signals by turning "off" inflammatory immune processes—are not being produced in sufficient numbers to work as they should (Miller & Chen, 2006). This is akin to a strong radio signal being sent out from a radio station (the body producing large amounts of cortisol under stress) but having very few receivers in people's homes (the glucocorticoid receptors in immune cells) to pick up the signal. There are functional implications for these cellular processes that drive asthma: peripheral blood mononuclear cells (PBMCs) harvested from asthmatic children with greater family stress are more resistant to hydrocortisone's effects on pro-inflammatory cytokine expression (e.g., IL-5 and IF-γ) relative to asthmatic patients reporting lower family stress (Miller, Gaudin, et al., 2009).

The possibility that epigenetic changes may play a contributing role to the development of inflammation has received significant attention in the past few years from human and animal researchers (Bjornsson et al., 2008; McGowan et al., 2009; Weaver et al., 2005). In classic terms, epigenetics refers to the heritable, but reversible, regulation of genetic functions. A major mechanism of epigenetic regulation that has been identified is DNA methylation. DNA methylation is a modification of DNA in which methyl groups are added to certain positions on the nitrogen bases, typically leading to the inhibiting or "silencing" of gene expression. With the ALOFT study, we are focusing on methylation of the glucocorticoid receptor gene NR3C1, a gene responsible for gene expression of the glucocorticoid receptors in immune cells (e.g., the "radio receivers" described previously). Recent work has shown that DNA methylation profiles can change over time (Bjornsson et al., 2008) and that such profiles can differ in monozygotic twins (Fraga et al., 2005). The relative instability of these epigenetic signatures makes them attractive candidates for studying the underlying mechanisms of complex disease such as asthma. Recent studies suggest that epigenetic regulation may in part mediate the complex gene–environment interactions that can lead to disease (Miller & Ho, 2008). These exciting new findings point to potential biological pathways through which family stress exacerbates physical health problems. The ALOFT study is investigating whether stressful family relationships foster epigenetic changes in immune cells— specifically hypermethylation (greater methylation) of glucocorticoid receptor promoter sites—and gene expression (e.g., reduced glucocorticoid receptor expression) that, in turn, explain how the tonically higher levels of cortisol associated with chronic stress may begin to shut down the immune system's "normal" response to cortisol, thus leading to greater incidence of inflammatory diseases such as asthma, cardiovascular disease, and arthritis.

CONCLUSION

The number of naturalistic studies of family relationships and cortisol is only beginning to catch up to the decades of cortisol studies conducted in the lab. However, the studies reviewed in this chapter hint at the huge strides that have been made in investigating how family interactions are linked to HPA axis functioning in daily life. Although this type of work can be challenging in terms of expense and both researcher and participant burden, the knowledge gained has led to a number of critical advances in our understanding of family relationships, stress, and health. On the psychological side, emerging technologies such as EAR are allowing us access to the inner workings of everyday family life that was never before possible. On the health side, advances in the biological sciences and a growing "team science" approach is bringing scientists from a variety of disciplines together to understand the effects of psychological factors on HPA functioning at a molecular level. What is most exciting is not what we have learned about these processes over the past 10 years, but what is still left to be learned about how family relationships "get under the skin" to impact physical health.

REFERENCES

Adam, E. K., & Gunnar, M. R. (2001). Relationship functioning and home and work demands predict individual differences in diurnal cortisol patterns in women. *Psychoneuroendocrinology, 26,* 189–208.

Ainsworth, M., Blehar, M., Waters, E., & Wall, S. (1978). *Patterns of attachment: A psychological study of the strange situation.* Hillsdale, NJ: Erlbaum.

Albers, E. M., Riksen-Walraven, J. M., Sweep, F. C. G. J., & de Weerth, C. (2008). Maternal behavior predicts infant cortisol recovery from a mild everyday stressor. *Journal of Child Psychology and Psychiatry, 49,* 97–103.

Barber, B. K., Stolz, H. E., & Olsen, J. A. (2005). Parental support, psychological control, and behavioral control: Assessing relevance across time, culture, and method. *Monographs of the Society for Research in Child Development, 70,* 1–137.

Barnett, R. C., Steptoe, A., & Gareis, K. C. (2005). Marital-role quality and stress-related psychobiological indicators. *Annals of Behavioral Medicine, 30,* 36–43.

Bevans, K., Cerbone, A., & Overstreet, S. (2008). Relations between recurrent trauma exposure and recent life stress and salivary cortisol among children. *Development and Psychopathology, 20,* 257–272.

Bjornsson, H. T., Sigurdsson, M. I., Fallin, M. D., Irizarry, R. A., Aspelund, T., Cui, H., ... Feinberg, A. P. (2008). Intra-individual change over time in DNA methylation with familial clustering. *Journal of the American Medical Association, 299,* 2877–2883.

Bolten, M. I., Wurmser, H., Buske-Kirschbaum, A., Papoušek, M., Pirke, K.-M., & Hellhammer, D. (2011). Cortisol levels in pregnancy as a psychobiological predictor for birth weight. *Archives of Women's Mental Health, 14,* 33–41.

Bowlby, J. (1969). *Attachment.* New York, NY: Basic Books.

Carlson, M., & Earls, F. (1997). Psychological and neuroendocrinological sequelae of early social deprivation in institutionalized children in Romania. *Annals of the New York Academy of Sciences, 807,* 419–428.

Carroll, J. S., & Doherty, W. J. (2003). Evaluating the effectiveness of premarital prevention programs: A meta-analytic review of outcome research. *Family Relations, 52,* 105–118.

Cicchetti, D., & Rogosch, F. A. (2001a). Diverse patterns of neuroendocrine activity in maltreated children. *Development and Psychopathology, 13,* 677–693.

Cicchetti, D., & Rogosch, F. A. (2001b). The impact of child maltreatment and psychopathology on neuroendocrine functioning. *Development and Psychopathology, 13*, 783–804.

Cohen, S., Janicki-Deverts, D., Doyle, W. J., Miller, G. E., Frank, E., Rabin, B. S., & Turner, R. B. (2012). Chronic stress, glucocorticoid receptor resistance, inflammation, and disease risk. *Proceedings of the National Academy of Sciences USA, 109*, 5995–5999.

Conner, T. S., Tennen, H., Fleeson, W., & Barrett, L. F. (2009). Experience sampling methods: A modern idiographic approach to personality research. *Social and Personality Psychology Compass, 3*, 292–313. doi: 10.1111/j.1751-9004.2009.00170.x.

Darling, N., Cumsille, P., & Martinez, M. L. (2008). Individual differences in adolescents' beliefs about the legitimacy of parental authority and their own obligation to obey: A longitudinal investigation. *Child Development, 79*, 1103–1118.

DeSantis, A. S., DiezRoux, A. V., Hajat, A., Aiello, A. E., Golden, S. H., Jenny, N. S.,… Shea, S. (2012). Associations of salivary cortisol levels with inflammatory markers: The Multi-Ethnic Study of Atherosclerosis. *Psychoneuroendocrinology, 37*, 1009–1018.

Dickerson, S. S., & Kemeny, M. E. (2004). Acute stressors and cortisol responses: A theoretical integration and synthesis of laboratory research. *Psychological Bulletin, 130*, 355–391.

Dishion, T. J., Poulin, F., & Skaggs, N. M. (2000). The ecology of premature autonomy in adolescence: Biological and social influences. In K. Kerns, J. Contreras, & A. Neal-Barnett (Eds.), *Family and peers: Linking two social worlds* (pp. 27–45). Westport, CT: Praeger /Greenwood.

Ditzen, B., Hahlweg, K., Fehm-Wolfsdorf, G., & Baucom, D. (2011). Assisting couples to develop healthy relationships: Effects of couples relationship education on cortisol. *Psychoneuroendocrinology, 36*, 597–607.

Ditzen, B., Hoppmann, C., & Klumb, P. (2008). Positive couple interactions and daily cortisol: On the stress-protecting role of intimacy. *Psychosomatic Medicine, 70*, 883–889.

Engert, V., Efanov, S. I., Dedovic, K., Dagher, A., & Pruessner, J. C. (2011). Increased cortisol awakening response and afternoon/evening cortisol output in healthy young adults with low early life parental care. *Psychopharmacology, 214*, 261–268.

Evans, G. W. (2003). A multimethodological analysis of cumulative risk and allostatic load among rural children. *Developmental Psychology, 39*, 924.

Evans, G. W., & Kim, P. (2007). Childhood poverty and health--Cumulative risk exposure and stress dysregulation. *Psychological Science, 18*, 953–957.

Fernald, L. C. H., & Gunnar, M. R. (2009). Poverty-alleviation program participation and salivary cortisol in very low-income children. *Social Science and Medicine, 68*, 2180–2189.

Fisher, P. A., Stoolmiller, M., Gunnar, M. R., & Burraston, B. O. (2007). Effects of a therapeutic intervention for foster preschoolers on diurnal cortisol activity. *Psychoneuroendocrinology, 32*, 892–905. doi: 10.1016/j.psyneuen.2007.06.008.

Fraga, M., Ballestar, E., Paz, M., Ropero, S., Setien, F., Ballestar, M.,… Esteller, M. (2005). Epigenetic differences arise during the lifetime of monozygotic twins. *Proceedings of the National Academy of Sciences USA, 102*, 10604–10609.

Frattaroli, J. (2006). Experimental disclosure and its moderators: A meta-analysis. *Psychological Bulletin, 132*, 823–865.

Glover, V., O'Connor, T. G., & O'Donnell, K. (2010). Prenatal stress and the programming of the HPA axis. *Neuroscience and Biobehavioral Reviews, 35*, 17–22.

Graber, J., Brooks-Gunn, J., & Petersen, A. C. (Eds.). (1996). *Transitions through adolescence: Interpersonal domains and context.* Hillsdale, NJ: Erlbaum.

Gunnar, M., & Quevedo, K. (2007). The neurobiology of stress and development. *Annual Review of Psychology, 58*, 145–173. doi: 10.1146/annurev.psych.58.110405.085605.

Gunnar, M. R., Morison, S. J., Chisholm, K., & Schuder, M. (2001). Salivary cortisol levels in children adopted from Romanian orphanages. *Development and Psychopathology, 13*, 611–628.

Gutman, L. M., & Eccles, J. S. (2007). Stage-environment fit during adolescence: Trajectories of family relations and adolescent outcomes. *Developmental Psychology, 43*, 522–537.

Halpern, C. T., Campbell, B., Agnew, C. R., Thompson, V., & Udry, J. R. (2002). Associations between stress reactivity and sexual and nonsexual risk taking in young adult human males. *Hormones and Behavior, 42*, 387–398.

Herrenkohl, T. I., Kosterman, R., Mason, W. A., Hawkins, J. D., McCarty, C. A., & McCauley, E. (2010). Effects of childhood conduct problems and family adversity on health, health behaviors, and service use in early adulthood: Tests of developmental pathways involving adolescent risk taking and depression. *Development and Psychopathology. Special Issue: Developmental Cascades: Part 1, 22*, 655–665.

Holmbeck, G. N., DeLucia, C., Essner, B., Kelly, L., Zebracki, K., Friedman, D., & Jandasek, B. (2010). Trajectories of psychosocial adjustment in adolescents with spina bifida: A 6-year, four-wave longitudinal follow-up. *Journal of Consulting and Clinical Psychology, 78*, 511–525.

Holt-Lunstad, J., Birmingham, W. A., & Light, K. C. (2008). Influence of a "warm touch" support enhancement intervention among married couples on ambulatory blood pressure, oxytocin, alpha amylase, and cortisol. *Psychosomatic Medicine, 70*, 976–985. doi: 10.1097/PSY.0b013e318187aef7.

Howard, T., Meyers, D., & Bleecker, E. (2003). Mapping susceptibility genes from allergic diseases. *Chest, 123*, 363S–368S.

Kiecolt-Glaser, J. K., & Newton, T. L. (2001). Marriage and health: His and hers. *Psychological Bulletin, 127*, 472–503.

Klumb, P., Hoppmann, C., & Staats, M. (2006). Work hours affect spouse's cortisol secretion-For better and for worse. *Psychosomatic Medicine, 68*, 742–746.

Kumari, M., Shipley, M., Stafford, M., & Kivimaki, M. (2011). Association of diurnal patterns in salivary cortisol with all-cause and cardiovascular mortality: Findings from the Whitehall II study. *Journal of Clinical Endocrinology and Metabolism, 96*, 1478–1485. doi: 10.1210/jc.2010-2137.

Laird, R. D., Criss, M. M., Pettit, G. S., Dodge, K. A., & Bates, J. E. (2008). Parents' monitoring knowledge attenuates the link between antisocial friends and adolescent delinquent behavior. *Journal of Abnormal Child Psychology, 36*, 299–310.

Laurenceau, J-P., Barrett, L. F., & Rovine, M. J. (2005). The interpersonal process model of intimacy in marriage: A daily-diary and multilevel modeling approach. *Journal of Family Psychology, 19*, 314.

Lee, T. H., Brattsand, R., & Leung, D. Y. M. (1996). Corticosteroid action and resistance in asthma. *American Journal of Respiratory Cell and Molecular Biology, 154*(Suppl), S1–S79.

Lerner, R. M. (2002). *Adolescence: Development, diversity, context, and application.* Upper Saddle River, NJ: Prentice Hall/Pearson Education.

Luecken, L. J., Suarez, E. C., Kuhn, C. M., Barefoot, J. C., Blumenthal, J. A., Siegler, I. C., et al. (1997). Stress in employed women: Impact of marital status and children at home on neurohormone output and home strain. *Psychosomatic Medicine, 59*, 352–359.

Maina, G., Saracco, P., Giolito, M. R., Danelon, D., Bogetto, F., & Todros, T. (2008). Impact of maternal psychological distress on fetal weight, prematurity and intrauterine growth retardation. *Journal of Affective Disorders, 111*, 214–220.

Markman, H. J., Rhoades, G., Delaney, R., & White, L. (2010). Extending the reach of research-based couples interventions: The role of relationship education. In K. Hahlweg, M. Grawe-Gerber & D. H. Baucom (Eds.), *Enhancing couples: The shape of couple therapy to come* (pp. 128—141). Gottingen, Germany: Hogrefe.

Marsman, R., Nederhof, E., Rosmalen, J. G. M., Oldehinkel, A. J., Ormel, J., & Buitelaar, J. K. (2012). Family environment is associated with HPA-axis activity in adolescents. The TRAILS study. *Biological Psychology, 89*, 460–466.

Matthews, K., Schwartz, J., Cohen, S., & Seeman, T. (2006). Diurnal cortisol decline is related to coronary calcification: CARDIA study. *Psychosomatic Medicine, 68,* 657–661. doi: 10.1097/01.psy.0000244071.42939.0e.

McEwen, B. S. (1998a). Protective and damaging effects of stress mediators. *New England Journal of Medicine, 388,* 171–179.

McEwen, B. S. (1998b). Stress, adaptation and disease: Allostasis and allostatic load. *Annals of the New York Academy of Sciences, 840,* 33–44.

McEwen, B. S., & Stellar, E. (1993). Stress and the individual: Mechanisms leading to disease. *Archives of Internal Medicine, 153,* 2093–2101.

McGowan, P. O., Sasaki, A., D'Alessio, A. C., Dymov, S., Labonté, B., Szyf, M., …Meaney, M. J. (2009). Epigenetic regulation of the glucocorticoid receptor in human brain associates with childhood abuse. *Nature Neuroscience, 12,* 342–348.

Mehl, M. R., Robbins, M. L., & Deters, F. (2012). Naturalistic observation of health-relevant social processes: The electronically activated recorder (EAR) methodology in psychosomatics. *Psychosomatic Medicine, 74,* 410–471.

Miller, G. E., & Chen, E. (2006). Stressful experience and diminished expression of genes encoding the glucocorticoid receptor and b2-adrenergic receptor in children with asthma. *Proceedings of the National Academy of Sciences USA, 103,* 5496–5501.

Miller, G. E., Chen, E., & Parker, K. J. (2011). Psychological stress in childhood and susceptibility to the chronic diseases of aging: Moving toward a model of behavioral and biological mechanisms. *Psychological Bulletin, 137,* 959–997.

Miller, G. E., Chen, E., & Zhou, E. S. (2007). If it goes up, must it come down? Chronic stress and the hypothalamic-pituitary-adrenocortical axis in humans. *Psychological Bulletin, 133,* 25–45.

Miller, G. E., Cohen, S., & Ritchey, A. K. (2002). Chronic psychological stress and the regulation of pro-inflammatory cytokines: A glucocorticoid-resistance model. *Health Psychology, 21,* 531–541.

Miller, G. E., Gaudin, A., Zysk, E., & Chen, E. (2009). Parental support and cytokine activity in childhood asthma: The role of glucocorticoid sensitivity. *Journal of Allergy and Clinical Immunology, 123,* 824–830.

Miller, G. E., Rohleder, N., & Cole, S. W. (2009). Chronic interpersonal stress predicts activation of pro—and anti-inflammatory signaling pathways 6 months later. *Psychosomatic Medicine, 71,* 57–62.

Miller, R., & Ho, S. (2008). Environmental epigenetics and asthma: Current concepts and call for studies. *American Journal of Respiratory and Critical Care Medicine, 177,* 567–573.

Nicolson, N. A., Davis, M. C., Kruszewski, D., & Zautra, A. J. (2010). Childhood maltreatment and diurnal cortisol patterns in women with chronic pain. *Psychosomatic Medicine, 72,* 471–480.

Obradović, J., & Hipwell, A. (2010). Psychopathology and social competence during the transition to adolescence: The role of family adversity and pubertal development. *Development and Psychopathology.Special Issue: Developmental Cascades: Part 1, 22,* 621–634.

Oskis, A., Loveday, C., Hucklebridge, F., Thorn, L., & Clow, A. (2009). Diurnal patterns of salivary cortisol across the adolescent period in healthy females. *Psychoneuroendocrinology, 34,* 307–316.

Papp, L. M., Pendry, P., & Adam, E. K. (2009). Mother-adolescent physiological synchrony in naturalistic settings: Within-family cortisol associations and moderators. *Journal of Family Psychology, 23,* 882–894.

Pendry, P., & Adam, E. K. (2007). Associations between parents' marital functioning, maternal parenting quality, maternal emotion and child cortisol levels. *International Journal of Behavioral Development, 31,* 218–231. doi: 10.1177/0165025407074634.

Pervanidou, P., Margeli, A., Lazaropoulou, C., Papassotiriou, I., & Chrousos, G. P. (2008). The immediate and long-term impact of physical and/or emotional stress from motor vehicle accidents on circulating stress hormones and adipo-cytokines in children and adolescents. *Stress: The International Journal on the Biology of Stress, 11*, 438–447.

Poulin, M. J., & Heckhausen, J. (2007). Stressful events compromise control strivings during a major life transition. *Motivation and Emotion, 31*, 300–311.

Reis, H. T., & Shaver, P. (1988). Intimacy as an interpersonal process. In S. Duck (Ed.), *Handbook of personal relationships* (pp. 367–389). Chichester, UK: Wiley.

Repetti, R. L., Robles, T. F., & Reynolds, B. M. (2011). Allostatic processes in the family. *Development and Psychopathology, 23*, 921–938.

Repetti, R. L., Taylor, S. E., & Seeman, T. E. (2002). Risky families: Family social environments and the mental and physical health of offspring. *Psychological Bulletin, 128*, 330–366. doi: 10.1037/0033-2909.128.2.330.

Repetti, R. L., Wang, S-W., & Saxbe, D. E. (2011). Adult health in the context of everyday family life. *Annals of Behavioral Medicine, 42*, 285–293.

Robles, T. F., & Kiecolt-Glaser, J. K. (2003). The physiology of marriage: Pathways to health. *Physiology and Behavior, 79*, 409–416.

Rueggeberg, R., Wrosch, C., Miller, G. E., & McDade, T. W. (2012). Associations between health-related self-protection, diurnal cortisol, and C-reactive protein in lonely older adults. *Psychosomatic Medicine, 74*, 937–944. doi: 10.1097/PSY.0b013e3182732dc6.

Ryan, R. M., Deci, E. L., Grolnick, W. S., & La Guardia, J. G. (2006). The significance of autonomy and autonomy support in psychological development and psychopathology. In D. Cicchetti & D. Cohen (Eds.), *Developmental psychopathology, Vol 1. Theory and method* (2nd ed., pp. 795–849). Hoboken, NJ: Wiley.

Sapolsky, R. M. (2000). Glucocorticoids and hippocampal atrophy in neuropsychiatric disorders. *Archives of General Psychiatry, 57*, 925–935.

Sapolsky, R. M., Romero, M., & Munck, A. U. (2000). How do glucocorticoids influence stress responses? Integrating permissive, suppressive, stimulatory, and preparative actions. *Endocrine Reviews, 21*, 55–89.

Saridjan, N. S., Huizink, A. C., Koetsier, J. A., Jaddoe, V. W., Mackenbach, J. P., Hofman, A.,...Tiemeir, H. (2010). Do social disadvantage and early family adversity affect the diurnal cortisol rhythm in infants? The Generation R study. *Hormones and Behavior, 57*, 247–254.

Saxbe, D. E. (2008). A field (researcher's) guide to cortisol: Tracking HPA axis functioning in everyday life. *Health Psychology Review, 2*, 163–190.

Saxbe, D. E., & Repetti, R. (2010a). No place like home: Home tours correlate with daily patterns of mood and cortisol. *Personality and Social Psychology Bulletin, 36*, 71–81.

Saxbe, D. E., & Repetti, R. L. (2010b). For better or worse? Coregulation of couples' cortisol levels and mood states. *Journal of Personality and Social Psychology, 98*, 92–103.

Saxbe, D. E., Repetti, R. L., & Graesch, A. P. (2011). Time spent in housework and leisure: Links with parents' physiological recovery from work. *Journal of Family Psychology, 25*, 271–281.

Saxbe, D. E., Repetti, R. L., & Nishina, A. (2008). Marital satisfaction, recovery from work, and diurnal cortisol among men and women. *Health Psychology, 27*, 15–25. doi: 10.1037/0278-6133.27.1.15.

Schoorlemmer, R. M., Peeters, G. M., van Schoor, N. M., & Lips, P. (2009). Relationships between cortisol level, mortality and chronic diseases in older persons. *Clinical Endocrinology, 71*, 779–786. doi: 10.1111/j.1365-2265.2009.03552.x.

Schreier, A., & Evans, G. W. (2003). Adrenal cortical response of young children to modern and ancient stressors. *Current Anthropology, 44*, 306–309.

Schulz, M. S., Cowan, P. A., Pape Cowan, C., & Brennan, R. T. (2004). Coming home upset: Gender, marital satisfaction, and the daily spillover of workday experience into couple interactions. *Journal of Family Psychology, 18*, 250–263.

Seckl, J. R., & Meaney, M. J. (2004). Glucocorticoid programming. In *Biobehavioral stress response: Protective and damaging effects* (pp. 63–84). New York, NY: New York Academy of Sciences.

Seidman, E., Lambert, L. E., Allen, L., & Aber, J. L. (2003). Urban adolescents' transition to junior high school and protective family transactions. *Journal of Early Adolescence, 23,* 166–193.

Selye, H. (1956). *The stress of life.* New York, NY: McGraw-Hill.

Sephton, S. E., Sapolsky, R. M., Kraemer, H. C., & Spiegel, D. (2000). Diurnal cortisol rhythm as a predictor of breast cancer survival. *Journal of the National Cancer Institute, 92,* 994–1000. doi: 10.1093/jnci/92.12.994.

Slatcher, R. B. (2010). Marital functioning and physical health: Implications for social and personality psychology. *Social and Personality Psychology Compass, 4,* 455–469. doi: 10.1111/j.1751-9004.2010.00273.x.

Slatcher, R. B., & Pennebaker, J. W. (2005). Emotional processing of traumatic events. In C. L. Cooper (Ed.), *The handbook of stress medicine and health* (pp. 293–307). Boca Raton, FL: CRC Press.

Slatcher, R. B., & Pennebaker, J. W. (2006). How do I love thee? Let me count the words: The social effects of expressive writing. *Psychological Science, 17,* 660–664.

Slatcher, R. B., & Robles, T. F. (2012). Preschoolers' everyday conflict at home and diurnal cortisol patterns. *Health Psychology, 31,* 834–838.

Slatcher, R. B., Robles, T. F., Repetti, R., & Fellows, M. D. (2010). Momentary work worries, marital disclosure and salivary cortisol among parents of young children. *Psychosomatic Medicine, 72,* 887–896.

Smith, T. W., Gallo, L. C., Goble, L., Ngu, L. Q., & Stark, K. A. (1998). Agency, communion, and cardiovascular reactivity during marital interaction. *Health Psychology, 17,* 537–545.

Smyth, J. M., Hockemeyer, J. R., & Tulloch, H. (2008). Expressive writing and post-traumatic stress disorder: Effects on trauma symptoms, mood states, and cortisol reactivity. *British Journal of Health Psychology, 13,* 85–93. doi: 10.1348/135910707x250866.

Story, L. B., & Repetti, R. (2006). Daily occupational stressors and marital behavior. *Journal of Family Psychology, 20,* 690–700.

Taylor, A., Glover, V., Marks, M., & Kammerer, M. (2009). Diurnal pattern of cortisol output in postnatal depression. *Psychoneuroendocrinology, 34,* 1184–1188.

Vedhara, K., Stra, J. T., Miles, J. N. V., Sanderman, R., & Ranchor, A. V. (2006). Psychosocial factors associated with indices of cortisol production in women with breast cancer and controls. *Psychoneuroendocrinology, 31,* 299–311.

Weaver, I. C. G., Champagne, F. A., Brown, S. E., Dymov, S., Sharma, S., Meaney, M. J., ... Szyf, M. (2005). Reversal of maternal programming of stress responses in adult offspring through methyl supplementation: Altering epigenetic marking later in life. *Journal of Neuroscience, 25,* 11045–11054.

Wolf, J. M., Nicholls, E., & Chen, E. (2008). Chronic stress, salivary cortisol, and alpha-amylase in children with asthma and healthy children. *Biological Psychology, 78,* 20–28. doi: 10.1016/j.biopsycho.2007.12.004.

CHAPTER 4

Divorce and Health Outcomes

From Social Epidemiology to Social Psychophysiology

DAVID A. SBARRA, WIDYASITA NOJOPRANOTO,
AND KAREN HASSELMO

A central premise of many of the chapters in this volume is that high-quality social relationships are essential to our psychological and physical health (e.g., Chapters 1 and 2, this volume). When our relationships flourish, so does our health. Although the question of causality remains to be fully addressed (Cohen & Janicki-Deverts, 2009; that is, do high-quality relationships play a causal role in promoting our health?), the statistical association between good relationships and good health is robust and as strong as many other important public health variables—for example, maintaining a normal body weight and getting regular excise (Holt-Lunstad, Smith, & Layton, 2010). In the current chapter, we extend this line of inquiry by reviewing the physical health correlates of ending a relationship through divorce. *What happens to our health when we divorce? Who fares well or poorly? What psychosocial mechanisms might account for the observed associations?*

The research emanating from our laboratory on the topic of divorce and health has profited by combining work in social epidemiology (Sbarra, 2009; Sbarra, Law, & Portley, 2011; Sbarra & Nietert, 2009) with work in social psychophysiology (Lee, Sbarra, Mason, & Law, 2011; Sbarra, Law, Lee, & Mason, 2009). In doing so, we examine the health correlates of divorce from both *macro* and *micro* perspectives, which is consistent with the application of multilevel theory in other domains of psychology (Anderson, 1998; Cacioppo, Berntson, Sheridan, & McClintock, 2000). By adopting an approach that shifts the resolution of analysis between these perspectives, we have attempted to integrate the tools of sociology and epidemiology—the study of large representative samples—with the tools of psychology and psychophysiology, which typically use smaller samples but with much finer measurement resolution. The epidemiological approach allows us to investigate the presence of broad-based effect sizes and ask the basic question of whether divorce increases risk for poor health (physical and mental). Then, our psychophysiological approach attempts to integrate these effects in the laboratory by investigating the potential mechanisms that convey risk.

This chapter begins with a basic review of the demography of divorce and then describes one of the most vexing problems in the literature on adult adjustment following the end of marriage. Namely, although many reports demonstrate that people are highly resilient in the face of divorce, other research indicates that divorced adults are at significant risk for both mental and physical health problems. What explains this apparent confusion in the literature? More important, what is the most accurate statement we can make about divorce and health risk given both patterns of effects? After discussing these issues, we review work emerging from the macro and micro perspectives described earlier. We end the chapter by outlining future directions in this area and trying to synthesize research findings across the varied levels of analysis.

MARITAL SEPARATION AND DIVORCE: WHO AND HOW MANY?

Marital separation and divorce in the United States began to rise dramatically in the 1960s, reaching a peak in 1981 at 5.3 per 1,000 people. Rates of divorce then began to fall, leveling off at near 4 per 1,000 people in 2000, and this rate has remained relatively stable for the last decade. Marriage and divorce rates vary widely by age and race; however, current estimates suggest that approximately 40% of marriages in the United States end in divorce (Kreider & Ellis, 2011). Among people who divorce, roughly 70% of women and 80% of men will remarry (Kreider & Ellis, 2011), and approximately 50%–60% of those who remarry will divorce again at least once (Ganong, Coleman, & Hans, 2006).

Although important, these statistics do not reflect the rates of nonmarital unions and dissolutions, which are the fastest growing family form in the United States (Kreider & Ellis, 2011). The formation and dissolution of these unions are more fluid, but the actual statistics are illusive as official record keeping is not in place. A byproduct of this shift to nonmarital unions is that a higher proportion of those who do marry are staying married. The latest data indicate that for more recent birth cohort years, the divorce rates have fallen. For example, for birth cohort years 1965–1969, the percentage of ever divorced falls to 18% for men and 22% for women 35 years old (Kreider & Ellis, 2011).

There are also period, demographic, and geographical differences found in the number of divorces (Teachman, Tedrow, & Hall, 2006). For example, the overall economy has a great impact on divorce rates. Divorces increase during periods of economic growth and fall in years of failing economy (Teachman et al., 2006). During war, divorces decrease; increases are observed when wars end and during times of relative peace (Ahrons, 1994). Religious affiliations are important as well. Divorce is lower among those religions whose doctrines oppose divorce (e.g., Catholics and Jews) and more frequent among those whose restrictions are more liberal (e.g., Protestants and those of mixed religious affiliations, agnostics, and atheists) (Rodrigues, Hall, & Fincham, 2006). Divorce is more common among people with no children than among parents. It is also higher in urban than rural areas and higher in early years of marriage compared to later years. Generally, divorce rates are highest in the West and some areas of the South and the lowest in the Northeast and sections of the Midwest (Rodrigues et al., 2006).

DIVORCE AND PSYCHOLOGICAL WELL-BEING: THE PROBLEM OF THE STATISTICAL MEAN

On average, do people fare well or poorly when their marriage ends via divorce? This question appears simple, but, as we argue elsewhere (Sbarra, Hasselmo, & Nojopranoto, 2012), the reporting of average (statistical mean) effects on the topic of divorce and health belies considerable and important variability in adults' functioning. As an illustration of the central problem in this literature, consider two studies that rely on data from the German Socio-Economic Panel Study (Lucas, 2005; Mancini, Bonanno, & Clark, 2011). Lucas (2005) used multilevel modeling to examine mean trajectories of life satisfaction prior to and following divorce. The primary findings from this report were that life satisfaction steadily decreases prior to divorce and that people do not return to their initial set point after the divorce (Lucas, 2005). Using data from *the same sample*, Mancini et al. (2011) applied a series of latent growth mixture models to identify potential subsamples, or classes, of how people respond to divorce. This study revealed that nearly 72% of adults reported high levels of life satisfaction prior to and following their divorce; 9% reported low levels of satisfaction that increased substantially following the divorce; and 19% reported a moderate decline in satisfaction over the study period (Mancini et al., 2011).

The difference between the main findings in these studies, which use almost entirely overlapping data, is substantial. The illustration serves as an important reminder that, in many instances, the statistical mean may be essentially meaningless for drawing veridical conclusions about the psychosocial and health sequelae of divorce. On average, people may fail to exhibit a return to their levels of life satisfaction prior to the divorce; at the same time *most people* may report little or no change in their subjective well-being. In this case, the difference between the statistical mean and the mode is important, and we must keep in mind that the statistical mean is highly sensitive to the influence of outliers. Thus, it is quite possible that the negative effects reported by Lucas (2005) are driven almost exclusively by the small group of people who report experiencing tremendous difficulties when their marriages end (Mancini et al., 2011). Perhaps the simplest conclusion from this complicated picture is that although divorce increases risk for poor outcomes *among some people*, most people are resilient when faced with the end of their marriage (Amato, 2010; Hetherington & Kelly, 2002), and this observation is entirely consistent with the general tendency toward resilience following many different types of negative and stressful life events (Bonanno, 2004). This conclusion suggests that we look carefully for moderating variables that attenuate or potentiate risk for adverse outcomes when marriage ends (see Mason & Sbarra, 2012).

With respect to *physical* health outcomes, this "statistical mean problem" is magnified because the available data are extremely impoverished. Although many studies examine moderators of psychological responses to divorce, we know little about the intrapersonal and interpersonal variables that help explain why some people suffer negative health consequences when marriage comes to an end (Mason & Sbarra, 2012). The primary explanation for this dearth of data is that representative epidemiological studies rarely measure psychosocial variables with any degree of complexity. Consequently, prospective studies that can speak to the long-term health correlates of divorce do not typically assess whether, for example, a person initiated the separation or was left by his or her partner, or whether distal health outcomes are associated with participants' longing for their ex-partner. Thus, the field can document broad-based effects by relying on epidemiological and sociological analyses, but the tools, and especially the measurement precision, of psychology are especially important for documenting the psychological, behavioral, and interpersonal moderators of risk for adverse health outcomes following divorce.

THE SOCIAL EPIDEMIOLOGY OF DIVORCE AND DEATH

Two very large meta-analyses document that divorce is associated with a significant increased risk for all-cause mortality. Integrating research in psychology, sociology, and epidemiology, Sbarra and colleagues (Sbarra et al., 2011) synthesized data from 32 prospective studies (involving more than 6.5 million people, 160,000 deaths, and over 755,000 divorces in 11 different countries). The overall risk hazard (RH) linking divorce and risk for early death was 1.23, which indicates that relative to married adults, divorced adults evidenced, on average and across all the studies in the review, a 23% greater risk of being dead each successive follow-up period. (The RH is a relative risk statistic; thus, this index does not translate into some type of calibrated metric that suggests divorced adults lose some definable number of years of life relative to married adults. Instead, the RH quantifies the difference in event occurrence between two groups at each successive measurement period in standard prospective research designs.) Although both men and women are at increased risk for early death following divorce, the meta-analysis revealed that divorced men evidenced greater risk for earlier death (RH = 1.31) than divorced women (RH = 1.13).

Based on the idea that the potential health effects that follow from divorce—if casual—take time to accrue (cf. Lorenz, Simons, & Conger, 1997), the Sbarra et al. (2011) meta-analysis focused exclusively on prospective studies, with average study length being 14 years. More recently, Shor, Roelfs, Bugyi, and Schwartz (2012) have taken a broader look at the potential association between divorce and death by studying every published report on this topic, including cross-sectional studies from very large census samples. Their final sample included 600 *million people* from more than 24 countries. Consistent with the results of the more narrowly focused meta-analysis, Shor et al. (2012) observed a significant average RH of 1.30, as well as significant differences between men (RH = 1.37) and women (RH = 1.22).

The fact that divorce is reliably associated with increased risk for early death raises a very interesting set of questions. Does marital separation play a causal role in hastening one's time to death among people who are otherwise healthy? Alternatively, is the association between divorce and death epiphenomenal and due to third variable confounds that increase risk for *both* divorce and death, for example, hostility (see Egger, Schneider, & Smith, 1998)? Sbarra et al. (2011) addressed these types of questions by considering four potential pathways linking marital separation and subsequent health outcomes: social selection, resource disruptions, health behavior changes, and psychological stress. In this chapter, we dig deeper into the question of remarriage. If, on average, divorce confers risk for poor distal health outcomes and this process is indeed causal, then we should also observe that remarriage eventually mitigates risk. The study of remarriage presents health outcome researchers with a natural A-B-A design, and an analysis of remarriage can help shed light on the nature on the divorce and death association.

DIVORCE, REMARRIAGE, AND HEALTH

A growing body of evidence suggests that remarriage may reduce morbidity and mortality following divorce or bereavement. (Some research does not make a distinction between these life events.) In a sample of adults in the United States who were followed over 10 years, Noda and colleagues (2009) found that after controlling for covariates (age, gender, smoking behavior, etc.), remarriage after bereavement or divorce was associated with a 50% reduction in risk of chronic obstructive pulmonary disease (COPD) over the decade study period. Sbarra and Nietert (2009) showed that 25 years after intake, approximately 50% of adults who had always been divorced or separated and never remarried remained alive; in contrast, roughly 65% of the remainder of the sample—consistently married, now remarried, or never married—remained alive. In addition, these authors found an increased risk for early mortality (by 55%) for participants who were separated or divorced at every assessment, versus both participants who were widowed at every assessment and participants who were single at every assessment.

Brockmann and Klein (2004) attempted to parse how the chronology of marriage, divorce, and widowing events may be associated with the protective or detrimental effects of these marital status transitions. In a sample of over 12,000 German adults followed over 14 years, they found evidence for the significance of the timing of marriages (at what age), accumulation of beneficial experiences from marriage over time, and the quick attenuation of the negative aspects of marital transitions on mortality risk. Men, however, were more strongly impacted by these transitions: Their mortality risk continues to decrease while women's risk stabilizes after 7 years of marriage, and even after remarriage a previous divorce increases men's mortality by 4% each year. Hughes and Waite (2002) examined a more comprehensive picture of marital transitions and the negative effects of divorce by studying the entire marital biography—divorces, remarriages, as well as current marital status—and the resulting associations on several dimensions of health (conditions that are chronic or that impact mobility, self-rated health, and mental health). These researchers found that there was a positive association between the number of years a person spent outside of marriage (widowed or separated/divorced) and the number of reported mobility issues or chronic conditions. However, these effects appeared to be conditional on the participant's current marital status: "*Being* married may protect or even improve health, *getting* divorced or becoming widowed may damage health, and *being* divorced or widowed may damage health" (p. 356). In other words, currently being divorced or widowed carries health risks, in addition to those accompanying the transition out of marriage itself.

Despite the potential risk mitigation remarriage may provide, subsequent divorce might increase one's risk for further negative health consequences. Kriegbaum and colleagues (2009), for example, found increased risk of premature death after experiencing one broken partnership, and also discovered further increases in risk after experiencing two or more broken partnerships. Other work has found similar results, with people divorced or widowed for a second time showing worse mental health than those who have experienced their first relationship disruption (Barrett, 2000). Finally, suggestive of a "cumulative effect" of living as a divorced adult, Lund and colleagues (2004) found an association between the number of years an adult had spent divorced and increasing mortality risk in a dose-dependent fashion. The negative effects remained significant, even though current marital status attenuated the strength of the associations between years divorced and increased mortality.

THE SOCIAL PSYCHOPHYSIOLOGY OF DIVORCE

As described earlier, it is critical to deconstruct the social epidemiology research on divorce using research tools that are better suited to studying mechanisms of action. As a discipline, social psychophysiology (Cacioppo, 1982) uses noninvasive measures of physiology (e.g., assessing autonomic nervous system functioning in response to emotionally evocative tasks) to study psychological and behavioral processes. When integrated with common research paradigms used in larger discipline of health psychology (see, for example, G. Miller, Chen, & Cole, 2009), these approaches provide a powerful means of examining the potential intervening variables that may link divorce with disease processes. If divorce exerts a causal effect on increased risk for early death, this life experience sets in motion a series of processes that contribute to the development and progression of disease pathophysiology. What are these processes?

This question is not unique to the divorce literature. One of the primary challenges facing health psychology is to identify biologically plausible pathways from psychosocial variables to disease outcomes (Miller et al., 2009). Miller et al. (2009) have advanced a conceptual approach to studying how biobehavioral responses to life events are associated with and may regulate (and be regulated by) molecular and cellular responses that are disease relevant. This approach highlights the role of *biological intermediaries*, or, as Miller et al. (2009) state, "Once a robust linkage between a psychosocial factor and a clinical health outcome is identified, the next step is to determine what biological processes convey those effects into the physical environment of disease pathogenesis" (p. 504).

Related to divorce, Miller et al.'s (2009) first criterion is satisfied. Beyond the meta-analytic findings we described earlier (Sbarra et al., 2011; Shor et al., 2012), other studies have demonstrated that divorce can result in a "proliferation of stress" that mediates the association between the end of marriage and poor self-rated health up to a decade later (Lorenz, Wickrama, Conger, & Elder, 2006). What is not yet known, however, are the biological intermediaries that translate the psychosocial stress of divorce into poor physical health. The field has some hints as to how these effects might operate but lack clear-cut, disease-relevant pathways. For example, Sbarra et al. (2009) demonstrated that high levels of divorce-related emotional intrusion are associated with elevated blood pressure, and that men who find thinking about their separation especially difficult evidence substantial blood pressure increases when asked to do so. Lee, Sbarra, Mason, and Law (2011) extended this work by showing that people who have a characteristic tendency to amplify their distress when faced with a relational threat (i.e., people who are high in attachment anxiety) *and* who spoke about their experiences in a highly personalized and experiential way also demonstrated significant increases in blood pressure when thinking about their separation experience.

In related research, Kiecolt-Glaser and colleagues (1987) demonstrated that relative to married adults, divorced adults had significantly higher antibody titers to the Epstein-Barr virus and lower percentage of natural killer cell activity, both of which indicate compromised immune functioning. Among the divorced group, a shorter separation period and continued attachment to a former spouse were associated with poorer physiological outcomes, suggesting that psychological variables specific to divorce adjustment (e.g., continued attachment to a former spouse) are associated with impaired immune functioning. Relative to women in stable marital relationships, women undergoing a stressful divorce also evidence greater evening cortisol levels (Powell et al., 2002).

These studies comprise the small body of research indicating that the end of marriage and divorce-related psychological variables are associated with biological functions that have direct relevance for distal health outcomes. One question is whether these effects are instantiated by the loss of (the benefits conferred in) a relationship or the onset of psychosocial stress. Sbarra and Hazan (2008) argued that the loss of psychophysiological coregulation—the biological and psychological interdependence between two partners that maintains a state of optimal functioning in both people—is itself incredibly stressful (cf. Hofer, 1984). Although the loss of coregulation and the onset of stress likely do not differ at the level of physiology—both lead to increases in neuroendocrine, autonomic, and immunological changes designed to deal with (real or perceived) threats in one's immediate environment—studying this distinction in the case of divorce will be meaningful. Said differently, do some people suffer after divorce because they have lost their primary source of support and, potentially, psychobiological regulation (Hofer, 1987), or is it the case that the burdens of marital separation (e.g., financial changes, new living arrangements, the psychological stress conferred by interparental conflict) drive these changes? Both pathways are plausible and likely exist, but future research can benefit by conceptualizing studies to investigate similarities and differences between the loss of relationship rewards and the onset of stress.

Divorce and Changes in Social Support: An Understudied Topic

One specific way in which the social psychophysiology of divorce literature can grow is to focus more squarely on social support. Do changes in social support explain changes in health-relevant biology after marital separation? Although no studies address this question directly, the available data do suggest the end of marriage is associated with considerable changes in social networks (Milardo, 1987). Social contacts and relationships become complicated after divorce, as changes in residence, finances, and even loyalties may change. For example, Rands (1988) found that 40% of divorced adults lose contact with parts of their social network following divorce and that these social networks constrict and become less dense. Some types of social contact increase after a marital separation (e.g., nonmutual friends, colleagues, etc.), but most people report major disruptions to their overall social network structure (Matthijs Kalmijn & van Groenou, 2005). Much of the literature on explicit social support processes after divorce focuses on familial relationships and, more specifically, on the relationships between parents and children. Lye and colleagues (1995), for example, examined the effects of divorce on parent–child relationships, specifically considering custodial structures and living arrangements in childhood. Because divorce (often followed by remarriage) disrupts normative family relationships (Hetherington, Bridges, & Insabella, 1998), the authors examined reported quality of relationships and frequency of visits with parents. They found that divorce negatively impacted perceived and received functional support, associated with lower quality relationships and less frequent reported contact with parents (Lye et al., 1995).

In a Dutch survey of adults with at least one living parent, Kalmijn (2007) investigated instrumental and emotional support provided to parents following divorce and found that fathers received less support from children than mothers; this effect held true regardless of whether the divorce occurred early or late in a child's life. Divorce was also associated with decreased weekly contact between older fathers and their adult children even when the divorce occurred after children had reached adulthood (although there were inconsistent effects among older divorced women). Finally, across several European countries divorce resulted in greater physical distance between father and children as well as reduced contact, potentially exacerbating the decrease in structural and functional support available to fathers (Kalmijn, 2008).

Taken together, this work suggests that divorce is associated with decreased social integration and functional support processes between parents and their children. These changes suggest reason for concern: Recent meta-analytic data from over 100 studies found that people who report unsatisfactory or poor social relationships evidence up to a 50% increase in the risk for early death compared to socially integrated adults (Holt-Lunstad et al., 2010; also see B. N. Uchino, 2004). Given the broad-based associations between social support/integration and health, we can turn to the large psychophysiology and health psychology literatures to examine precisely how changes in social support may impact health following divorce. Through what pathways does social support affect health outcomes? Although much remains to be learned about the specific mechanisms through which social support impacts physiological functioning, changes in three physiological systems—cardiovascular, endocrine, and immune—demonstrate strong links to both structural and functional support, most likely through stress-related processes (see Uchino, 2006).

Most studies examining the association between social support and stress-related health outcomes have focused on cardiovascular functioning. For example, partner-specific social interactions are associated with lower ambulatory blood pressure (Gump, Polk, Kamarck, & Shiffman, 2001)—high levels of which predict cardiovascular risk. Here we see that high-quality interactions, especially with a romantic partner, are associated with a decrease in blood pressure. In contrast, other studies show that interactions with ambivalent (as opposed to generally supportive) friends and family are associated with negative health outcomes (Holt-Lunstad, Uchino, Smith, & Hicks, 2007; Uchino et al., 2012). People who directly interacted with or had more ties to ambivalent others—people whom we feel both positive and negative about— showed the greatest levels of blood pressure reactivity to stress (Holt-Lunstad et al., 2007) as well as shorter telomere length (Uchino et al., 2012), which are the protective nucleotide sequences that cap each of our chromosomes (shortened telomere length is believed to evidence hastened cellular aging and increased disease risk—see Epel et al., 2004).

With respect to divorce, these findings point to two potentially fruitful lines of future research. First, given the noted disruptions in social networks that follow marital separation and considering the results of Gump et al. (2001), we can ask whether divorced adults are at increased risk for poor health outcomes because they are chronically *underexposed* to the salubrious physiological processes that are conferred by frequent contact with a romantic partner. Alternatively, the social support literature indicates that ambivalent feelings toward an interaction partner are unique predictors of blood pressure reactivity and other health-relevant variables. It is easy to imagine a situation in which divorced partners—perhaps those who are attempting to negotiate successful coparenting agreements—might experience more ambivalence toward each than outright conflict (see Sbarra & Emery, 2005). These two perspectives represent a testable means of exploring the loss of reward/presence of stress ideas discussed earlier, and it would be worthwhile for future studies to pit these competing hypotheses against each other in a study of divorced adults.

FUTURE DIRECTIONS: INTEGRATING ACROSS LEVELS OF ANALYSIS

What is the best way to integrate research findings from the epidemiological and the psychological/psychophysiological study of divorce? One approach, which we alluded to earlier, is to use the epidemiological findings to guide more mechanistic studies that are rooted in psychological science. In addition to deconstructing the overall meta-analytic effect linking divorce and risk for early death, one area that is ripe for future research is the study of gender differences, and this topic provides an excellent means of outlining future directions in the study of divorce and health. As noted earlier, both Sbarra et al. (2011) and Shor et al. (2012) found significant differences between men and women in the risk for early death when marriages end; these differences are not trivial and translate into an approximately 58% greater risk for early death among men following divorce than among women.

Translating epidemiological findings (Sbarra & Nietert, 2009) into psychological research, Sbarra et al. (2009) pursued the idea that differences in emotional coping resources might explain why divorced men are at increased risk for poor health relative to divorced women. Relative to women, men tend to use more problem-focused and less emotion-focused coping processes for dealing with acute stressors, and men also appear to rely less on social support (Ptacek, Smith, & Dodge, 1994). In addition, to the extent that differences in language use reflect variability in psychological states (Pennebaker & King, 1999), a recent study of over 14,000 text files found that women are much more likely than men to use language that refers to social and emotional processes, whereas men are more likely to use words than refer to objects and are impersonal in nature (e.g., occupations, money, and sports; Newman, Groom, Handelman, & Pennebaker, 2008). Together, this set of findings is consistent with observations that, when married, women maintain close affiliative relationships with a number of confidants beyond their partner alone, whereas men tend to rely on their partner as their sole source of emotional support (Phillipson, 1997).

Sbarra et al. (2009) used this logic to hypothesize that men who reported feeling uncomfortable managing their emotions (when asked to think about their divorce experience) should evidence the greatest cardiovascular reactivity when asked to do so. This is just what they observed: Regardless of how emotionally difficult women found thinking about their separation, doing so provoked little change in their minute-to-minute blood pressure responses; in contrast, men who reported finding the task emotionally difficult and requiring considerable emotion regulatory effort evidenced significant increases in blood pressure relative to less distressed men (Sbarra et al., 2009).

This study may provide some insight into why men suffer more than women when relationships end through divorce, but it only touches the surface of the psychological research questions that can be brought to bear on this problem. First, how long do findings of this nature last? Are these transient laboratory effects, or can they be observed in experience sampling and/or ambulatory physiology studies? Thus, an essential question here is generalizability: Is it the case that men suffer more than women because they have more difficultly, on average, than women coping with (i.e., regulating) intense emotions, which can uniquely potentiate the stress of marital separation for men? If this is the case, then we need to see studies documenting that (a) women are able to solicit and use social support more easily than men after a separation, and (b) that emotion regulatory difficulties in men are linked with health-relevant biological processes over a long-term period.

Beyond these questions, competing hypotheses must be considered and evaluated. The most obvious competing hypothesis with respect to gender differences and health following divorce is that changes in health behaviors are largely responsible for the distal differences between men and women. This perspective argues that differences in emotional functioning between men and women (and, by extension, the availability and use of social support) are not as important as differences in health behaviors, and, perhaps especially, health behavior changes that unfold after marriage ends. The social control model of health behaviors refers to the idea that "relationships may provide social control of health behaviors indirectly by affecting the internalization of norms for healthful behavior, and directly by providing informal sanctions for deviating from behavior conducive to health" (Umberson, 1987, p. 309). When marriages dissolve, social control changes dramatically; married adults report that their spouse is the most frequent person to remind them about their health and health behaviors, whereas separated/divorced adults report that the most frequent reminders for good health come from unrelated adults in their life (Umberson, 1992).

Men appear to enjoy particular benefits from the social control of health behaviors, and women are much more likely to attend to men's heath behaviors than the other way around (Umberson, 1992). However, it is not yet clear whether the loss of socially regulated health behaviors can explain why men are at unique risk for poor health when marriage ends. In epidemiological research, a set of health behavior variables (including tobacco use, alcohol consumption, eating a regular breakfast, rates of exercise, and body mass index) significantly reduced differences between married and divorced adults' perceived general health and subjective complaints, as well as the difference in the number of chronic medical conditions among women (Joung, Stronks, Van de Mheen, & Mackenbach, 1995). However, the effects were not largely different for men and women: The set of health behaviors led to an 11% reduction in the difference between married and divorced men's ratings of subjective health and a 14% reduction in the difference between married and divorced women's ratings of subjective health (also see Ikeda et al., 2007).

To summarize, epidemiological research indicates that men suffer a greater risk for early death than women when marriage ends by divorce, and the essential question is why. We have offered two possible explanations—one focused on gender differences in emotional coping and one focused on gender differences in health behaviors. Both explanations require further study and, in particular, psychological studies that are designed to assess whether, when, and why men and women behave differently when their marriages end. Research of this nature will play a large role in uniting research findings in epidemiology and psychology, and thus enhance what is known about divorce, gender, and health.

Toward a Greater Understanding of Biological Intermediaries

As we noted earlier when reviewing research on the social psychophysiology of divorce, only a few studies have assessed health-relevant biological responding in divorcing or divorced samples. To move the field forward, we must think strategically about the biological intermediaries that link the experience of divorce with disease pathophysiology. This approach need not be distinct from the models outlined by Miller et al. (2009), which we discussed earlier. In their review, Miller et al. (2009) provide an illustration of "the mechanistic chain of events through which the social world 'gets inside the body' to influence disease pathogenesis" (p. C-1). When outlining the model for cardiovascular disease, these authors argue for a pathway from chronic stress and/or depression, to glucocorticoid resistance (presumed to operate through chronically elevated cortisol levels; Cohen et al., 2012; Miller, Cohen, & Ritchey, 2002), to increases in systemic inflammation, to arterial plaque growth and instability, to, ultimately, myocardial infarction or stroke (Miller et al., 2009). Within this chain of events, it is important to have studies that link each step in the process. Applied to the study of divorce, the field will benefit by identifying whether separation-specific variables (e.g., longing for an ex-partner, self-identity disruptions, separation-related emotional intrusion) are associated with autonomic, neuroendocrine, or immunological responses (i.e., the first and second steps in Miller et al.'s (2009) mechanistic chain of events toward disease endpoints) over and above more generalized emotional distress or psychological stress.

This task is critical for detailing whether divorce instantiates a set of unique psychological responses that drive biological changes or whether this life event is best considered among a class of other life events that simply increases our risk for chronic stress and mood disturbances. The field knows much more about the ways in which these latter topics are translated into biological risk (although, admittedly, this work is still relatively nascent). Determining whether there is anything unique about the psychological and behavioral responses to divorce that link separation to health-relevant biological responding is an important step in identifying the psychobiological chain of events that link marital dissolution to risk for early death.

One psychological variable that may prove to be an especially important link to health-relevant biological intermediaries is self-concept clarity. Romantic relationships play a large role in shaping our self-concept (Agnew, 2000; Aron, Aron, Tudor, & Nelson, 1991), and it follows that self-concept reorganization is an important task when recovering from a romantic separation (Lewandowski, Aron, Bassis, & Kunak, 2006). People who are successful in reorganizing their sense of self often cope well with a separation, whereas people who struggle to define their sense of self in the wake of a separation report considerable psychological distress (Mason, Law, Bryan, Portley, & Sbarra, 2011; Slotter & Gardner, 2012; Slotter, Gardner, & Finkel, 2010). Furthermore, recent evidence suggests that improvements in one's self-concept following a nonmarital breakup— that is, the increasing belief that you know who you are and have clarity in this sense of self without your former partner—predict improvements in overall psychological well-being, but not the other way around (Mason et al., 2011); thus, improvements in psychological well-being following a romantic separation appear to depend on a person's ability to reorganize his or her sense of self.

On what basis do we believe self-concept clarity will be uniquely associated with health-relevant biological responses after a marital separation? A large body of research indicates that self-conscious emotions, and especially perceptions of social evaluative threat (Dickerson & Kemeny, 2004), are associated with heightened sympathetic and neuroendocrine responding in standardized laboratory paradigms. In a now classic study, Cole, Kemeny, and Taylor (1997) demonstrated that HIV+ men who were highly threat sensitive (defined, in part, by basing their sexual identity on positive evaluations from others) evidenced a faster time to the onset of AIDS and HIV mortality compared to men who did not base their self-identity construals on others' evaluations of them. A follow-up study demonstrated that up to 90% of the association between social inhibition and viral load among HIV+ men could be accounted for by autonomic nervous system activity (predominately sympathetic nervous system responses; Cole, Kemeny, Fahey, Zack, & Naliboff, 2003). These findings suggest that self-concept disruptions, and perhaps especially the self-relevant implications of extent to which divorce becomes a social evaluative threat (e.g., by causing people to experience shame or a sense that their social standing is disrupted), may represent an important and understudied starting point for understanding the mechanistic chain of events that ultimately links marital separation with long-term disease progression.

CONCLUSIONS

This chapter reviewed research on divorce and health from the perspectives of social epidemiology and social psychophysiology. The former literature indicates that there is a robust association between divorce and risk for early mortality, and that this association is (a) stronger for divorced men than divorced women, and (b) may be mitigated by remarriage but appears most highly associated with years spent as a divorced adult. The latter social psychophysiology literature is beginning to suggest mechanistic clues for understanding how broad-based epidemiological effects might unfold over time. For example, we reviewed studies demonstrating that men's but not women's blood pressure responses were associated with the amount of emotion regulatory effort expended when thinking about their relationship history and separation experience. Thus, how men regulate emotion related to the stress of divorce is associated with biological responding that has clear relevance for long-term health outcomes. We also suggested that the study of social support following divorce is ripe for psychophysiological investigations. Finally, the chapter closed with more speculative ideas about how to integrate research from the epidemiological and psychophysiological perspectives. We outlined competing hypotheses that might explain why men are at unique health risk relative to women and ways to build more complete "mechanistic chains of events" that link divorce-related psychological and behavioral responses to biological processes that are associated with disease progression and more distal health outcomes. The field (and, ultimately, divorced adults) will benefit greatly by initiating these and related lines of inquiry.

REFERENCES

Agnew, C. R. (2000). Cognitive interdependence and the experience of relationship loss. In J. H. Harvey & E. D. Miller (Eds.), *Loss and trauma: General and close relationship perspectives* (pp. 385–398). New York, NY: Brunner-Routledge.

Ahrons, C. R. (1994). *The good divorce*. New York, NY: HarperPerrennial.

Amato, P. R. (2010). Research on divorce: Continuing trends and new developments. *Journal of Marriage and Family, 72,* 650–666.

Anderson, N. B. (1998). Levels of analysis in health science: A framework for integrating sociobehavioral and biomedical reseacrch. *Annals of the New York Academy of Sciences, 840,* 563–576.

Aron, A., Aron, E. N., Tudor, M., & Nelson, G. (1991). Close relationships as including other in the self. *Journal of Personality and Social Psychology, 60,* 241–253.

Barrett, A. E. (2000). Marital trajectories and mental health. *Journal of Health and Social Behavior, 41*, 451–464.

Bonanno, G. A. (2004). Loss, trauma, and human resilience: Have we underestimated the human capacity to thrive after extremely aversive events? *American Psychologist, 59*, 20–28.

Brockmann, H., & Klein, T. (2004). Love and death in Germany: The marital biography and its effect on mortality. *Journal of Marriage and Family, 66*, 567–581.

Cacioppo, J. T. (1982). Social psychophysiology: A classic perspective and contemporary approach. *Psychophysiology, 19*, 241–251.

Cacioppo, J. T., Berntson, G. G., Sheridan, J. F., & McClintock, M. K. (2000). Multilevel integrative analyses of human behavior: Social neuroscience and the complementing nature of social and biological approaches. *Psychological Bulletin, 126*, 829–843.

Cohen, S., & Janicki-Deverts, D. (2009). Can we improve our physical health by altering our social networks? *Perspectives on Psychological Science, 4*, 375–378.

Cohen, S., Janicki-Deverts, D., Doyle, W. J., Miller, G. E., Frank, E., Rabin, B. S., & Turner, R. B. (2012). Chronic stress, glucocorticoid receptor resistance, inflammation, and disease risk. *Proceedings of the National Academy of Sciences USA, 109*, 5995–5999.

Cole, S. W., Kemeny, M. E., Fahey, J. L., Zack, J. A., & Naliboff, B. D. (2003). Psychological risk factors for hiv pathogenesis: Mediation by the autonomic nervous system. *Biological Psychiatry, 54*, 1444–1456.

Cole, S. W., Kemeny, M. E., & Taylor, S. E. (1997). Social identity and physical health: Accelerated HIV progression in rejection-sensitive gay men. *Journal of Personality & Social Psychology, 72*, 320–335.

Dickerson, S. S., & Kemeny, M. E. (2004). Acute stressors and cortisol responses: A theoretical integration and synthesis of laboratory research. *Psychological Bulletin, 130*, 355–391.

Egger, M., Schneider, M., & Smith, G. (1998). Meta-analysis spurious precision? Meta-analysis of observational studies. *British Medical Journal, 316*, 140.

Epel, E. S., Blackburn, E. H., Lin, J., Dhabhar, F. S., Adler, N. E., Morrow, J. D., & Cawthon, R. M. (2004). Accelerated telomere shortening in response to life stress. *Proceedings of the National Academy of Sciences USA, 101*, 17312.

Ganong, L., Coleman, M., & Hans, J. (2006). Divorce as a prelude to stepfamily living and the consequences of redivorce. In M. Fine & J. Harvey (Eds.), *Handbook of divorce and relationship dissolution* (pp. 409–434). New York, NY: Earlbaum.

Gump, B. B., Polk, D. E., Kamarck, T. W., & Shiffman, S. M. (2001). Partner interactions are associated with reduced blood pressure in the natural environment: Ambulatory monitoring evidence from a healthy, multiethnic adult sample. *Psychosomatic Medicine, 63*, 423–433.

Hetherington, E. M., Bridges, M., & Insabella, G. M. (1998). Five perspectives on the association between marital transitions and children's adjustment. *American Psychologist, 53*, 167–184.

Hetherington, E. M., & Kelly, J. (2002). *For better or for worse: Divorce reconsidered.* New York, NY: Norton & Company.

Hofer, M. A. (1984). Relationships as regulators: A psychobiological perspective on bereavement. *Psychosomatic Medicine, 46*, 183–197.

Hofer, M. A. (1987). Early social relationships: A psychobiologist's view. *Child Development, 58*, 633–647.

Holt-Lunstad, J., Smith, T., & Layton, J. (2010). Social relationships and mortality risk: A meta-analytic review. *PLoS Medicine, 7*, e1000316. doi:10.1371/journal.pmed.1000316.

Holt-Lunstad, J., Uchino, B. N., Smith, T. W., & Hicks, A. (2007). On the importance of relationship quality: The impact of ambivalence in friendships on cardiovascular functioning. *Annals of Behavioral Medicine, 33*, 278–290.

Hughes, M. E., & Waite, L. J. (2002). Health in household context: living arrangements and health in late middle age. *Journal of Health and Social Behavior, 43*, 1–21. Ikeda, A., Iso, H., Toyoshima, H., Fujino, Y., Mizoue, T., Yoshimura, T.,...Tamakoshi, A. (2007). Marital status and mortality among japanese men and women: The Japan collaborative cohort study. *BMC Public Health, 7*, 73.

Joung, I. M., Stronks, K., Van de Mheen, H., & Mackenbach, J. P. (1995). Health behaviours explain part of the differences in self reported health associated with partner/marital status in The Netherlands. *Journal of Epidemiology and Community Health, 49*, 482–488.

Kalmijn, M. (2007). Gender differences in the effects of divorce, widowhood and remarriage on intergenerational support: Does marriage protect fathers? *Social Forces, 85*, 1079–1104.

Kalmijn, M. (2008). The effects of separation and divorce on parent–child relationships in ten european countries. In C. Saraceno (Ed.), *Families, ageing and social policy: Intergenerational solidarity in european welfare states* (pp. 170–193). Cheltenham, PA: Edward Elgar.

Kalmijn, M., & van Groenou, M. B. (2005). Differential effects of divorce on social integration. *Journal of Social and Personal Relationships, 22*, 455–476.

Kiecolt-Glaser, J. K., Fisher, L. D., Ogrocki, P., Stout, J. C., Speicher, C. E., & Glaser, R. (1987). Marital quality, marital disruption, and immune function. *Psychosomatic Medicine, 49*, 13–34.

Kreider, R. M., & Ellis, R. (2011). *Number, timing, and duration of marriages and divorces: 2009.* Washington, DC: US Department of Commerce, Economics and Statistics Administration, US Census Bureau.

Kriegbaum, M., Christensen, U., Lund, R., & Osler, M. (2009). Job losses and accumulated number of broken partnerships increase risk of premature mortality in Danish men born in 1953. *Journal of Occupational and Environmental Medicine, 51*, 708.

Lee, L. A., Sbarra, D. A., Mason, A. E., & Law, R. W. (2011). Attachment anxiety, verbal immediacy, and blood pressure: Results from a laboratory analog study following marital separation. *Personal Relationships, 18*, 285–301.

Lewandowski, G. W., Jr., Aron, A., Bassis, S., & Kunak, J. (2006). Losing a self-expanding relationship: Implications for the self-concept. *Personal Relationships, 13*, 317–331.

Lorenz, F. O., Simons, R. L., & Conger, R. D. (1997). Married and recently divorced mothers' stressful events and distress: Tracing change across time. *Journal of Marriage and the Family, 59*, 219–232.

Lorenz, F. O., Wickrama, K. A., Conger, R. D., & Elder, G. H., Jr. (2006). The short-term and decade-long effects of divorce on women's midlife health. *Journal of Health and Social Behavior, 47*, 111–125.

Lucas, R. E. (2005). Time does not heal all wounds: A longitudinal study of reaction and adaptation to divorce. *Psychological Science, 16*, 945–950.

Lund, R., Holstein, B. E., & Osler, M. (2004). Marital history from age 15 to 40 years and subsequent 10-year mortality: A longitudinal study of danish males born in 1953. *International Journal of Epidemiology, 33*, 389.

Lye, D. N., Klepinger, D. H., Hyle, P. D., & Nelson, A. (1995). Childhood living arrangements and adult children's relations with their parents. *Demography, 32*, 261–280.

Mancini, A. D., Bonanno, G. A., & Clark, A. E. (2011). Stepping off the hedonic treadmill. *Journal of Individual Differences, 32*, 144–152.

Mason, A. E., Law, R. W., Bryan, A. E. B., Portley, R. M., & Sbarra, D. A. (2011). Facing a breakup: Electromyographic responses moderate self-concept recovery following a romantic separation. *Personal Relationships.* doi: 10.1111/j.1475-6811.2011.01378.x.

Mason, A. E., & Sbarra, D. (2012). Romantic separation, loss, and health: A review of moderators. In M. Newman & N. Roberts (Eds.), *Handbook of health and social relationships* (pp. 95–120). Washington, DC: American Psychological Association.

Milardo, R. M. (1987). Changes in social networks of women and men following divorce: A review. *Journal of Family Issues, 8,* 78–96. doi: 10.1177/019251387008001004.

Miller, G., Chen, E., & Cole, S. (2009). Health psychology: Developing biologically plausible models linking the social world and physical health. *Annual Review of Psychology, 60,* 501–524.

Miller, G. E., Cohen, S., & Ritchey, A. K. (2002). Chronic psychological stress and the regulation of pre-inflammatory cytokines: A glucocorticoid-resistance model. *Health Psychology, 21,* 531–541.

Newman, M. L., Groom, C. J., Handelman, L. D., & Pennebaker, J. W. (2008). Gender differences in language use: An analysis of 14,000 text samples. *Discourse Processes, 45,* 211–236.

Noda, T., Ojima, T., Hayasaka, S., Hagihara, A., Takayanagi, R., & Nobutomo, K. (2009). The health impact of remarriage behavior on chronic obstructive pulmonary disease: Findings from the US longitudinal survey. *BMC Public Health, 9,* 412.

Pennebaker, J. W., & King, L. A. (1999). Linguistic styles: Language use as an individual difference. *Journal of Personality and Social Psychology, 77,* 1296–1312.

Phillipson, C. (1997). Social relationships in later life: A review of the research literature. *International Journal of Geriatric Psychiatry, 12,* 505–512.

Powell, L. H., Lovallo, W. R., Matthews, K. A., Meyer, P., Midgley, A. R., Baum, A., . . . Ory, M. G. (2002). Physiologic markers of chronic stress in premenopausal, middle-aged women. *Psychosomatic Medicine, 64,* 502–509.

Ptacek, J. T., Smith, R. E., & Dodge, K. L. (1994). Gender differences in coping with stress: When stressor and appraisals do not differ. *Personality and Social Psychology Bulletin, 20,* 421–430.

Rands, M. (Ed.). (1988). *Changes in social networks following marital separation and divorce.* Newbury Park, CA: Sage.

Rodrigues, A. E., Hall, J. H., & Fincham, F. D. (2006). What predicts divorce and relationship dissolution. In M. A. Fine & J. Harvey (Eds.), *Handbook of divorce and relationship dissolution* (pp. 85–112). New York, NY: Earlbaum.

Sbarra, D. A. (2009). Marriage protects men from clinically meaningful elevations in c-reactive protein: Results from the national social life, health, and aging project (NSHAP). *Psychosomatic Medicine, 71,* 532–540.

Sbarra, D. A., & Emery, R. E. (2005). Co-parenting conflict, nonacceptance, and depression among divorced adults: Results from a 12-year follow-up study of child custody mediation using multiple imputation. *American Journal of Orthopsychiatry, 75,* 73–75.

Sbarra, D. A., Hasselmo, K., & Nojopranoto, W. (2012). Divorce and death: A case study for health psychology. *Social and Personality Psychology Compass, 12,* 905–919.

Sbarra, D. A., & Hazan, C. (2008). Coregulation, dysregulation, and self-regulation: An integrative analysis and empirical agenda for understanding attachment, separation, loss, and recovery. *Personality and Social Psychology Review, 12,* 141–167.

Sbarra, D. A., Law, R. W., Lee, L. A., & Mason, A. E. (2009). Marital dissolution and blood pressure reactivity: Evidence for the specificity of emotional intrusion-hyperarousal and task-rated emotional difficulty. *Psychosomatic Medicine, 71,* 532–540.

Sbarra, D. A., Law, R. W., & Portley, R. M. (2011). Divorce and death: A meta-analysis and research agenda for clinical, social, and health psychology. *Perspectives on Psychological Science, 6,* 454–474.

Sbarra, D. A., & Nietert, P. J. (2009). Divorce and death: Forty years of the Charleston heart study. *Psychological Science, 20,* 107–113.

Shor, E., Roelfs, D. J., Bugyi, P., & Schwartz, J. E. (2012). Meta-analysis of marital dissolution and mortality: Reevaluating the intersection of gender and age. *Social Science and Medicine, 75*(1), 46–59.

Slotter, E. B., & Gardner, W. L. (2012). How needing you changes me: The influence of attachment anxiety on self-concept malleability in romantic relationships. *Self and Identity*, *11*, 386–408.

Slotter, E. B., Gardner, W. L., & Finkel, E. J. (2010). Who am I without you? The influence of romantic breakup on the self-concept. *Personality and Social Psychology Bulletin*, *36*, 147–160.

Teachman, J., Tedrow, L., & Hall, M. (2006). The demographic future of divorce and dissolution. In M. A. FIne & J. H. Harvey (Eds.), *Handbook of divorce and relationship dissolution* (pp. 59–82). New York, NY: Earlbaum.

Uchino, B., Cawthon, R., Smith, T., Light, K., McKenzie, J., Carlisle, M., … Bowen, K. (2012). Social relationships and health: Is feeling positive, negative, or both (ambivalent) about your social ties related to telomeres? *Health Psychology*, *31*, 789–796. doi: 2010.1037/a0026836.

Uchino, B. N. (2004). *Social support and physical health: Understanding the health consequences of relationships*. New Haven, CT: Yale University Press.

Uchino, B. N. (2006). Social support and health: A review of physiological processes potentially underlying links to disease outcomes. *Journal of Behavioral Medicine*, *29*, 377–387.

Umberson, D. (1987). Family status and health behaviors: Social control as a dimension of social integration. *Journal of Health and Social Behavior*, *28*, 306–319.

Umberson, D. (1992). Gender, marital status and the social control of health behavior. *Social Science and Medicine*, *34*, 907–917.

PART THREE

Marital, Family, and Social Relationships, and Health and Well-Being

CHAPTER 5

It Sometimes Takes Two

Marriage as a Mechanism for Managing Chronic Illness

MARY ANN PARRIS STEPHENS, RACHEL C. HEMPHILL,
KAREN S. ROOK, AND MELISSA M. FRANKS

Many chronic conditions of mid to late life, such as diabetes and heart disease, can be managed effectively through lifestyle behaviors like diet and exercise, but individuals experiencing these conditions frequently find it challenging to make and maintain lifestyle modifications. Among married couples, it is common for spouses to try to assist their ill partners (i.e., patients) with achieving recommended changes in lifestyle behaviors, yet not all forms of spousal involvement may be equally welcome or effective. In this chapter, we aim to illuminate ways in which spouses of chronically ill patients attempt to regulate (through influence and support) their partners' adherence to recommended health behaviors, as well as the effects of these efforts on patients' behavior change. Central to our discussion is our conceptualization of chronic illness as a family problem—more specifically, a couple (or dyadic) problem—rather than solely a problem of the individual with the disease diagnosis. To set the stage, this chapter first highlights the demands that chronic illnesses place on individuals and their close others. We then turn our focus to theoretical and empirical literature bearing on direct and indirect social mechanisms by which the marital relationship may serve as a means of managing the demands of chronic illness. In doing so, this chapter draws heavily on the programmatic research that we and our colleagues have conducted on spouses' involvement in the dietary behavior of their partners with type 2 diabetes.

CHRONIC ILLNESS IN MID TO LATE LIFE

Chronic illness is one of the foremost public health concerns of the 21st century. Nearly half of all adults in the United States are living with at least one chronic condition—80% of those aged 65 years and older—and chronic diseases now account for 7 out of 10 deaths each year (Aldrich & Benson, 2008; Centers for Disease Control and Prevention [CDC], 2009). Many individuals living with chronic illness experience significant decrements in physical functioning and emotional well-being as a result of these conditions (e.g., Stewart et al., 1989). In addition to their toll on human life, chronic illnesses place an enormous burden on the health care system, representing over 75% of all health care costs (CDC, 2009).

Evidence of the sobering impact of chronic diseases in the United States and worldwide lends great urgency to the identification of effective strategies for preventing and treating these conditions. Yet several characteristics of chronic conditions make attainment of these goals challenging. Unlike acute infectious diseases, chronic diseases typically have complex etiologies involving multiple causes or risk factors. Many of these risk factors are lifestyle behaviors such as poor diet, smoking, excessive drinking, and lack of physical activity, which take a gradual toll on physical health. As such, the onset of chronic conditions is often slow and insidious, sometimes developing over 20 to 30 years, and diagnosis typically takes place in mid to late adulthood. Once developed, chronic conditions endure over a prolonged period of time and are often incurable, degenerative, and likely to function as risk factors in their own right for other conditions (CDC, 2009; Ford et al., 2009).

Because individuals with chronic illness typically live with their condition for many years, often for the rest of their lives, it is crucial for patients to adhere to treatment regimens that can prevent or delay complications and disease progression. Treatment regimens for chronic conditions are often complex and involve a variety of health professionals, including physicians, dietitians, physical therapists, and psychologists (e.g., American Diabetes Association [ADA], 2012). Much of the treatment for chronic illnesses, however, occurs in the home and relies on patients to assume personal responsibility for implementation. That is, patients must take on a very active role in their treatment by engaging in regular and sustained self-care (Bodenheimer, Lorig, Holman, & Grumbach, 2002; Gonder-Frederick, Cox, & Ritterband, 2002). Though the level and type of self-care required vary across conditions, treatment regimens for some of the most common chronic illnesses (e.g., heart disease, diabetes, cancer) share many components, including regular medication routines and changes in lifestyle behaviors like physical activity, stress management, and healthy eating.

One aspect of treating chronic conditions that makes them particularly challenging is that patients are often required to modify the very lifestyle behaviors that increased their vulnerability to the disease in the first place. For example, individuals diagnosed with heart disease will typically be instructed to increase physical activity, but their sedentary lifestyle was likely a contributing factor in the development of the disease. Such patients would need to overcome a well-established pattern of sedentary behavior in order to initiate physical exercise. They would then also need to monitor progress and sustain a regular exercise regimen for the rest of their lives. Given these circumstances, it is not surprising that patients with chronic illness often have difficulty continuously adhering to their treatment regimens (e.g., DiMatteo, 2004a; Green, Bazata, Fox, & Grandy, 2007).

Type 2 Diabetes

In our empirical work discussed later in this chapter, we and our colleagues have focused on the management of type 2 diabetes, a chronic disease of the endocrine system characterized by an inability to properly produce or utilize the hormone insulin. This disorder has become a primary public health concern in recent decades due to its steadily rising prevalence. If current trends continue, one in every three Americans will have diabetes by 2050 (CDC, 2011). Presently, nearly 27% of Americans aged 65 or older already have diabetes, and an estimated 90%–95% of these cases are type 2, rather than type 1 (CDC, 2011). Serious complications associated with type 2 diabetes, such as heart disease, kidney failure, and stroke, can often be prevented or delayed through modifications of lifestyle behaviors; however, many patients struggle to maintain the strict adherence required to manage this disease successfully (CDC, 2011; Gonder-Frederick et al., 2002; Moreau et al., 2009).

The treatment regimen for type 2 diabetes is particularly complex and challenging. In order to manage day-to-day symptoms and prevent or delay serious long-term complications, patients must continuously adhere to multiple health behaviors. Specifically, on a daily basis patients with type 2 diabetes must monitor their blood glucose levels, often several times a day; administer medications, which may include oral medications and/or insulin injections; engage in physical activity; and follow a healthy diet plan (ADA, 2012; Gherman et al., 2011).

Social Context of Diabetes Management

Adhering to this complex treatment regimen poses a significant challenge, yet many patients with type 2 diabetes do not face the burdens of disease management alone. Chronic disease may occur in a family context, and conditions like type 2 diabetes that usually develop during adulthood frequently occur in the context of the marital relationship (Fisher et al., 1998, 2000). Accordingly, a growing number of researchers have begun to conceptualize chronic illness as a family or couple (i.e., dyadic) problem, rather than solely a problem of the ill individual (e.g., Berg & Upchurch, 2007; Coyne & Smith, 1991; Cutrona, 1996; Revenson, 2003; Skerrett, 1998). In support of this conceptualization, research indicates that among married couples, one partner's chronic illness is a source of emotional distress for both partners and often requires changes to their established family roles and routines (DeLongis & O'Brien, 1990; Feldman & Broussard, 2006; Franks, Hemphill, Seidel, Stephens, & Rook, 2012; Rohrbaugh et al., 2002). Furthermore, married partners often view the patient's chronic illness as a shared burden that requires their joint coping efforts, and many spouses take an active role in patients' disease management (Berg & Upchurch, 2007; Franks et al., 2006; Kayser, Watson, & Andrade, 2007; Stephens et al., 2013). Managing chronic illness is thus not solely a matter of individual efforts to adhere to treatment regimens but also frequently includes spouses' efforts to regulate patients' adherence behaviors. Accordingly, we turn to theories of self-regulation and social regulation to provide a framework for considering the social nature of chronic disease management and the ways in which spouses may facilitate (or hinder) patients' management of type 2 diabetes.

SELF-REGULATION AND SOCIAL REGULATION

Medical recommendations for the treatment of many chronic diseases, including type 2 diabetes, usually assume that patients have sole responsibility for implementing the treatment plan. Individuals who can self-regulate possess an ability to alter their behaviors in line with standards or expectations (including prescribed treatment regimens) in order to pursue long-term goals. Self-regulatory processes involve deliberate, conscious, and effortful attempts to refrain from engaging in one behavior so that it is possible to engage in a different behavior (Baumeister, Vohs, & Tice, 2007). Taking responsibility for managing one's own disease means that patients must continuously make choices and engage in activities that are consistent with treatment recommendations, sometimes forgoing a preferred or well-established behavior in order to engage in a recommended health behavior (e.g., taking a walk after dinner instead of watching the evening news).

Some theorists have posited that resources needed for self-regulation are finite (Baumeister et al., 2007). Such resources are believed to be depleted by repeated exertion of self-regulatory efforts, which in turn reduces the resources available for subsequent actions that require self-regulation. The capacity to self-regulate is likened to a muscle that becomes tired when it is overused. Research has shown that self-regulation required to continuously resist temptation degrades over time and that the likelihood of success on subsequent attempts at self-control decreases (Muraven & Baumeister, 2000). Furthermore, inadequate self-regulatory resources have been linked to a variety of maladaptive behaviors, including those that compromise health, such as overeating, alcohol abuse, and smoking (Baumeister et al., 2007).

Strictly adhering to the complex treatment regimen for type 2 diabetes requires an individual to exert self-regulatory efforts every day. Engaging in these deliberate, conscious, and effortful actions on a daily basis is likely to deplete the capacity needed to sustain adherent behavior. For example, resisting temptations to consume unhealthy food may exhaust one's ability to continue overriding these temptations. When resources to resist poor food choices have been depleted, success in other arenas (e.g., staying physically active) may also be jeopardized. Thus, even patients who adhere to recommended lifestyle changes most of the time will occasionally lose the capacity to maintain some or all activities prescribed by the treatment plan.

It has been further theorized that self-regulatory resources threatened by repeated exertion may be buttressed, bolstered, or replenished through interactions with close network members (Baumeister et al., 2007). Network members may affirm or strengthen individuals' ongoing self-regulatory efforts, enabling them to remain on track with treatment recommendations (Rook, August, Sorkin, Stephens, & Franks, unpublished data). Alternatively, following lapses in adherence, network members may help to restore or replenish an individual's ability to self-regulate and thus to get back on track with the treatment plan. Thus, harkening back to the metaphor of self-regulation as a muscle, an individual's self-regulatory resources may be protected from overuse, and ultimately, exhaustion, if another person helps carry the load. Moreover, when an individual's self-regulatory resources have been exhausted and a lapse in behavior ensues, as resources begin to recover, a network member may channel them toward the desired behavior. In this chapter, we review theory and research on how social network members may regulate, control, or influence an individual's self-regulatory resources and health behavior.

Theories of social control have proposed both indirect and direct mechanisms by which ties with close social network members may function to regulate others' behavior. Indirect mechanisms emphasize the obligations and responsibilities that particular social roles entail, and the self-imposed restraints on risk-taking behavior that are prompted by the desire to fulfill those role obligations. From this perspective, individuals are thought to be motivated, consciously or unconsciously, to engage in healthy behaviors or avoid unhealthy behaviors because failure to do so might otherwise compromise their ability to fulfill their role obligations (Lewis & Rook, 1999). For example, a father might decide to quit smoking so that he can fulfill his commitments to raise his child to young adulthood and to protect his child from the harmful effects of secondary smoke. In research that has tested this indirect mechanism of social control, role incumbency has generally served as a proxy for feelings of role obligation. Consistent with this idea, research has found that individuals who are married or are parents are more likely to engage in positive health behaviors (such as regular physical activity and cancer screening), and to avoid riskier behaviors (such as smoking and heavy drinking), compared to individuals not occupying these roles (Eng, Kawachi, Fitzmaurice, & Rimm, 2005; Schoenborn & Adams, 2010; Umberson, 1987; 1992; van Jaarsveld, Miles, Edwards, & Wardle, 2006).

Direct mechanisms of social control emphasize explicit requests or demands from a network member to change one or more behaviors, such as increasing sound health behaviors or abstaining from risky behaviors (Lewis & Rook, 1999). For example, a wife might try to motivate her husband to lose weight by reminding him not to have second helpings at dinner, which may refocus his self-regulatory efforts. Strategies of direct forms of social control range from encouraging a partner to engage in healthier behaviors to the more caustic tactics of coercion (Lewis

& Rook, 1999; Tucker, 2002; Umberson, 1987). Milder forms of social control (e.g., trying to persuade a partner to engage in healthier behaviors) often elicit improvement in health behaviors (Lewis & Rook, 1999; Stephens et al., 2009; Tucker, Orlando, Elliott, & Klein, 2006), whereas more coercive forms of control (e.g., criticizing or pressuring a partner to make changes) are often ineffective or counterproductive in changing behavior (Fekete, Geaghan, & Druley, 2009; Lewis & Rook, 1999; Stephens et al., 2009; Tucker et al., 2006). Thus, although spouses may intend to facilitate patients' maintenance of lifestyle modifications, the effectiveness of their attempts to achieve this goal depends on the manner in which it is carried out.

Social regulation of health behaviors may be implicated in the well-established finding that married partners are often similar (i.e., concordant) in their lifestyle behaviors. Partners have been found to exhibit significant levels of similarity on a variety of characteristics and behaviors, including those in the health domain (e.g., Buss, 1984; Dufouil & Alpérovitch, 2000; Feng & Baker, 1994; Price & Vandenburg, 1980). In particular, partners tend to eat the same foods, engage in comparable levels of physical activity, and have similar smoking and drinking habits (e.g., Conn & Armer, 1995; Falba & Sindelar, 2008; Pai, Godboldo-Brooks, & Edington, 2010).

Although concordance in married partners' health behaviors may be due in part to assortative mating (i.e., individuals select partners for marriage based on similarities in specific traits; Whyte, 1990), considerable research evidence suggests that similarities in health behaviors arise through processes of convergence, whereby partners become more similar over time due to shared exposure to environmental factors and/or their influence on one another (e.g., Falba & Sindelar, 2008; Meyler, Stimpson, & Peek, 2007). Multiple studies have observed a pattern of increasing similarity over time in a range of married partners' health habits, particularly smoking and diet. Specifically, individuals are more likely to initiate and succeed in making positive change in a health behavior when their partner already practices the desired behavior or engages in positive behavior change at the same time (Falba & Sindelar, 2008; Franks, Pienta, & Wray, 2002; Homish & Leonard, 2008; Kemmer, Anderson, & Marshall, 1998; Price & Vandenburg, 1980; Pyke, Wood, Kinmonth, & Thompson, 1997; Tambs & Moum, 1992).

It is possible that convergence in partners' health habits arises through direct forms of social regulation, such as social control strategies. Alternatively, health-related concordance may come about through less active forms of social influence. For example, dietary interventions targeting wives also affect the eating habits of their husbands, presumably through husbands' acceptance of wives' changes to household eating practices (Sexton et al., 1987; Shattuck, White, & Kristal, 1992; White et al., 1991). Taken together, research on concordance in married partners' health behaviors strongly reinforces our assumption that marriage serves as a regulatory mechanism for managing lifestyle behaviors involved with treatment of chronic illness.

SPOUSES' REGULATORY EFFORTS IN DIETARY ADHERENCE IN THE CONTEXT OF TYPE 2 DIABETES

To better understand how marriage might serve as a mechanism for managing type 2 diabetes, our research has examined couples' interactions surrounding dietary habits. We selected diet as our focus for two primary reasons. First, adherence to a healthy diet is a crucial, but particularly difficult, component of diabetes management (Beverly, Miller, & Wray, 2008; Woodcock & Kinmonth, 2001). Patients must regularly make healthy food choices, carefully control portion sizes, space meals throughout the day, and coordinate food intake with medication/insulin injection in order to keep blood glucose levels within acceptable ranges (ADA, 2008; Choudary, 2004). Only one third of patients, however, report usually or always following an eating plan prescribed by a physician (Green et al., 2007). In one of our recent studies, patients indicated following a healthy eating plan fewer than 5 days a week, on average (Hemphill, Stephens, Rook, Franks, & Salem, 2013). Such failure to make proper dietary choices on a regular basis could have serious consequences for patients' day-to-day well-being and long-term health. Thus, improving dietary adherence is a major target of diabetes education and research. Our second reason for focusing on diet was that dietary choices offer a rich context for investigating social interactions that may serve a regulatory function in chronic illness. Not only do couples eat many of their meals together, but they also share diet-related activities such as menu planning and grocery shopping (Franks, Sahin, et al., 2012; Kemmer et al., 1998), and research has consistently documented concordance in marital partners' dietary practices (Meyler et al., 2007).

Next we describe studies conducted under two of our larger dyadic projects focusing on spousal involvement in managing the diabetic partners' dietary adherence, the "Couples Coping With Diabetes" and "The 2-partner Diabetes Management" (T2DM) projects. Both projects used virtually identical criteria for enrolling patients and their spouses. To be eligible, patients had to be at least 50 years of age (55 in the T2DM project), married or in a marriage-like relationship, and have a medical diagnosis of type 2 diabetes. Spouses had to be nondiabetic, and the couples had to live together in the same household.

Couples Coping With Diabetes Project

Our "Couples Coping With Diabetes" project (Stephens, Rook, Franks, Khan, & Iida, 2010) collected data via mailed questionnaires completed independently by each partner ($n = 191$ couples). In one study we conducted with these data, we explored two types of social control strategies used by spouses to urge patients with type 2 diabetes to improve adherence to the recommended diet: encouragement and warning. Encouragement refers to actions by a spouse that are intended to promote patients' healthier food choices, whereas warning refers to actions by a spouse that are intended to caution the patient about the consequences of eating a poor diet. Our dyadic design assessed spouses' use of encouragement and warning reported by spouses and by patients.

We first elicited each partner's open-ended descriptions of actions engaged in by spouses to try to encourage or warn the patient. Descriptions of spousal encouragement were organized by the research team into 10 categories. These categories were created and coded by the research team to reflect specific actions recorded by participants. Approximately three quarters of all responses were classified into four of these categories:

- *Actively involved in diet* refers to spouses buying and preparing foods that are consistent with the recommended diet, as well as regulating or making suggestions about sizes of food portions (e.g., "S/he helps me make cooking choices that are on my diet"; "I just try to fix meals of the correct foods").
- *Adopted recommended diet* refers to spouses integrating the recommended diet into his or her own habits or making the recommended diet a normal part of family life (e.g., "S/he went on the diet with me"; "I also ate the same things s/he ate").
- *Suggested healthy foods* refers to spouses' recommendations that patients add more healthy foods to their diet (e.g., "S/he encourages me to buy more fresh veggies and fruit"; "I say that this is better for him/her than that").
- *Complimented dietary management* refers to spouses acknowledging or reinforcing patients' dietary adherence or results of adherence (e.g., "S/he tells me that I'm looking better as I lose weight"; "I commended him/her on how much energy s/he has to take long walks").

Likewise, descriptions of spousal warning were organized into 11 categories and three quarters of all descriptors were classified into five of these:

- *Actively involved in diet* refers to spouses buying and preparing foods that are consistent with the recommended diet, as well as controlling or making suggestions about food portions (e.g., "S/he makes sure I eat vegetables and fruit and not candy and chips"; "I say, 'That's not good for you'").
- *Emphasized diabetes complications* refers to spouses underscoring linkages between dietary nonadherence and diabetes complications (e.g., "S/he warns that I will lose limbs as a result of eating too many sweets"; "I warn of possible heart attack because of weight and high blood sugar").
- *Demanded dietary adherence* refers to spouses explicitly cautioning their partners not to eat (or to eat less of) unhealthy foods (e.g., "S/he tells me that one piece of cake is enough"; "I tell him/her to stop snacking on nuts or corn chips").
- *Discussed dietary information* refers to spouses seeking information about dietary management (e.g., health magazines, health Web sites) and discussing this information with patients (e.g., "We read a lot of literature to educate ourselves"; "I point out nutritional values of most foods as well as total carbs, chemicals, and such").

- *Raised doubts or concerns* refers to spouses directly questioning patients' poor food choices or indirectly questioning food choices by asking about blood sugar or weight (e.g., "S/he asks if I should be eating that"; "I ask if s/he has checked blood values lately").

Most patients and spouses in this study were able to generate descriptions and give examples of behaviors that spouses had recently tried as a means to influence the patients' dietary choices. Over one third of all open-ended descriptions of spouses' attempts to influence patients' adherence (whether in reference to encouragement or warning) were characterized by spouses being *actively* involved in patients' dietary choices. Although active involvement was cited by participants as an example of both encouragement and warning, it was mentioned nearly twice as often when describing encouragement. Moreover, the manner in which spouses appeared to be actively involved varied by the control strategy used, with descriptions of warning being more negative and demanding than those described as encouragement.

Using these same data, we next investigated the correspondence between patients' and spouses' reports of the frequency with which spouses had recently engaged in encouragement and warning. Each partner retrospectively rated the frequency with which the spouse had used each strategy in the prior month, using a 5-point scale ranging from 0 (never) to 4 (very often/at least one time per day). Analyses were based on a subset of couples ($n = 109$) in which both partners reported that the spouse had engaged in both encouragement and warning in the past month.

The bivariate correlation between patient and spouse reports of encouragement was $r = .49$, and for warning, it was $r = .40$. These coefficients represent medium effect sizes between partners' frequency ratings. Such correspondence indicates that perspectives of patients and spouses on spouses' use of these control strategies overlap to some degree (16%–24%).

The mean frequency of spousal encouragement in the past month reported by patients was 2.6 ($SD = 0.9$, range = 1–4), and the mean frequency reported by spouses was 2.2 ($SD = 1.0$, range = 1–4). For spousal warning in the past month, the mean frequency reported by patients was 2.3 ($SD = 1.0$, range = 1–4), and the mean frequency reported by spouses was 1.9 ($SD = 0.9$, range = 1–4). Significant differences between patients' and spouses' perspectives emerged in the mean frequency with which they reported that each strategy had been used. On average, patients perceived that the spouse had been engaged in both kinds of control strategies more often than did spouses. One reason for differences in perceptions of frequency may be that most patients had been coping with diabetes for a relatively long period of time (approximately 11 years, on average), so spouses' actions in relation to patients' dietary choices may have become routine and automatic. As a result, spouses may not have labeled their actions as encouragement or warning, or they may not have been aware of how often they had used these strategies of influence.

Within this same subset of couples, we examined associations between the frequency of spousal encouragement and warning and patients' adherence to dietary recommendations. Although spousal encouragement and warning were reported by each partner, dietary adherence was assessed only from the perspective of patients. Patients were asked to report how well in the past month they had (1) eaten healthy foods that helped them manage their diabetes, (2) avoided unhealthy foods that interfered with their diabetes management, and (3) stuck to a diet that was recommended by their health care provider. Responses were rated on a 4-point scale from 0 (not at all) to 3 (very much). The mean adherence score was 2.2 (SD = 0.6, range = 0.67–3).

Regression analysis was used to predict patients' reports of dietary adherence from spousal encouragement and warning (reported by both patients and spouses). Spousal encouragement as reported by spouses was significantly and positively associated with patients' reports of dietary adherence, even after adjusting for the severity of patients' diabetes symptoms and each partner's reported marital quality. Patients' reports of spousal encouragement were, however, not associated with their own reports of dietary adherence. Likewise, spousal warning as reported by spouses was significantly and inversely associated with patients' reports of their dietary adherence (same covariates as previous analysis). As with encouragement, patients' reports of spousal warning were not associated with their own reports of dietary adherence.

These findings showed that spousal encouragement and warning were associated with patients' adherence to the recommended diet, but in opposite directions. Consistent with prior dyadic research on various strategies of social control (Lewis & Butterfield, 2007; Tucker & Anders, 2001), our findings revealed that spousal encouragement was associated with better dietary adherence, whereas spousal warning was associated with poorer adherence. Although patients in our study perceived that spousal warning and encouragement occurred more often than spouses perceived, it was the *spouses'* perceptions of their own influence attempts, and not patients' perceptions, that were consequential for patients' adherence. These findings suggest that patients may not have been fully aware of specific ways in which the spouse engaged in social control or the effectiveness of such control. It is entirely possible that some attempts to regulate patients' dietary choices were essentially "invisible" to patients (Bolger, Zuckerman, & Kessler, 2000; Shrout, Herman, & Bolger, 2006), or that patients and spouses were referring to different specific actions when they considered the frequency of encouragement and warning (Cutrona, 1996).

This study was conducted to identify ways that spouses might appropriately and effectively regulate patients' dietary choices. Findings revealed that patients' dietary behavior is typically best served when spouses use more positive and less coercive influence attempts. Moreover, our findings suggest that patients are not always aware of the particular spousal influence attempts that are most (or least) effective in regulating their adherence to the recommended diet and that spouses' perceptions of their own actions may be more useful in predicting patients' dietary adherence.

The 2-Partner Diabetes Management Project

Findings from our Couples Coping With Diabetes project revealed that spousal efforts to regulate patients' disease management have the potential to both facilitate and hinder patients' dietary adherence. Building upon these findings, we conducted our T2DM project to get a clearer picture of the *day-to-day* involvement of spouses in their partners' disease management and how these daily interactions relate to patients' adherence behaviors (Stephens et al., 2013). This project relied on end-of-day diaries completed independently by each partner ($n = 129$ couples) for 24 consecutive days. Using these daily diaries, we investigated two strategies of spouses' diet-related control, persuasion and pressure, as well as spouses' use of support for patients' dietary adherence. The larger project used a 3-wave panel design with assessments at baseline (T1), six months following baseline (T2), and 12 months following baseline (T3). End-of-day diary assessments were conducted for 24 consecutive days at T1 and T3. Data reported in this chapter come from the T1 diary period.

We provided each couple with a laptop computer, which was left in their home throughout the diary period. The diary software was designed for easy access by older adults and people with minimal computer experience. Diary content was displayed in large font, one diary item was presented on each screen, and there were multiple options for registering responses (i.e., mouse, arrow keys, or number pad). Patients and spouses completed diaries every evening between 8:00 p.m. and 11:59 p.m. for 24 consecutive days. Each daily record was time and date specific and could only be accessed during this 4-hour window. Patients and spouses were instructed to complete diaries separately and were given individual passwords to their own daily records to encourage independent responding.

At the end of each day during the diary period, patients were instructed to record the extent to which they had engaged in each of five behaviors that day: (1) followed a healthful eating plan, (2) made some unhealthy food choices that got you off track with your diet (reverse coded), (3) ate five or more servings of fruits and vegetables, (4) avoided high-fat foods such as red meat or full-fat dairy products, and (5) spaced carbohydrates evenly throughout the day. Using a 3-point scale, patients indicated the extent to which they had engaged in each behavior that day (1 = not at all, 2 = somewhat, 3 = very much). The mean across all items was 2.4 ($SD = 0.3$), suggesting that the average patient on the average day adhered to the recommended diet between somewhat and very much.

In addition to average levels of adherence, it is informative to consider day-to-day variability in patients' adherence to dietary recommendations. The finite nature of self-regulatory resources suggests that even patients who are generally successful at controlling their dietary choices may experience lapses. Figure 5.1 displays adherence trajectories for three patients who exhibit differing levels of variability (and means) across the 24-day diary period. The dashed line represents a patient who successfully adhered to a healthy diet on most days in the diary period, with

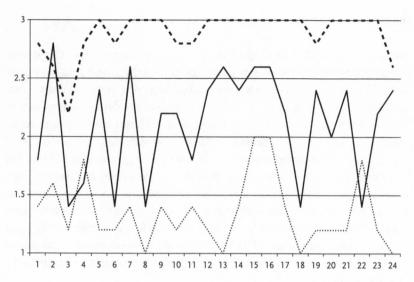

Figure 5.1: Day-to-day variability in dietary adherence for three patients in the T2DM study.

relatively little variation from day to day. The dotted line represents a patient who displayed more day-to-day variation in adherence but was generally unsuccessful at following dietary recommendations. The solid line represents a patient who experienced more frequent and sizable ups and downs in dietary adherence from one day to the next. The primary purpose of our study was to determine the extent to which spouses' daily involvement in patients' diet (diet-related persuasion, pressure, and support) could account for such variability in patients' dietary adherence.

Our social control constructs of persuasion and pressure are similar to those of encouragement and warning that we examined in the prior study. Specifically, diet-related persuasion involved a spouse's attempts to motivate the partner to make improvements in his or her dietary behaviors (e.g., encouraging the partner to change). Diet-related pressure involved a spouse's attempts to coerce the partner to make improvements in dietary choices (e.g., persistent reminders; Stephens et al., 2009). Based on theories of self-regulation and social control, in this study, we predicted that more spousal persuasion on a given day would be related to higher levels of patients' dietary adherence, whereas more pressure from the spouse on a given day would be related to lower levels of dietary adherence.

Using persuasive strategies, spouses attempt to refocus patients' attention and behavior in order to motivate them to improve dietary choices. Such communications might include reminding the partner of proper dietary choices and behavior and reiterating the importance of dietary adherence for long-term health goals. By underscoring standards for health behavior and emphasizing long-term health goals, patients may once again be motivated to engage in healthy behavior. Spouses might also involve patients in activities that trigger appropriate eating behavior (e.g., planning an enjoyable meal that aligns with patients' recommended diet).

Thus when spouses attempt to persuade by redirecting patients' thinking (e.g., reiterating standards and expectations) and behavior (e.g., creating opportunities to resume and practice healthy behavior), patients are likely to be re-energized to engage in these deliberate, conscious, and effortful actions on their own.

Like persuasion, the intent of spouses' pressuring is to get patients to improve their dietary choices. Unlike persuasion, however, the effects of such actions are typically undesirable and frequently unsuccessful (Fekete et al., 2009; Stephens et al., 2013; Thorpe, Lewis, & Sterba, 2008; Tucker et al., 2006). Spouses might criticize or express annoyance when patients make choices that deviate from dietary recommendations. Some forms of dissatisfaction with patients' actions might be less obvious, for example, raising doubts about the wisdom of patients' choices. Whether expressed explicitly or more subtly, spousal pressure has the potential to arouse negative emotions, generate resistance to spouses' requests or demands, and create psychological reactance whereby patients ignore the requests or engage in the opposite behavior (Franks et al., 2006).

In addition to social control, support from family members represents another crucial social resource for adhering to the complex treatment regimen associated with type 2 diabetes (e.g., Gonder-Frederick et al., 2002; Goodall & Halford, 1991). Whereas social control aims to get patients to improve their health behaviors, support provided for health-promoting activities (i.e., health-related support) aims to reinforce patients' *maintenance* of ongoing health behaviors (Franks et al., 2006). Receiving health-related support from family members (most often spouses) appears to foster patients' adherence to the diabetes regimen, including diet (e.g., Garay-Sevilla et al., 1995; Glasgow & Toobert, 1988; Williams & Bond, 2002). In fact, many patients identify spousal support for dietary adherence as a primary form of assistance that is particularly useful in managing diabetes (Trief et al., 2003).

In this study, we expected that more diet-related support from the spouse on a given day would be associated with higher levels of patients' dietary adherence. We assume that spouses' support for ongoing behavior is likely to buttress or reinforce patients' self-regulatory resources that could be threatened or depleted by repeated exertion. Spouses might engage in instrumental actions such as purchasing healthy snacks for the household that could reduce patients' temptation to eat poorly. Moreover, expressions of understanding and affirmation by the spouse could enhance patients' satisfaction with the marriage and reinforce their obligations to stay healthy for the sake of the partner. Supporting patients' healthy food choices, therefore, may increase the likelihood that patients will continue making choices and engaging in activities that are consistent with treatment recommendations, sometimes forgoing a preferred, but less healthy, behavior in order to do so.

At the end of each day, spouses reported various ways in which they had been involved in patients' dietary choices. Using a 3-point scale, spouses indicated the extent to which they had engaged in a given behavior that day (1 = not at all, 2 = somewhat, 3 = very much). For diet-related persuasion, spouses reported the extent to which they had tried to convince or motivate the patient to improve dietary choices that day by attempting to persuade the patient to follow the recommended diet, doing something to get the patient to improve food choices, and/or letting the patient know that poor food choices were worrisome ($M = 1.5, SD = 0.3$). For diet-related pressure, spouses reported the extent to which they had tried to force or coerce the patient to improve dietary choices that day by expressing irritation about the patient's poor food choices, criticizing the patient's poor food choices, and/or questioning or expressing doubts about the patient's poor food choices ($M = 1.2, SD = 0.3$). For diet-related support, spouses reported the extent to which they had provided support to the patient in adhering to dietary recommendations that day by showing appreciation for the patient sticking with the recommended diet, doing something to help the patient stick with the recommended diet, and/or showing that he or she understands the importance of the patient following a healthy meal plan ($M = 1.9, SD = 0.4$).

Figure 5.2 displays the proportion of spouses who reported engaging in each type of involvement over the diary period (the x-axis represents the 24 days of the diary period, divided into quartiles for ease of presentation). A strong majority of spouses (82%) supported patients' healthy food choices on more than three quarters of diary days. In stark contrast, a considerable majority of spouses (66%) tried to pressure patients to improve their dietary choices on less than one quarter of all diary days. The proportion of spouses who tried to persuade patients to improve dietary choices was fairly evenly distributed across quartiles, but the largest proportion (43%) used this control strategy on more than three quarters of diary days.

Using multilevel modeling (MLM), we examined patients' reports of their daily dietary adherence as a function of spouses' reports of their daily use of persuasion, pressure, and support for patients' dietary choices (Stephens et al., 2013). We adjusted for four time-varying covariates: day in the diary period, severity of patients' daily

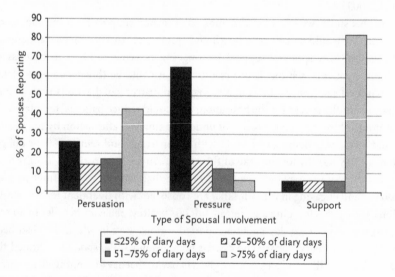

Figure 5.2: Spouses' diet-related involvement during the diary period.

symptoms from comorbid (i.e., nondiabetes) symptoms, diabetes-specific distress, and dietary adherence on the prior day. Time-invariant covariates included patients' gender, age, race/ethnicity, and diabetes symptom severity in the past month.

Consistent with our predictions, MLM results revealed that the effect of spousal pressure on adherence was negative and marginally significant ($p = .09$) and that the effect of spousal support was positive and significant ($p < .001$). These findings suggest that on days when spouses engaged in pressure more than they usually did, patients reported a marginal decrease in dietary adherence relative to the prior day. In contrast, on days when spouses provided support more than usual, patients reported a significant increase in dietary adherence. The effect of spousal persuasion on adherence was negative (rather than positive as we predicted) and was marginally significant ($p = .08$). As with pressure, on days when spouses engaged in more persuasion than usual, patients' adherence slightly declined relative to the prior day.

Associations between daily spousal support and pressure with patients' adherence behavior showed patterns similar to those of prior studies, including those using cross-sectional designs (e.g., Tucker et al., 2006), longer time frames (e.g., Franks et al., 2006), and patient-only reports (e.g., Fekete et al., 2009). The relatively homogeneous results regarding support and pressure across heterogeneous methods, operational definitions, and populations testify to the broad generality of the growing empirical and theoretical literature on these particular forms of health-related spousal involvement. Indeed, one of the most consistent findings in the literature on social control in chronic illness is that forceful attempts to urge improvement in health behaviors are usually counterproductive. Spouses may try to regulate patients' health behaviors in order to help patients minimize health risks, but when spouses are perceived as coercive, patients may resist making appropriate changes. Findings from both studies we reviewed in this chapter demonstrated that patients whose spouses pressured (or warned) them to make better food choices remained nonadherent to the recommended diet and, in some cases, engaged in even poorer food choices.

Although social control theories assume that interactions involving social influence will facilitate better health behaviors (Lewis & Butterfield, 2005), when health behavior change is unwanted or difficult, being prompted by others to undertake such change can provoke resistance or refusal to change the targeted health behavior (Rook, Thuras, & Lewis, 1990). Whether spousal control promotes improvements in health behaviors or triggers resistance may depend, in part, on patients' normative beliefs, or expectations, about the appropriate role for a spouse in helping to regulate his or her partner's disease management.

EXPECTATIONS FOR SPOUSAL INVOLVEMENT

Normative beliefs and expectations about what network members *should* give and receive serve as guideposts for interaction in all social relationships (Clark, Patarki,

& Carver, 1996). When these norms are perceived as being violated, such as when a spouse's attempts at regulating the partner's health behaviors are not expected or welcome, feelings of resentment or disappointment may arise (Clark & Reis, 1988). By extension, patients who believe that a spouse should be involved in regulating the partner's illness management may be less likely to react with hostility and resistance to their spouse's efforts to exert health-related social control. Using data from our Couples Coping With Diabetes project, we conducted a study to examine the proposition that patients would be less resistant to their spouses' pressure for dietary change to the extent that they believe it is normative (i.e., expected) for a spouse to be involved in the partner's health (Rook, August, Stephens, & Franks, 2011). Because expectations about the role of a spouse may differ by gender (Berg & Upchurch, 2007), we also investigated the possibility that the moderating effect of these expectations would differ for men versus women.

Patients were asked to indicate the extent to which they agreed (1 = strongly disagree to 6 = strongly agree) with five statements about the responsibility spouses should have in managing their partners' health. Statements included "It is a wife's [husband's] duty to be involved in helping her husband [his wife] manage his [her] health" and "It is important that a husband [wife] protect his wife's [her husband's] health, even if it causes them to quarrel." Patients, on average, had fairly strong beliefs that a spouse should be involved in managing the partner's health ($M = 4.2, SD = 1.1$).

We assessed two strategies spouses may use to pressure patients to make improvements in their dietary choices: (1) issuing warnings about the harmful consequences of eating a poor diet and (2) attempting to restrict patients from making poor food choices. Patients rated each item on a 5-point scale (0 = never to 4 = very often) and these items were averaged to form a composite measure of spousal pressure ($M = 1.5, SD = 1.21$).

Behavioral resistance to spousal control attempts was measured using two sets of four items adapted from Tucker and Anders (2001). Each set of items asked participants how they had responded when the spouse had engaged in each form of control (e.g., "How did you respond when your wife (husband) tried to warn/restrict your diet?"). The four items in each set assessed the following: (1) ignoring the spouse's request, (2) doing the opposite of what (s)he wanted the patient to do, (3) hiding or disguising eating behavior, and (4) going along with the spouse's request (reverse coded). Each item was rated on a 6-point scale (1 = not at all to 6 = very much). The four items that tapped patients' responses to their spouses' efforts to warn them about their diet and the four items that tapped patients' responses to their spouses' efforts to restrict their diet were averaged to form a composite measure of behavioral resistance ($M = 2.0, SD = .79$).

Prior to investigating our proposition that patients would exhibit less resistance to spouses' diet-related control the more strongly they expected spouses to be involved in their partner's health, we assessed whether those expectations differed for male versus female patients. Female patients reported lower expectations that a spouse should be involved in managing the partner's health than did male patients (p <.001). Specifically, the mean expectation rating reported by female patients was 3.65 (SD = 1.08), and for male patients it was 4.46 (SD = 1.01).

We then used regression analysis to examine the moderating effects of expectations for spousal involvement in health on the relationship between spousal pressure and patients' resistance to pressure, and whether this effect differed for female and male patients. A three-way interaction emerged as significant, after adjusting for patients' age and marital quality. The behavioral resistance exhibited by female patients was moderated by their expectations for spousal involvement. Women who more strongly believed that a spouse should be involved in the partner's health exhibited less behavioral resistance to their own spouses' pressure, as compared to women whose beliefs about spousal involvement were not as strong. No moderating effect of spousal expectations was found for male patients.

The counterproductive effects of spouses' coercive efforts to get patients to improve their dietary choices appear to be mitigated by expectations about spousal involvement for women but not for men. Female patients who more strongly believed that a husband has a responsibility to be involved in his wife's health were less resistant to their spouses' control attempts, in comparison to female patients whose beliefs about spousal involvement were not as strong. By contrast, male patients' resistance to their wives' social control was largely unaffected by the strength of their beliefs about how involved a wife should be in her husband's health. Men appear to have generally higher expectations for spousal involvement. Thus, even men with somewhat lower expectations may have experienced their wife's involvement as normative and felt little inclination to resist her social control attempts.

Women's gender role identity focuses on communal values, nurturing, and caring and is consistent with expectations of greater involvement in others' health behaviors (Lewis, Butterfield, Darbes, & Johnston-Brooks, 2004; Umberson, 1992). Women tend to cast a "wider net of concern" than do men, being more aware of others' needs and more involved in providing care to others (Kessler, McLeod, & Wethington, 1985). In contrast, men's active involvement in others' health behaviors may be viewed as less consistent with male gender role identity, which centers on agency and independence. Consistent with gender role expectations, most men may expect their wives to be heavily involved in their illness management, whereas women may not expect their husbands to be involved.

Consistent with prior research, our findings for women show that unwelcome involvement by others in one's health is likely to arouse resistance to making changes in one's behavior (e.g., Markey, Gomel, & Markey, 2008). Spouses' coercion and criticism may be perceived as an inappropriate or insensitive intrusion into one's autonomy, thereby triggering psychological reactance or feelings of betrayal (e.g., Brehm & Brehm, 1981). The resulting defiant or resistant behavior (e.g., ignoring spouses' requests to improve food choices) may be one way by which female patients tried to regain a sense of independence and autonomy.

Our findings indicate that spouses' use of social control to influence their ill partners' health behaviors operates successfully only in certain contexts, such as when partners expect spouses to be involved with the day-to-day requirements of disease management. Examining gender and social network members' expectations for their involvement in each other's health helps to identify some conditions under which social control has beneficial versus detrimental effects on behavior. As such, this study broadens our understanding of how spouses' efforts at social control may ultimately affect their partners' physical health.

DISCUSSION AND CONCLUSIONS

Having to exert deliberate, conscious, and effortful actions every day to adhere to a complex dietary regimen is likely to exhaust the capacity of patients with type 2 diabetes to maintain adherent behavior. One key assertion of our program of research is that chronic illness management involves both self-regulatory and social regulatory processes to sustain behaviors over the long term. We conceptualize the management of diabetes by married individuals as a couple (or dyadic) problem, and thus, our work shifts the focus for dietary adherence from the patient alone to both partners in the marital relationship. Our studies of patients with type 2 diabetes and their spouses provide evidence that some marital interactions can enable ongoing dietary adherence, whereas other interactions can interfere with adherence.

In a study from our T2DM project, we found that on days when spouses provided more support than usual, patients' dietary adherence increased relative to the prior day. Our findings regarding day-to-day support and adherence align well with prior research on more general forms of social support (i.e., support that is not specific to a given behavior) and adherence processes (e.g., Garay-Sevilla et al., 1995; Glasgow & Toobert, 1988; Williams & Bond, 2002). When spouses showed appreciation for, and understanding about, the needs of patients to adhere to the recommended diet and took action to help patients adhere, patients maintained (and in some cases, improved) their daily dietary adherence. Thus, day-to-day spousal support of patients' healthy dietary practices may have buttressed or reinforced patients' self-regulatory resources that could be threatened by repeated exertion (Baumeister et al., 2007). Preservation of these resources, in turn, may have made it possible for patients to continue making choices and engaging in activities that are consistent with treatment recommendations.

Findings from two of our studies underscore the harmful consequences of coercive strategies as a way to elicit improvement in patients' dietary choices. Specifically, spouses were less likely to achieve the outcome of improving patients' diet when they questioned, criticized, expressed irritation about, or warned about the harmful consequences of patients' poor food choices. These findings mirror prior research on the unintended behavioral consequences of negative strategies of social control (e.g., Fekete et al., 2009; Tucker et al., 2006). Perhaps forceful attempts to influence a partner's dietary choices are usually counterproductive because they elicit negative emotions, as well as resistant behaviors. As such, these strategies may further deplete self-regulatory resources that ultimately reduce patients' capacity to return to more adherent behavior.

The mixed pattern of findings for diet-related persuasion has been a perplexing aspect of our work on patients with type 2 diabetes and their spouses. In our Couples Coping With Diabetes project, spouses' efforts to promote patients' healthier food choices through encouragement were associated with better dietary adherence. In contrast, our T2DM project revealed that spouses' attempts to persuade patients to improve dietary choices were not effective in eliciting the desired change. Rather than increasing patients' dietary adherence, adherent behavior tended to decrease on days when spouses tried to convince or motivate patients to improve dietary choices or expressed concern about patients' choices.

Similar to our work, prior research on persuasion (often referred to as positive control) among the chronically ill has produced mixed results (Fekete et al., 2009; Stephens et al., 2009; Thorpe et al., 2008). Taken together, findings suggest that patients with chronic illness often react negatively even to mild forms of control. Patients may be sensitive to any attempt by the spouse to alter their health behavior due to the difficulty of initiating, monitoring, and maintaining behavior change long term. Thus, the self-regulatory resources exhausted by adherence to a complex treatment regimen do not appear to be easily re-energized when spouses try to redirect patients' attention to the diet or motivate them to get back on track with the treatment plan.

It is possible that even what we conceptualized as a "softer side" of social regulation (i.e., persuasion) is perceived by patients as intrusive or threatening. No matter how influence attempts are communicated, some patients may view any effort by their spouse to get them to change as insulting, judgmental, or meddlesome. Further investigations of patients' expectations and desires for, as well as appraisals of, spouses' social regulation attempts could shed light on the likely effectiveness of such attempts. In addition, efforts to elicit compliance may be seen by patients as one-way communication that overlooks the patients' perspective. It is possible that patients experience real barriers to their own dietary adherence or that they have ideas about how the spouse could be more helpful. Two-way communication that allows for patients and spouses to collaborate in problem solving (Berg & Upchurch, 2007) may be a fruitful direction for future inquiry regarding lapses in adherence.

Another important issue to consider is that of temporal ordering. Based on theories of control (Lewis & Rook, 1999; Tucker & Anders, 2001) and support (e.g., DiMatteo, 2004b; Gallant, 2003), our theoretical model posits that spousal involvement in patients' dietary management helps determine the extent to which patients adhere to the prescribed diet. It is possible, however, that when spouses become aware of patients' poor adherence, they begin pressuring or persuading patients to improve dietary choices. It is also possible that the links between spouses' involvement and patient adherence are dynamic and reciprocal. Longitudinal investigations of control (e.g., Franks et al., 2006; Stephens et al., 2009) and support (e.g., Skinner, John, & Hampson, 2000), however, have reported findings consistent with our theoretical model and increase the confidence that can be placed in the temporal order of events we propose.

In this chapter, we have explored ways in which spouses of chronically ill patients attempt to regulate their partners' adherence to recommended health behaviors through social control and support, as well as the effects of these efforts on patients' behavior change. Spouses' control and support efforts represent some of the primary social interactions by which marriage serves as a mechanism for managing chronic illness. However, our work, combined with work of our colleagues, clearly demonstrates that not all forms of spousal involvement are equally welcome or effective in eliciting healthy change. Given the important role of lifestyle behaviors in managing a variety of chronic conditions, the serious health consequences that could result from poor adherence, and the difficulty that many patients have in making and maintaining recommended lifestyle modifications, it is crucial to identify effective ways for spouses to intervene when patients experience lapses or setbacks in their treatment routines.

REFERENCES

Aldrich, N., & Benson, W. F. (2008). Disaster preparedness and the chronic disease needs of vulnerable older adults. *Preventing Chronic Disease, 5,* 1–7.

American Diabetes Association. (2008). Nutrition recommendations and interventions for diabetes: A position statement of the American Diabetes Association. *Diabetes Care, 31,* S61–S78.

American Diabetes Association. (2012). Standards of medical care in diabetes—2012. *Diabetes Care, 35,* S11–S63.

Baumeister, R. F., Vohs, K. D., & Tice, D. M. (2007). The strength model of self-control. *Current Directions in Psychological Science, 16,* 351–355.

Berg, C. A., & Upchurch, R. (2007). A developmental-contextual model of couples coping with chronic illness across the adult life span. *Psychological Bulletin, 133,* 920–954.

Beverly, E. A., Miller, C. K., & Wray, L. A. (2008). Spousal support and food-related behavior change in middle-aged and older adults living with type 2 diabetes. *Health Education and Behavior, 2008,* 707–720.

Bodenheimer, T., Lorig, K., Holman, H., & Grumbach, K. (2002). Patient self-management of chronic disease in primary care. *Journal of the American Medical Association, 288,* 2469–2475.

Bolger, N., Zuckerman, A., & Kessler, R. C. (2000). Invisible support and adjustment to stress. *Journal of Personality and Social Psychology, 79,* 953–961.

Brehm, S. S., & Brehm, J. W. (1981). *Psychological reactance: A theory of freedom and control.* New York, NY: Academic Press.

Buss, D. M. (1984). Marital assortment for personality dispositions: Assessment with three different data sources. *Behavior Genetics, 14,* 111–123.

Centers for Disease Control and Prevention, National Center for Chronic Disease Prevention and Health Promotion. (2009). *Chronic diseases: The power to prevent, the call to control: At a glance 2009.* Retrieved January 2014, from http://www.cdc.gov/chronicdisease/resources/publications/aag/chronic.htm.

Centers for Disease Control and Prevention, National Center for Chronic Disease Prevention and Health Promotion. (2011). *Diabetes: Successes and opportunities for population-based prevention and control: At a glance 2011*. Retrieved January 2014, from http://www.cdc.gov/chronicdisease/resources/publications/AAG/ddt.htm.

Choudary, P. (2004). Review of dietary recommendations for diabetes mellitus. *Diabetes Research and Clinical Practice, 65*, S9–S15.

Clark, M. S., Patarki, S. P., & Carver, V. H. (1996). Some thoughts and findings on self-presentation of emotions in relationships. In G. J. O. Fletcher & J. Fitness (Eds.), *Knowledge structures in close relationships: A social psychological approach* (pp. 247–274). Mahwah, NJ: Erlbaum.

Clark, M. S., & Reis, H. T. (1988). Interpersonal processes in close relationships. *Annual Review of Psychology, 39*, 609–672.

Conn, V. S., & Armer, J. S. (1995). Older spouses: Similarity in health promotion behaviors. *Journal of Family Nursing, 1*, 397–414.

Coyne, J. C., & Smith, D. A. (1991). Couples coping with a myocardial infarction: A contextual perspective on wives' distress. *Journal of Personality and Social Psychology, 61*, 404–412.

Cutrona, C. E. (1996). *Social support in couples: Marriage as a resource in times of stress*. Thousand Oaks, CA: Sage.

DeLongis, A., & O'Brien, T. (1990). An interpersonal framework for stress and coping: An application to the families of Alzheimer's patients. In M. A. P. Stephens, J. H. Crowther, S. E. Hobfall, & D. L. Tennenbaum (Eds.), *Stress and coping in later-life families* (pp. 221–239). New York, NY: Hemisphere.

DiMatteo, M. R. (2004a). Variations in patients' adherence to medical recommendations: A quantitative review of 50 years of research. *Medical Care, 42*, 200–209.

DiMatteo, M. R. (2004b). Social support and patient adherence to medical treatment: A meta-analysis. *Health Psychology, 23*, 207–218.

Dufouil, C., & Alpérovitch, A. (2000). Couple similarities for cognitive functions and psychological health. *Journal of Clinical Epidemiology, 53*, 589–593.

Eng, P. M., Kawachi, I., Fitzmaurice, G., & Rimm, E. B. (2005). Effects of marital transitions on changes in dietary and other health behaviours in US male health professionals. *Journal of Epidemiology and Community Health, 59*, 56–62.

Falba, T. A., & Sindelar, J. L. (2008). Spousal concordance in health behavior change. *Health Services Research, 43*, 96–116.

Fekete, E., Geaghan, T. R., & Druley, J. A. (2009). Affective and behavioural reactions to positive and negative health-related control strategies in HIV+ men. *Psychology and Health, 24*, 501–515.

Feldman, B. N., & Broussard, C. A. (2006). Men's adjustment to their partners' breast cancer: A dyadic coping perspective. *Health and Social Work, 31*, 117–127.

Feng, D., & Baker, L. (1994). Spouse similarity in attitudes, personality, and psychological well-being. *Behavior Genetics, 24*, 357–364.

Fisher, L., Chesla, C. A., Bartz, R. J., Gilliss, C., Skaff, M. A., Sabogal, F., ... Lutz, C. P. (1998). The family and type 2 diabetes: A framework for intervention. *The Diabetes Educator, 24*, 599–607.

Fisher, L., Chesla, C. A., Skaff, M. A., Gilliss, C., Mullan, J. T., Bartz, R. J., ... Lutz, C. P. (2000). The family and disease management in Hispanic and European-American patients with type 2 diabetes. *Diabetes Care, 23*, 267–272.

Ford, E. S., Bergmann, M. M., Kröger, J., Schienkiewitz, A., Weikert, C., & Boeing, H. (2009). Healthy living is the best revenge: Findings from the European Prospective Investigation into Cancer and Nutrition–Potsdam Study. *Archives of Internal Medicine, 169*, 1355–1362.

Franks, M. M., Hemphill, R. C., Seidel, A. J., Stephens, M. A. P., & Rook, K. S. (2012). Setbacks in diet adherence and emotional distress: A study of older patients with type 2 diabetes and their spouses. *Aging and Mental Health, 16,* 902–910.

Franks, M. M., Pienta, A. M., & Wray, L. A. (2002). It takes two: Marriage and smoking cessation in the middle years. *Journal of Aging and Health, 14,* 336–354.

Franks, M. M., Sahin, Z. S., Seidel, A. J., Shields, C. G., Oates, S. K., & Boushey, C. J. (2012). Table for two: Diabetes distress and diet-related interactions of married patients with diabetes and their spouses. *Families, Systems, and Health, 30,* 154–165.

Franks, M. M., Stephens, M. A. P., Rook, K. S., Franklin, B. A., Keteyian, S. J., & Artinian, N. T. (2006). Spouses' provision of health-related support and control to patients participating in cardiac rehabilitation. *Journal of Family Psychology, 20,* 311–318.

Gallant, M. P. (2003). The influence of social support on chronic illness self-management: A review and directions for research. *Health Education and Behavior, 30,* 170–195.

Garay-Sevilla, M. E., Nava, L. E., Malacara, J. M., Huerta, R., de León, J. D., Mena, A., & Fajardo, M. E. (1995). Adherence to treatment and social support in patients with non-insulin dependent diabetes mellitus. *Journal of Diabetes and Its Complications, 9,* 81–86.

Gherman, A., Schnur, J., Montgomery, G., Sassu, R., Veresiu, I., & David, D. (2011). How are adherent people more likely to think? A meta-analysis of health beliefs and diabetes self-care. *The Diabetes Educator, 37,* 392–408.

Glasgow. R. E., & Toobert, D. J. (1988). Social environment and regimen adherence among type II diabetic patients. *Diabetes Care, 11,* 377–386.

Gonder-Frederick, L. A., Cox, D. J., & Ritterband, L. M. (2002). Diabetes and behavioral medicine: The second decade. *Journal of Consulting and Clinical Psychology, 70,* 611–625.

Goodall, T. A., & Halford, W. K. (1991). Self-management of diabetes mellitus: A critical review. *Health Psychology, 10,* 1–8.

Green, A. J., Bazata, D. D., Fox, K. M., & Grandy, S. (2007). Health-related behaviours of people with diabetes and those with cardiometabolic risk factors: Results from SHIELD. *International Journal of Clinical Practice, 61,* 1791–1797.

Hemphill, R. C., Stephens, M. A. P., Rook, K. S, Franks, M. M., & Salem, J. K. (2013). Older adults' beliefs about the timeline of type 2 diabetes and adherence to dietary regimens. *Psychology and Health, 28,* 139–153.

Homish, G. G., & Leonard, K. E. (2008). Spousal influence on general health behaviors in a community sample. *American Journal of Health Behavior, 32,* 754–763.

Kayser, K., Watson, L. E., & Andrade, J. T. (2007). Cancer as a "we-disease": Examining the process of coping from a relational perspective. *Families, Systems, and Health, 25,* 404–418.

Kemmer, D., Anderson, A. S., & Marshall, D. W. (1998). Living together and eating together: Changes in food choice and eating habits during the transition from single to married/cohabiting. *Sociological Review, 46,* 48–72.

Lewis, M. A., & Butterfield, R. M. (2005). Antecedents and reactions to health-related social control. *Personality and Social Psychology Bulletin, 31,* 146–427.

Lewis, M. A., & Butterfield, R. M. (2007). Social control in marital relationships: Effect of one's partner on health behaviors. *Journal of Applied Social Psychology, 37,* 298–319.

Lewis, M. A., Butterfield, R. M., Darbes, L. A., & Johnston-Brooks, C. (2004). The conceptualization and assessment of health-related social control. *Journal of Social and Personal Relationships, 21,* 669–687.

Lewis, M. A., & Rook, K. S. (1999). Social control in personal relationships: Impact on health behaviors and psychological distress. *Health Psychology, 18,* 63–71.

Kessler, R. C., McLeod, J. D., & Wethington, E. (1985). The costs of caring: A perspective on the relationship between sex and psychological distress. In I. G. Sarason & B. R. Sarason (Eds.), *Social support: Theory, research, and applications* (pp. 491–507). Boston, MA: Martinus Nijhoff.

Markey, C. N., Gomel, J. N., & Markey, P. M. (2008). Romantic relationships and eating regulation. *Journal of Health Psychology, 13,* 422–432.

Meyler, D., Stimpson, J. P., & Peek, M. K. (2007). Health concordance within couples: A systematic review. *Social Science and Medicine, 64,* 2297–2310.

Moreau, A., Aroles, V., Souweine, G., Flori, M., Erpeldinger, S., Figon, S.,...Ploin, D. (2009). Patient versus general practitioner perception of problems with treatment adherence in type 2 diabetes: From adherence to concordance. *European Journal of General Practice, 15,* 147–153.

Muraven, M., & Baumeister, R. F. (2000). Self-regulation and depletion of limited resources: Does self-control resemble a muscle? *Psychological Bulletin, 126,* 247–259.

Pai, C., Godboldo-Brooks, A., & Edington, D. W. (2010). Spousal concordance for overall health risk status and preventive service compliance. *Annals of Epidemiology, 20,* 539–546.

Price, R. A., & Vandenberg, S. G. (1980). Spouse similarity in American and Swedish couples. *Behavior Genetics, 10,* 59–71.

Pyke, S. D. M., Wood, D. A., Kinmonth, A., & Thompson, S. G. (1997). Change in coronary risk and coronary risk factor levels in couples following lifestyle intervention. *Archives of Family Medicine, 6,* 354–360.

Revenson, T. A. (2003). Scenes from a marriage: Examining support, coping, and gender within the context of chronic illness. In J. Suls & K. A. Wallston (Eds.), *Social psychological foundations of health and illness* (pp. 530–559). Malden, MA: Blackwell.

Rohrbaugh, M. J., Cranford, J. A., Shoham, V., Nicklas, J. M., Sonnega, J. S., & Coyne, J. C. (2002). Couples coping with congestive heart failure: Role and gender differences in psychological distress. *Journal of Family Psychology, 16,* 3–13.

Rook, K. S., August, K. J., Stephens, M. A. P., & Franks, M. M. (2011). When does spousal social control provoke negative reactions in the context of chronic illness? The pivotal role of patients' expectations." *Journal of Social and Personal Relationships, 28,* 772–789.

Rook, K. S., Thuras, P. D., & Lewis, M. A. (1990). Social control, health risk taking, and psychological distress among the elderly. *Psychology and Aging, 5,* 327–334.

Schoenborn, C. A., & Adams, P. F. (2010). Health behaviors of adults: United States, 2005-2007. *Vital and Health Statistics, 10,* 1–132.

Sexton, M., Bross, D., Hebel, R., Schumann, B. C., Gerace, T. A., Lasser, N., & Wright, N. (1987). Risk-factor changes in wives with husbands at high risk of coronary heart disease (CHD): The spin-off effect. *Journal of Behavioral Medicine, 10,* 251–261.

Shattuck, A. L., White, E., & Kristal, A. R. (1992). How women's adopted low-fat diets affect their husbands. *American Journal of Public Health, 82,* 1244–1250.

Shrout, P. E., Herman, C. M., & Bolger, N. (2006). The costs and benefits of practical and emotional support on adjustment: A daily diary study of couples experiencing acute stress. *Personal Relationships, 13,* 115–134.

Skerrett, K. (1998). Couple adjustment to the experience of breast cancer. *Families, Systems, and Health, 16,* 281–298.

Skinner, T. C., John, M., & Hampson, S. E. (2000). Social support and personal models of diabetes as predictors of self-care and well-being: A longitudinal study of adolescents with diabetes. *Journal of Pediatric Psychology, 25,* 257–267.

Stephens, M. A. P., Fekete, E. M., Franks, M. M., Rook, K. S., Druley, J. A., & Greene, K. (2009). Spouses' use of pressure and persuasion to promote osteoarthritis patients' medical adherence after orthopedic surgery. *Health Psychology, 28,* 48–55.

Stephens, M. A. P., Franks, M. M., Rook, K. S., Iida, M., Hemphill, R. C., & Salem, J. K. (2013). Spouses' attempts to regulate day-to-day dietary adherence among patients with type 2 diabetes. *Health Psychology, 32*(10), 1029–1037. doi: 10.1037/a0030018.

Stephens, M. A. P., Rook, K. S., Franks, M. M., Khan, C., & Iida, M. (2010). Spouses use of social control to improve diabetic patients' dietary adherence. *Families, Systems, and Health, 28*, 199–208.

Stewart, A. L., Greenfield, S., Hays, R. D., Wells, K., Rogers, W. H., Berry, S. D., ... Ware, J. E. (1989). Functional status and well-being of patients with chronic conditions. *Journal of the American Medical Association, 262*, 907–913.

Tambs, K., & Moum, T. (1992). No large convergence during marriage for health, lifestyle, and personality in a large sample of Norwegian spouses. *Journal of Marriage and the Family, 54*, 957–971.

Thorpe, C. T., Lewis, M. A., & Sterba, K. R. (2008). Reactions to health-related social control in young adults with type 1 diabetes. *Journal of Behavioral Medicine, 31*, 93–103.

Trief, P. M., Sandberg, J., Greenberg, R. P., Graff, K., Castronova, N., Yoon, M., & Weinstock, R. S. (2003). Describing support: A qualitative study of couples living with diabetes. *Families, Systems, and Health, 21*, 57–67.

Tucker, J. S. (2002). Health-related social control within older adults' relationships. *Journal of Gerontology: Psychological Sciences, 57*, P387–P395.

Tucker, J. S., & Anders. S. L. (2001). Social control of health behaviors in marriage. *Journal of Applied Social Psychology, 31*, 467–485.

Tucker, J. S., Orlando, M., Elliott, M. N., & Klein, D. J. (2006). Affective and behavioral responses to health-related social control. *Health Psychology, 25*, 715–722.

Umberson, D. (1987). Family status and health behaviors: Social control as a dimension of social integration. *Journal of Health and Social Behavior, 28*, 306–319.

Umberson, D. (1992). Gender, marital status and the social control of health behavior. *Social Science and Medicine, 34*, 907–917.

van Jaarsveld, C. H. M., Miles, A., Edwards, R., & Wardle, J. (2006). Marriage and cancer prevention: Does marital status and inviting both spouses together influence colorectal cancer screening participation? *Journal of Medical Screening, 13*, 172–176.

White, E., Hurlich, M., Thompson, R. S., Woods, M. N., Henderson, M. M., Urban, N., & Kristal, A. (1991). Dietary changes among husbands of participants in a low-fat dietary intervention. *American Journal of Preventive Medicine, 7*, 319–325.

Whyte, M. K. (1990). *Dating, mating, and marriage.* Hawthorne, New York: Aldine de Gruyter.

Williams, K. E., & Bond, M. J. (2002). The roles of self-efficacy, outcome expectancies and social support in the self-care behaviours of diabetics. *Psychology, Health and Medicine, 7*, 127–141.

Woodcock, A., & Kinmonth, A. L. (2001). Patient concerns in their first year with type 2 diabetes: Patient and practice nurse views. *Patient Education and Counseling, 42*, 257–270.

CHAPTER 6

The Couple and Family Discord Model of Depression

Updates and Future Directions

STEVEN R. H. BEACH

The marital discord model was proposed in 1990 by Beach, Sandeen, and O'Leary (1990) as a broad integration of available social and clinical research highlighting the role of intimate relationships in the management of depressed patients. The model highlighted interpersonal stress processes and the potentially discontinuous nature of marital discord, two aspects of the model that have been further developed in recent years. This original model also highlighted the importance of erosion of support in understanding the connection between marital difficulties and depressive episodes. In the 20-plus years since the model was introduced, there has been considerable development, yielding a model that is more inclusive of family relationships and is more developed at a theoretical and at a practical level. Whereas the original model focused on marital relationships, recent research has expanded to include parenting relationships as well as broadening the model to include a range of romantic couple relationships. This has allowed the model to become increasingly relevant to a diverse range of families and has occasioned a shift in terminology, leading the model to be renamed in the current chapter as the couple and family discord model of depression (CFDM).

To provide context for the CFDM, the chapter begins with a brief description of the prevalence and impact of the depressive disorders. This is followed by a review of the patterns of association between family relationships and depression that provides support for the basic tenets of the model, with a focus on problems in marriage and romantic relationships as well as an examination of associations with problems in parenting relationships. After examining data relevant to the model, the clinical context and the impact of relational interventions for depression are explored. After discussing clinical implications, recent advances related to the incorporation of genetic and epigenetic research into the CFDM are considered, underscoring the continuing conceptual expansion of the CFDM.

The depressive disorders are common and consequential in the general population. Indeed, they are among the most prevalent of Axis I disorders in adulthood, with an estimated 32 to 35 million adults in the United States having met criteria for an episode of major depression in their lifetime (Kessler et al., 2003). Because of its prevalence across the life span, depression is associated with substantial annual economic costs (Greenberg et al., 2003) and has the potential to disrupt social ties for both sufferers and family members. It is not surprising, therefore, that depressed individuals often report problems with family relationships, and that concerns about family relationships are prominent for many depressed persons. Likewise, ability to fulfill work, family, or other major responsibilities often is compromised, with severe or very severe impairment in over 70% of cases (Kessler et al., 2003). Therefore, those engaged in offering clinical services to depressed individuals are likely to confront several types of family relational problems in the context of working with depressed individuals, and these may often be a focus of clinical attention. Unfortunately, clinicians working from an individual or biological perspective sometimes conclude that family concerns are epiphenomenal, underscoring the importance of a well-developed conceptual model to guide clinical intervention. The CFDM adopts a broad social-contextual perspective and suggests that consideration of couple and family relational problems may be central to effective intervention and long-term maintenance of gains for many depressed individuals.

ASSOCIATION OF RELATIONSHIP PROBLEMS WITH DEPRESSION

If the CFDM has merit as an organizing framework for clinical work, there should be ample evidence of covariation between problems in intimate relationships or parenting relationships and depression. Fortunately, these associations have been well examined.

Intimate Partner Relationship Problems

In an early compilation of cross-sectional research with community samples, Whisman (2001a) reported a moderate, negative association of approximately .4 between marital quality and depressive symptomatology for both women and men, indicating a significant association overall, and a small, but significant gender difference, with women showing a slightly stronger effect. Similarly, summarizing contrasts between individuals with a diagnosis of depression and nondepressed comparison samples, Whisman (2001b) noted a significantly lower average marital satisfaction for those with a diagnosis of depression, indicating that the average depressed individual was maritally distressed. More recent studies have replicated and extended the finding of an association between intimate partner problems and depression (e.g., Horwtiz, Briggs-Gowan, Storfer-Isser, & Carter, 2007; Whisman, 2007), and a recent meta-analysis of 66 studies examining the cross-sectional association between marital quality and well-being, primarily measured in terms of depressive symptoms, found a weighted mean effect size of .37 (Proulx, Helms, & Buehler, 2007), providing a strong conceptual replication of the earlier Whisman (2001a) results.

The consistent finding that the marital relationships of depressed men and women are often (but not always) distressed is reinforced by related research on the broader construct of life satisfaction showing that marital satisfaction is the strongest predictor of overall life satisfaction across many specific domains of life satisfaction (Fleeson, 2004). Further suggesting the importance of positive, stable intimate relationships, marital dissolution is strongly associated with increases in depression and depressive symptoms for both men and women (Wade & Pevalin, 2004), and marital dissolution due to death of a partner is associated with a ninefold increase in major depression and a fourfold increase in depressive symptoms among recently bereaved older adults. The effect of bereavement is especially pronounced for those lacking social support. Accordingly, there is a substantial foundation, across a range of samples and methods, supporting the basic premise of the model that problems in intimate partner relationships are often, but not always, associated with depression.

Covariation and Lagged Relationships Across Time

If depression and discord in intimate partner relationships are causally connected, one would also expect to see covariation in the way the two constructs change across time. To examine the possibility of covariation in depression and reported relationship satisfaction across time, Davila, Karney, Hall, and Bradbury (2003) used growth curve analyses and reported bidirectional influence and strong covariation in change over time. Similar results were obtained from a multistage stratified sample of couples from Detroit, Michigan, among whom intimate partner relational problems were associated with increased risk of depression (McLeod & Eckberg, 1993). Likewise, in a population-based sample in the Netherlands, intimate partner relational problems were associated with increased incidence of dysthymia and major depressive episodes (Overbeek et al., 2006). Finally, in a population-based sample of more than 900 married adults who did not meet criteria for 12-month major depressive episode (MDE) at baseline, intimate partner relational problems were associated with a 2.7-fold increased risk for MDE during the following 12 months (Whisman & Bruce, 1999). An examination of physical conflict in marital relationships also demonstrated that it increased depressive symptoms over time, even after controlling for earlier depressive symptoms and earlier level of relationship dissatisfaction (Beach et al., 2004; see also Chapter 7, this volume), suggesting that relationship aggression may need to be examined directly in the context of depression.

Association of Partner Relational Problems With Parenting Problems

Attention to parenting relationships is a natural extension of the marital discord model of depression. Problems in intimate partner relationships influence both parental adjustment and parenting behavior toward children (Cummings & Davies, 2002; Erel & Burman, 1995; Krishnakumar & Buehler, 2000), and intimate partner relational problems have received considerable attention in the research literature on parenting and child outcomes. Healthy family relationships are characterized by low levels of stress and conflict in the parents' relationship and are linked to mental health and adjustment in both children and adults; unhealthy family relationships, however, are characterized by high levels of stress and conflict in the parents' relationship with each other and have been linked to a wide range of parenting problems, including poor discipline (Gerard, Krishnakumar, & Beuhler, 2006), negativity (Belsky, Youngblade, Rovine, & Vollig, 1991), and low warmth (Davies, Sturge-Apple, & Cummings, 2004). In addition, increased psychopathology among children (e.g., Cummings, Davies, & Campbell, 2000) and declines in overall well-being among children (Booth & Amato, 2001) may increase parent–child conflict, potentially increasing parents' vulnerability to depressive symptoms (e.g., Jones, Beach, & Forehand, 2001). Conversely, longitudinal declines in parental marital conflict are associated with better adjustment among young adults (Amato, Lomis, & Booth, 1995). Accordingly, there is a substantial foundation in the broader literature for the expectation that parenting problems will display a pattern of association with depression that is similar to that found for problems in intimate partner relationships; that is, greater parenting problems are associated with more depression among parents.

Parenting Problems and Depression

Depressed parents report considerable distress in their parenting relationships and display reduced efficacy in parenting behavior. In a summary of 46 observational studies of the parenting behavior of depressed women, Lovejoy, Gracyk, O'Hare, and Neuman (2000) found evidence that depressed mothers reliably displayed more withdrawn behavior and made greater use of negative parenting behavior. Creating the potential for a vicious cycle between parenting and depression that may parallel the vicious cycles observed within the intimate partner relationship (Davila, Bradbury, Cohan, & Tochluk, 1997), there is evidence that difficulties in the parent–child relationship can increase parents' vulnerability to depressive symptoms (e.g., Jones et al., 2001), as well as confer risk for future problems among offspring of depressed parents

(Goodman, 2007). Consistent with the literature on couple relationships, many, but not all, depressed persons experience difficulties in parenting, and problems in this domain may influence depressive symptoms in a reciprocal manner. Accordingly, both intimate partner problems and parenting problems are associated with depression, have the potential to engender reciprocal effects, and have the potential to create vicious cycles that help to maintain depressive episodes. In view of their potential theoretical as well as practical importance, next we turn to a brief review of the literature documenting the potential relevance of relationship problems as predictors of treatment response in the context of treatments for depression.

RELATIONSHIP PROBLEMS AS PREDICTORS OF RESPONSE TO TREATMENT

The empirical evidence of strong concurrent covariation between intimate partner discord, parenting difficulties, and depression suggests the likelihood that clinicians will be confronted with many cases in which a depressed individual expresses concerns about important aspects of his or her social environment, particularly a romantic relationship, a parenting relationship, or both. An important practical issue is whether such problems can be ignored until depressive symptoms have been addressed through individual or biological interventions, or whether these problems may be relevant for treatment planning and for maximizing treatment outcomes over time. Early literature suggested that relationship difficulties at the beginning of treatment are associated with poorer symptomatic improvement for depression at posttreatment (Rounsaville, Weisman, Prusoff, & Herceg-Baron, 1979) and at follow-up (Rounsaville, Prusoff, & Weisman, 1980). More recent work suggests the importance of relationships for ultimate treatment outcome across a number of individual treatment modalities (Goering, Lancee, & Freeman, 1992), as well as for those receiving antidepressant medication (Kung & Elkin, 2000; Whisman, 2001b). Likewise, when key marital, family, or other interpersonal issues are not resolved over the course of treatment, this may increase the risk for relapse (cf. Hooley, 2007). So, from the standpoint of optimal treatment response and maintenance of gains over time, it behooves clinicians to consider each depressed patient's concurrent difficulties in marital and parenting relationships as they plan for treatment. This raises the further issue of whether there are potential interventions to address these domains when problems are present. If so, the result presents an opportunity to test the CFDM experimentally.

CAN WE TEST THE MODEL EXPERIMENTALLY?

Given the large number of depressed individuals experiencing marital or parenting problems, the likelihood that marital and family difficulties dampen response to standard, individually oriented interventions for depression should be worrisome. However, at the same time, to the extent that we can identify programs that are efficacious in resolving these problems, it creates an opportunity to test the CFDM within an experimental context. That is, we can examine the impact on depression of creating change in the putative causal domains of intimate partner and parenting problems. If problems in these areas are helping maintain depressive symptoms, interrupting that cycle with efficacious interventions should interrupt the underlying vicious cycle and so have a beneficial effect on depressive symptoms. Given the potential for increased power using experimental approaches and likelihood of enhanced clarity regarding causal processes (McClelland & Judd, 1993), this also creates an excellent opportunity for conceptual advancement.

Identifying and Using Well-Established, Efficacious Interventions

Are efficacious interventions for intimate partner problems and parenting problems available? Happily, there are well-specified approaches for both intimate partner problems and for parenting problems. Behavioral couples therapy, cognitive-behavioral couples therapy, emotion-focused therapy, and insight-oriented marital therapy have all been examined and supported as efficacious interventions for intimate partner problems (Snyder, Castellani, & Whisman, 2006). Evidence also has accumulated to support the efficacy of integrative couples therapy (Christensen, Atkins, Baucom, & Yi, 2010). Similarly, a large number of studies indicate that parent management training (Patterson, Reid, & Dishion, 1992) is efficacious for alleviating parenting problems. Indeed, parent management training, a program that modifies the coercive and maladaptive patterns of parent–child interaction that are characteristic of families of children with oppositional behavior, has been shown to be an efficacious treatment for children with disruptive behavior disorders (e.g., oppositional defiant disorder and conduct disorder; see Kazdin, 2005 for a review).

Efficacious Couples-Based Programs to Alleviate Depressive Symptoms

The existence of efficacious interventions allows for direct examination of the central hypothesis of the CFDM that changing the social context will have an impact on depressive symptoms. In an initial look at this relationship, three older studies compared behavioral marital therapy (BMT) to individual therapy with similar results. In the first study, Jacobson, Dobson, Fruzzetti, Schmaling, and Salusky (1991) randomly assigned 60 married, depressed women to BMT, individual cognitive therapy (CT), or a treatment combining BMT and CT. Couples were not selected for the presence of marital discord and so later could be subdivided into those who were more and less maritally distressed. Second, Beach and O'Leary (1992) randomly assigned 45 couples in which the wife was depressed to one of three conditions: (1) conjoint BMT; (2) individual CT; or (3) a 15-week waiting list condition. To be included in the study, both partners had to score in the discordant range of the DAS and report ongoing marital discord. Finally, Emanuels-Zuurveen and Emmelkamp (1996) assigned 27 depressed, maritally distressed outpatients to either individual cognitive-behavioral therapy or communication-focused marital therapy. The sample for this study included both depressed husbands ($n = 13$) and depressed wives ($n = 14$). Across the three studies, behavioral marital therapy proved to be as effective as the established individual therapy comparison conditions, yielding equivalent outcomes when depressive symptoms were examined as the dependent variable. In the one study that included a control group, the marital therapy group outperformed the control group (Beach & O'Leary, 1992). In the one study that included both distressed and nondistressed couples, the distressed couples responded to a greater degree (Jacobson et al., 1991). In the one study that included both men and women, gender did not moderate outcome (Emanuels-Zuurveen & Emmelkamp, 1996). Thus, supporting a major premise of the couple and family discord model, marital therapy was found to be significantly better than a waitlist control in reducing depressive symptoms (Beach & O'Leary, 1992), and it was as good as an established alternative therapeutic approach.

The effects documented using BMT as an intervention for marital problems have been replicated and extended using other approaches to couples therapy. Research examining couples-based cognitive therapy (couples CT) reported positive results (Teichman, Bar-El, Shor, Sirota, & Elizur, 1995), finding that depressed couples assigned to couples CT had fewer depressive symptoms at the end of treatment than those assigned to individual cognitive therapy or to the waitlist condition. Couples-based interpersonal psychotherapy (IPT-CM) was also examined in one small pilot study (Foley, Rounsaville, Weissman, Sholomskas, & Chevron, 1989), demonstrating equal improvement in depression for those in IPT-CM as for those assigned to the individual format as well as marginally greater improvement in marital satisfaction. Likewise, systemic couples therapy was examined in an outcome study by Leff and colleagues (2000), where it was found that the couples therapy approach resulted in lower levels of attrition and lower self-reported depressive symptoms in the systemic intervention group than in the medication-only group across the 2-year follow-up period. Emotion-focused therapy (EFT) has also been shown to be efficacious in the treatment for depression in several case studies (e.g., Whiffen, 2004) and in the context of treatment of other problems. In addition, EFT was examined in one small treatment outcome study focused on clinically depressed women in distressed marriages (Desaulles, Johnson, & Denton, 2003), demonstrating equal efficacy as antidepressant medication in reducing depressive symptoms. Finally, in a recent study, Bodenmann and colleagues (2008) trained spouses of depressed patients to help them process stressful events more effectively, and they contrasted this marital condition with both CT and individual IPT. As in other similar studies, the marital condition was as effective as the alternative, individual approaches to therapy in reducing depressive symptoms (see Bodenmann, et al., 2008), again supporting the view that couples-based intervention strategies are as efficacious in the treatment of depression as currently used approaches.

These studies are sufficient to demonstrate that efficacious forms of couples therapy can be safely and usefully applied to a depressed population and that doing so will alleviate depressive symptoms among those experiencing relationship problems, a conclusion recently underscored by a meta-analytic examination of the data (Barbato & D'Avanzo, 2008). At the same time, research focused on training partners to provide effective social support in the context of marriage (Bodenmann et al., 2008; Cohen, O'Leary, & Foran, 2010) and to repair attachment disruption (Whiffen, 2004) suggests the potential to expand and further strengthen the impact of interventions on depression by focusing on positive, supportive relationship dynamics.

Parent Training Also Alleviates Depressive Symptoms

One can also examine efficacious approaches to parent training to see whether they may have an impact on the parent's depressive symptoms. In an early examination of parent training in the context of depressive symptoms, Forehand, Wells, and Griest (1980) examined the effects of a parent training program in a sample of 15 clinic-referred children and their mothers, finding that mothers in the clinic-referred, but not the nonclinic group, evidenced a significant reduction in depressive symptoms from pretreatment to posttreatment. Hutchings Lane, and Kelly (2004) examined the efficacy of behavioral parent training ($n = 21$) compared to standard mental health service treatment ($n = 13$) for parents of 2- to 10-year-old children who presented for conduct problems, finding that mothers in the parenting intervention reported significantly lower levels of depression at 6-month and 4-year follow-ups than did mothers in the standard treatment group (Hutchings et al., 2004). Likewise, Triple P (Positive Parenting Program), a universal prevention program developed by researchers in Australia to enhance child behavior and parenting efficacy, was found to be associated with significant declines in parental depressive symptoms pretreatment to posttreatment (Gallart & Matthey, 2005).

Building on these findings, Beach et al. (2008) examined the effects of a prevention-oriented, parenting intervention on 163 mothers with elevated depression scores. Compared with the control group, participation in the parenting program was associated with reduced depressive symptoms, enhanced parenting skills, and improvements in youth behavior. Changes in parenting behaviors (consistent discipline, child monitoring, open communication), but not in youth intrapersonal competencies, were found to significantly mediate intervention effects on mothers' depression. Results support the link between reduced depressive symptoms and stronger family relationships, particularly the importance of enhanced parenting efficacy in alleviating depressive symptoms.

Examining parenting at an earlier stage of development, Gelfand, Teti, Seiner, and Jameson (1996) evaluated a multicomponent intervention program in which registered nurses visited depressed mothers of infants at their homes to assess mothers' parenting skills, enhance mothers' self-confidence, and reinforce mothers' existing parenting techniques. Mothers diagnosed with major depression were assigned to the parenting intervention group ($n = 37$; needs assessment, modeling of warm mother–infant interactions, reinforcement of positive parenting skills) or the usual mental health care group ($n = 36$; ongoing treatment with referral source). Gelfand and colleagues (1996) found that mothers in the intervention group demonstrated significantly greater improvement in depressive symptoms than did those in usual care.

Sanders and McFarland (2000) also examined behavioral parenting training for parental depression. Forty-seven families in which the mother met diagnostic criteria for major depression and in which at least one child met diagnostic criteria for either conduct or oppositional-defiant disorder were randomly assigned to either the traditional Behavioral Family Intervention (a program using instruction, role playing, feedback, and coaching in the use of social-learning principles) or a cognitively enhanced BFI condition (in addition to traditional BFI skills, focused on identifying and interrupting dysfunctional child-related cognitions and automatic thoughts, and strategies to increase relaxation). Although both interventions were associated with significant change in child behavior problems, significantly more mothers in the CBFI condition (72%) than in the BFI condition (35%) were nondepressed at follow-up.

Jointly, the studies reviewed here suggest that parenting approaches are promising for alleviating parental depressive symptoms as well as for enhancing child outcomes. In addition, it appears that developmentally appropriate parenting interventions may have beneficial effects on parental depression across a wide range of child ages. As with marital interventions, it appears that changes associated with the intervention mediate the impact of the intervention on depression.

THEORETICAL CONCLUSIONS AND PRACTICAL IMPLICATIONS

The results of efficacious programs for couple problems and for parenting problems provide experimental support for the couple and family discord model of depression (CFDM). In each study an approach designed to enhance interpersonal functioning had an effect on depressive symptoms while ruling out some third variables and maturation. Accordingly, the practical recommendation that depressed persons may often benefit from receiving treatment for interpersonal problems in romantic relationships or in parenting relationships is strongly supported, particularly if couple or parenting problems are still present at the end of a course of treatment for depression. Fortunately, there are many interventions designed to help with couple and family problems that have documented efficacy. They have been shown to produce change in nondepressed, as well as depressed, individuals in the key stress-generating domains of marital and parenting relationships and to influence long-term outcomes for depression. Therefore, there is good reason to think that such interventions are of particular importance for depressed persons who report that the onset of their problems with spouses or their children preceded and perhaps caused their current episode of depression.

Theoretically, these results suggest a firm foundation for the CFDM. A theoretical problem of considerable importance, however, is whether there is a "cut point" for severity of problems that might indicate a discontinuity in the nature of the problems being experienced and so warrant referral for marital or family treatment. The obvious, and perhaps more intuitive, alternative for psychologists interested in measurement would be that marital and parenting problems are distributed as Gaussian distributions with no clear cut point separating "distress" and "nondistressed." Because this distinction has implications for the underlying nature of marital distress (e.g., Gottman, Murray, Swanson, Tyson, & Swanson, 2002), as well as for the nature of the link between marital distress and depression, it has garnered some attention. Fortunately, recent developments in the assessment of marital discord as a dichotomous variable (see Beach, Fincham, Amir, & Leonard, 2005; Whisman, Beach, & Snyder, 2008) provide considerable help in addressing this question.

Are Relationship Problems Distributed Discontinuously?

The CFDM portrays interpersonal problems as waxing and waning, with points at which problems transition from "ordinary" problems into more substantial clusters of problems that may require therapeutic attention because they cause greater suffering. This suggests a point of rarity or discontinuity in the distribution of distress scores, with some individuals reporting multiple, mutually supporting problem areas that render problem solution more difficult and that may have an especially strong association with depressive symptoms. To the extent that individuals beyond the point of rarity can be identified, they would represent a group at increased risk of vicious cycles between depression and interpersonal problems of the sort hypothesized to drive the CFDM, and so should be ideal candidates for a therapeutic focus on couple and family problems. However, identifying the optimal cut point for distinguishing "distressed" and "nondistressed" can be challenging. Increasing the challenge for couples treatment is the expectation that a recommendation for couples treatment will be based on a "couple-level" designation as discordant, not merely a classification of one spouse as distressed.

A statistical technique that has been helpful in identifying a nonarbitrary cut point is taxometrics (Waller & Meehl, 1998). This approach addresses the question of whether couples can be dichotomized into two groups that differ qualitatively and not just quantitatively. Research using this approach found that couples could be classified as "discordant" versus "nondiscordant" (Beach et al., 2005), indicating the presence of a natural break point, that is, point of discontinuity, between the two groups. A follow-up study involving 1,020 couples that were representative of the US population with respect to race and ethnicity, educational level, and occupation replicated this conclusion (Whisman et al., 2008), again suggesting that there is an identifiable group of couples in need of referral. Because the analyses in this latter study were conducted using the Marital Satisfaction Inventory-Revised (MSI-R) (Snyder, 1997), the authors were able to develop interview-based and self-report screening scales (Whisman et al., 2008). In keeping with theoretical expectations, recent research with an older sample of community couples married at least 10 years found that taxon membership was associated with depressive symptoms for both wives and husbands. In addition, for wives, the association between taxon membership and symptoms of depression remained statistically significant even after controlling for the continuously distributed measures of relationship quality (Whisman, Beach, & Snyder, unpublished data).

Accordingly, it appears that problems in couple and parenting domains are (1) related to depression both concurrently and over time, (2) influential with regard to therapeutic response to individually oriented treatments, (3) responsive to efficacious treatments, and (4) responsive even in the context of an ongoing depressive episode. Furthermore, the group most in need of therapeutic services can be designated as a discrete group. These observations have considerable practical importance as well as theoretical importance, allowing for the development of intervention guidelines as well as providing a foundation for further expansion of the model to include genetic and biological processes.

USING ESTABLISHED EFFECTS TO BETTER UNDERSTAND GENETIC EFFECTS AND GENETIC MODERATION

Although the CFMD has expanded in several directions, and it has always been clear that the model was assumed to fit some individuals better than others, insufficient attention has been paid to characterizing the individual differences that may influence response to marital problems. In particular, there are likely to be important individual differences with genetic roots that may help link marital and parenting problems to the biological processes that influence or mediate some symptoms of depression. Recently, this oversight has begun to be addressed. One approach has been to examine well-established variable nucleotide tandem repeats (VNTRs). VNTRs are genes that have sections of repeated genetic code. In many cases the repeated code is functional and has an impact on the gene product or on level of gene expression. We have focused on two candidate genes, the serotonin transporter (5HTT) and the dopamine receptor (DRD4). These VNTRs are the best known of a group with mounting evidence suggesting that they play a role in individual differences in response to contextual processes, including family processes (Belsky &

Pluess, 2009). In particular, there may be several VNTRs (and some other types of genetic polymorphisms) that increase responsiveness to environmental influences and environmental stress (for a review and overview of theory, see Belsky & Pluess, 2009; for a general critique of GxE research, see Duncan & Keller, 2011).

First, we briefly review the case for genetically linked, individual differences in response to stress generation, and then present the results of a recent investigation. As noted earlier, stress generation is a key process in the maintenance of depression by interpersonal problems (Hammen, 2006), and so genetic moderation would suggest individual differences in a core aspect of the model. Second, we examine the effect of genetic variation on response to intervention, focusing on the impact of a child's *5HTT* status as a moderator of a parent's change in depression in response to a parenting intervention. We note that the genetic variables *DRD4* and *5HTT* are probably best viewed as "heuristic" at the current stage of understanding of genetic moderation effects, and we expect that future iterations of research on genetic moderation will likely utilize "gene networks" or other approaches to better characterize broad sources of genetic influence rather than focusing on single genes acting alone. Accordingly, our single-gene analyses are best viewed as an initial approximation that may be supplanted by future research. Nonetheless, the exercise is likely useful in that the particular polymorphisms utilized in research to date are well understood and point to directions for future model development. In addition, interest in biological mechanisms has increased interest in the ways that the processes captured within the CFDM may "get under the skin" and so come to be reflected in epigenetic change. Although there is, as yet, limited data on this process, we briefly review the current research and present a recent study in order to convey the potential excitement of these developments for social and clinical researchers.

DRD4 and Individual Differences in Stress Generation

One pathway connecting relationship problems and depression within the CFDM is stress generation. Indeed, many of the persistent effects of problems in close relationships can be seen as reflecting stress generation processes that perpetuate and sometimes amplify negative affect, making conflict in family relationships more toxic than would otherwise be the case (Hammen, 2006). Recently, however, a number of studies have suggested that some genetic factors may amplify the impact of context (Belsky & Pluess, 2009). So, combining the conceptual structure of stress generation with recent developments in the understanding of genetic susceptibility, we proposed that contextual effects may be amplified due to their influence on interpersonal processes and that genetic factors may influence the magnitude of such effects, thus leading to amplified stress generation processes. The dopamine D4 receptor (*DRD4*) is a candidate gene of particular interest in this regard because of its effects on attention and negative arousal. *DRD4* contains a 48 bp variable nucleotide repeat (VNTR) polymorphism in exon III of chromosome 11 that is highly polymorphic, with 2 to 11 repeats. Individuals with at least one DRD4 allele containing 7 or more repeats (7R+) of the 48 bp section of the gene that is repeated show reduced gene expression (Schoots & Van Tol, 2003) and altered signaling in the frontal cortex (Wang, Zhong, & Yan, 2002), as well as greater emotional and behavioral reactivity to environmental deprivation and heightened anxiety in response to unconditioned stimuli (Falzone et al., 2002). Accordingly, we proposed and tested a three-stage model combining the stress generation framework (e.g., Hammen, 2006) with a genetic susceptibility perspective (Belsky & Pluess, 2009), proposing that positive and negative contexts would influence negative arousal, which in turn would influence parent–child interactions, which would then influence subsequent negative arousal, with each stage of the process amplified by the presence of the DRD4 7R+ allele.

As predicted, a significant moderation effect emerged, reflecting the interaction of external stress and DRD4 on negative arousal. Examination of simple slopes indicated that the slope for the impact of stressful circumstances on negative arousal for respondents with DRD4 7R+ alleles was significantly different from zero, but the slope for respondents who had no 7R+ allele was not significantly different from zero. This yielded the cross-over pattern predicted by the differential susceptibility hypothesis. Presence of a DRD4 7R+ allele was associated with significantly greater negative arousal when the context was more negative but was associated with significantly lower negative arousal when the context was less negative and more positive.

To examine the next stage of the model, that is, to document stress generation effects, we examined the impact of negative arousal on change in parent–child interaction. As predicted, there was a significant interaction of negative arousal with DRD4 in the prediction of change in parent–child interaction. Analysis of simple slopes indicated that the slope for the impact of negative arousal on quality of observed parent–child interaction for respondents with one or more DRD4 7R+ alleles was significantly different from zero, but the slope for respondents with no DRD4 7R+ alleles was not significantly different from zero.

Although the presence of a DRD4 7R+ allele was associated with significantly more problematic, negative parent–child interactions when negative arousal was elevated, there was no significant difference for those with and without a DRD4 7R+ allele when negative arousal was low. Accordingly, there was an effect of genetic variability on stress generation, but no evidence for a particularly positive response to low levels of negative arousal.

To test the expectation that the observed shifts in the interpersonal context could carry effects forward over long periods of time, thus maintaining the effects of an initially stressful environment, we examined the impact of negative parenting on negative arousal 10 years after the collection of the initial baseline data and 8 years after collection of the Wave 2 parent–child interaction data. Again, there was a significant interaction. Parent–child interaction and DRD4 interacted to predict later negative arousal. The slope relating earlier parent–child interaction to later negative arousal for those with at least one *DRD4* 7R+ allele was significantly different from zero, but the slope for respondents with no *DRD4* 7R+ alleles was not significantly different from zero. In this case, the differing slopes resulted in a significant crossover effect.

To summarize, as predicted by the contextual amplification model, chronic contextual stressors and supports were associated with level of negative arousal at baseline, and the impact of context on negative arousal was significantly greater for those with at least one 7R+ allele at *DRD4*. Moreover, as predicted in the second stage of the contextual amplification model, negative arousal in parents was associated with a shift toward more negative and less positive parent–child interaction only among those with at least one 7R+ allele at *DRD4*. Completing the hypothesized process, level of positive versus negative parent–child interactions was associated with change in negative arousal over time. Thus, as predicted by the contextual amplification model, the role of the 7R+ allele of *DRD4* was apparent at each of three separate stages of the stress generation process, resulting in amplification at each step. The results of the investigation suggest the potential importance of including individual differences linked to genetic factors within the expanded CFDM. Genetic features may be particularly important in understanding some aspects of the development and maintenance of depressive episodes and the way in which couple and family relationships are implicated in maintenance of negative affect over time.

Recent research has also implicated 5HTT in the stress generation process (Starr, Hammen, Brennan, & Najman, 2012). The serotonin transporter (*5HTT*) is a key regulator of serotonergic neurotransmission, localized to 17p13 and consisting of 14 exons and a single promoter. Variation at the 5HTTLPR (*5HTT* linked polymorphic region) results in two main variants, a short and a long allele; presence of the short allele results in lower serotonin transporter availability. The short variant has 12 copies, and the long variant 14 copies, of a 22 bp repeat element, and the short allele appears to exert a similar effect on temperament for both males and females (Munafo, Clark, & Flint, 2004). Although the short allele is more common among European Americans than African Americans, it is present with a relatively high frequency in the African American population as well (40.4% European American vs. 25.4% African American; Gelernter, Kranzler, & Cubells, 1997), allowing for examination in both ethnic groups.

Starr and colleagues (2012) found that *5HTT* genotype interacted with depression at age 15 to predict dependent stressful events at age 20. In line with expectations, those with one or more short (i.e., "s") alleles showed a stronger effect of depression on later dependent and interpersonal events than did those who carried only the long ('l') allele, suggesting another potential route for genetic factors to influence developmental processes relevant to the CFDM. Similarly, it is of interest to consider how genetic variation may relate to response to intervention, a topic to which we now turn.

5HTT and Response to Treatment

A growing body of research suggests that some individual differences linked to genetic factors may also influence response to intervention (Brody, Beach, et al., 2013). Stimulating interest in variation at 5HTT, children with one or two copies of the 5HTT "short" allele may exhibit more self-control difficulties (Miller & Brown, 1991; Rutter et al., 1997), higher activity levels, shorter attention spans, and more frequent negative affect (Auerbach, Faroy, Ebstein, Kahana, & Levine, 2001; Propper & Moore, 2006). As a consequence, learning the principles of competence-promoting parenting may be particularly useful to depressed parents of youths with the short 5HTT allele. Based on this rationale, we used genetic data obtained from 109 youths to examine differential program impact on caregiver depression as a function of youth genetic risk (Beach et al., 2009). All families self-identified as African American and in each family, the caregiver initially scored in the depressed range of the CESD.

Consistent with effects described in the analysis of overall treatment effects in the full sample described earlier (Beach et al., 2008), the treatment effect was significant, with caregivers who participated in the Strong African American Families (SAAF) program demonstrating significantly greater reductions in depressive symptoms than controls despite beginning the study equally depressed and having similar demographic characteristics (Beach et al., 2009). No significant main effect emerged for youth genetic risk, but the risk × intervention interaction was significant, indicating that presence of a youth carrying the 5HTT short allele moderated treatment impact on the parent. In particular, SAAF's benefit in reducing depressive symptoms was minimal for caregivers of youth with two copies of the longer allele for 5HTT, but for caregivers of youth with one or two copies of the short allele, assignment to SAAF was associated with long-term reductions in parent's CES-D, whereas assignment to the control condition was not. Thus, SAAF was more beneficial in reducing depression among caregivers of youth with a short 5HTT allele than for caregivers of youth who did not carry the short allele.

Conclusions

Although it is preliminary in many respects, an emerging literature suggests that genetic factors may be important in expanding various elements of the CFDM. In particular, it appears likely that individual differences linked to genetic variability may be consequential in moderating environmental influences on affect, moderating the influence of affect on stress generation and subsequent relationship problems, and moderating the impact of interventions designed to interrupt stress generation and alleviate family problems in the context of depression. The results are preliminary because it is likely that effects will ultimately prove to be more complex and involve more genetic elements than have been studied in the research reviewed herein. In particular, in future research a focus on broader gene networks related to outcomes of interest may better capture genetic main effects as well as more accurately describe genetic moderation effects. However, the observation of genotypic effects suggests a variety of important pathways to be further explored, and it has also increased interest in potential connections between processes central to the CFDM and various biological changes that may allow external stress to "get under the skin" (Taylor, Reppetti, & Seeman, 1997), leading to consideration of epigenetic change processes.

Can Family Environment Reprogram Genetic Effects?

The presence of genetic effects on processes related to the CFDM raises questions about the potential relevance of family of origin experiences that may alter genetic activity and downstream production of gene products. Because genetic variability is thought to influence outcomes primarily through its impact on gene product activity and level of gene expression, it follows that if there are other sources of influence on gene activity and gene expression, these might also be relevant to the CFDM. Because of documented impact on gene activity and expression, "epigenetic change" is of increasing interest to researchers. Accordingly, we turn next to an examination of emerging research on epigenetic change in family context.

Epigenetic change refers to alterations in DNA that have the potential to influence gene expression or activity and that can be transmitted from a parent cell to a daughter cell without involving changes in the base pairs that make up the genetic code. In some, but certainly not all, cases these alternations may be transmitted to offspring as well, leading subsequent generations to display a somewhat different phenotype (for an example, see "the agouti mouse"). When epigenetic changes lead to changes in gene expression, these may give rise to downstream outcomes of interest such as changes in developmental trajectories.

Methylation at a particular location typically has the effect of reducing the expression of gene products associated with that particular location. At the same time, methylated DNA is more readily bound by proteins that initiate chromatin remodeling, which ultimately generates a different shape for the methylated regions of DNA, often further reducing the activity of the gene. Given the potential to substantially affect gene transcription, methylation of regions with known gene regulatory importance, such as promoter regions of genes, may be of particular interest for behavioral scientists attempting to understand the role of the early family environment in programming long-term behavioral propensities. It is significant, therefore, that CpG pairs, that is, cytosine-phosphate sequences that are particularly prone to methylation, which are the targets of methylation, are not randomly distributed across the human genome. Rather, CpG pairs are typically concentrated in areas known as "CpG islands," that is, areas with a high density of CpG residues.

In turn, CpG islands are often found in close proximity to gene promoters, or gene transcription start sites, that is, regions known to be important in regulating gene expression. This suggests that examination of methylation of promoter regions may be particularly fruitful as attempts are made to unravel the way in which environments affect behavior via epigenetic reprogramming.

As a preliminary examination of the plausibility of methylation change as a function of family stressors, Beach Brody, Todorov, Gunter, and Philibert (2011) conducted an investigation of the impact of child abuse on changes in methylation in the promoter region of *5HTT*. We examined the CpG island associated with the promoter of *5HTT* because this is a highly conserved and phylogenetically old component of the serontonergic regulatory system, and decreased responsiveness of the serotonin system has been observed to produce behavioral effects in humans (Carver, Johnson, & Joormann, 2008). We proposed that hypermethylation of the promoter region of *5HTT* might be one mechanism by which the experience of child sex abuse contributes to an intermediate phenotype characterized by antisocial and other risky behavior.

DNA was prepared from lymphoblast cell lines derived from 155 females who had been separated from their biological parents at birth. Methylation in the promoter region of *5HTT* was determined through quantitative mass spectroscopy, and the resulting values were averaged to produce an average CpG ratio for each participant that described methylation across the region. Simple associations and path analyses were examined to characterize the relationships among childhood sex abuse by a family member, overall level of methylation, and subsequent antisocial behavior in adulthood. Because the sample was drawn from an adoption study, we were also able to control the effect of biological parent psychopathology as well as *5HTT* genotype, and so control for genetic main effects. Replicating prior work (Beach, Brody, Todorov, Gunter, & Philibert, 2010), a significant effect of childhood sex abuse on methylation of the *5HTT* promoter region emerged for women. In addition, a significant effect of methylation at *5HTT* on symptoms of antisocial personality disorder (ASPD) emerged for women, and this effect fully mediated the direct effect of child sex abuse on symptoms of ASPD.

We concluded that child sex abuse may create long-lasting changes in a behavioral phenotype by producing changes in methylation of the promoter region of 5HTT in women and these changes may account for some of the long-term effects of this experience. In particular, we concluded that hypermethylation in key gene promoters, such as the promoter region for *5HTT*, may be one mechanism linking childhood sex abuse to changes in risk for adult antisocial behavior in women. At the same time, it should be noted that broader examination of methylation across the genome will be necessary to identify the larger patterns of epigenetic change associated with child sex abuse. Likewise, because child adversity is often multifaceted, it is likely that some effects on methylation are attributable to associated aspects of adversity rather than to sex abuse per se. In addition, it appears likely that there are somewhat different impacts for males and females. Accordingly, although the results are encouraging in many respects, they indicate the need for exploration of this pathway in greater detail in the future.

Although epigenetic research within a family framework is in its infancy, it seems possible that epigenetic change attributable to childhood experiences, particularly adverse childhood events (ACEs) occurring in a family context, may sometimes alter biological processes and shift behavioral phenotypes. Accordingly, epigenetic changes may be as important as genotype in understanding developmental outcomes and in predicting response to intervention. In addition, epigenetic change may help explain long-term environmental effects and in some cases may help account for observed gene–environment interaction effects. These possible connections suggest considerable future activity in research focused on family context and epigenetic change. Assessment of epigenetic change also affords researchers an additional option for assessment that does not depend on self-report but that may capture experience of ACEs, opening new opportunities for research on the long-term impact of ACEs on personal and relationship adjustment, again suggesting considerable potential for epigenetic assessment in future expansion of the CFDM.

SUMMARY

The foregoing overview of research related to the CFDM is meant to provide both a retrospective view of theoretical development in the model as well as a prospective view of future directions for theoretical development. We expect Lewin's dictum that "There is nothing so practical as a good theory" to hold true as the theoretical aspects of the CFDM continue to develop. Greater theoretical development will bring with it additional practical implications. At a minimum, it seems clear that a future expanded version of the CFDM will incorporate both individual differences linked to genetic factors and epigenetic changes that produce lasting changes in vulnerability. Remaining open to diverse pathways and incorporating both behavioral processes (such as stress generation) and biological processes (such as gene methylation) has the potential to identify ways in which biological and behavioral pathways may reinforce each other or interact, thereby identifying new directions for both prevention of depression and stimulating the development of new interventions designed to help those already experiencing a depressive episode.

In addition to the areas covered in the current chapter, there are also clear opportunities for future growth in the theoretical connections between the CFDM and interpersonal models associated with other mental health disorders (see Introduction and Chapter 12, this volume), as well as considerable potential for expanded points of contact with models of family influence on children's depression (see Chapter 8, this volume). Equally exciting is the potential for connections between the CFDM and research on inflammatory responses to relationship stress (Chapter 1, this volume) as well as impact on psychophysiological responses (Chapter 4, this volume). Work in these areas promises to identify additional physiological mechanisms and pathways relevant to the CFDM (see also Brody, Yu, et al., 2013). Likewise, a broader model that is more fully integrated with the literature on biological mechanisms is more likely to have implications for models of cardiac health (Chapter 2, this volume) and other aspects of physical health (Chapter 3, this volume).

Hopefully, the foregoing review indicates that research on the CFDM remains active, with new theoretical horizons coming into view on multiple fronts, and new practical implications being developed and tested. As a consequence, we are hopeful that the CFDM will remain useful as an organizing heuristic for both researchers and clinicians. In particular, we hope it will remain a useful translational tool, connecting cutting-edge research to recommendations for practical intervention.

AUTHOR'S NOTE

Manuscript development was supported by award number 1P30DA027827 from the National Institute on Drug Abuse. The content is solely the responsibility of the author and does not necessarily represent the official views of the National Institute on Drug Abuse or the National Institutes of Health.

REFERENCES

Amato, P. R., Loomis, L. S., & Booth, A. (1995). Parental divorce, marital conflict, and offspring well-being during early adulthood. *Social Forces, 73,* 895–916. doi:10.1093/sf/73.3.895.

Auerbach, J. G., Faroy, M., Ebstein, R., Kahana, M., & Levine, J. (2001). The association of the dopamine D4 receptor gene (DRD4) and the serotonin transporter promoter gene (5-HTTLPR) with temperament in 12-month-old infants. *Journal of Child Psychology and Psychiatry and Allied Disciplines, 42,* 777–783. doi:10.1111/1469-7610.00774.

Barbato, A., & D'Avanzo, B. (2008). Efficacy of couple therapy as a treatment for depression: A meta-analysis. *Psychiatric Quarterly, 79,* 121–132. doi:10.1007/s11126-008-9068-0.

Beach, S. R. H., Brody, G. H. Todorov, A. A., Gunter, T. D., & Philibert, R. A. (2011). Methylation at *5HTT* mediates the impact of child sex abuse on women's antisocial behavior: An examination of the Iowa Adoptee Sample. *Psychosomatic Medicine, 73,* 83–87. doi:10.1097/PSY.0b013e3181fdd074.

Beach, S. R. H., Brody, G. H., Todorov, A., Gunter, T., & Philibert, R. A. (2010). Methylation at SLC6A4 is linked to family history of child abuse: An examination of the Iowa Adoptee Sample. *American Journal of Medical Genetics: Part B Neuropsychiatric Genetics, 153B,* 710–713.

Beach, S. R. H., Kim, S., Cercone-Keeney, J., Gupta, M., Arias, I., & Brody, G. (2004). Physical aggression and depressive symptoms: Gender asymmetry in effects? *Journal of Social and Personal Relationships, 21,* 341–360. doi:10.1177/0265407504042836.

Beach, S. R. H., Kogan, S. M., Brody, G. H., Chen, Y., Lei, M. & Murry, V. M. (2008). Change in maternal depression as a function of the Strong African American Families Program. *Journal of Family Psychology, 22,* 241–252. doi:10.1037/0893-3200.22.2.241.

Beach, S. R. H., Brody, G. H., Kogan, S. M., Philibert, R. A., Chen, Y., & Lei, M. (2009). Change in caregiver depression in response to parent training: Genetic moderation of intervention effects. *Journal of Family Psychology, 23,* 112–117.

Beach, S. R. H., Fincham, F. D., Amir, N., & Leonard, K. E. (2005). The taxometrics of marriage: Is marital discord categorical? *Journal of Family Psychology, 19,* 276–285. doi:10.1037/0893-3200.19.2.276.

Beach, S. R. H., & O'Leary, K. D. (1992). Treating depression in the context of marital discord: Outcome and predictors of response for marital therapy versus cognitive therapy. *Behavior Therapy, 23,* 507–258. doi:10.1016/S0005-7894(05)80219-9.

Beach, S. R. H., Sandeen, E. E., & O'Leary, K. D. (1990). *Depression in marriage: A model for etiology and treatment.* New York, NY: Guilford Press.

Belsky, J., & Pluess, M. (2009). Beyond diathesis stress: Differential susceptibility to environmental influences. *Psychological Bulletin, 135,* 885–908. doi:10.1037/a0017376.

Belsky, J., Youngblade, L., Rovine, M., & Vollig, B. (1991). Patterns of marital change and parent–child interaction. *Journal of Marriage and the Family, 53,* 487–498. doi:10.2307/352914.

Bodenmann, G., Plancherel, B., Beach, S. R. H., Widmer, K., Gabriel, B., Meuwly, N., … Schramm, E. (2008). Effects of coping-oriented couple therapy on depression: A randomized clinical trial. *Journal of Consulting and Clinical Psychology, 76,* 944–954. doi:10.1037/a0013467.

Booth, A., & Amato, P. R. (2001). Parental predivorce relations and offspring postdivorce well-being. *Journal of Marriage and Family, 63,* 197–212.

Brody, G. H., Beach, S. R. H., Hill, K. G., Howe, G. W., Prado, G., & Fullerton, S. M. (2013).Using genetically informed, randomized prevention trials to test etiological hypotheses about child and adolescent drug use and psychopathology. *American Journal of Public Health,* 103 Suppl 1:S19--24. doi: 10.2105/AJPH.2012.301080. Epub 2013 Aug 8.

Brody, G. H., Yu, T., Chen, Y–F., Kogan, S. M., Evans, G. W., Beach, S. R.H., … Philibert, R. A. (2013). Cumulative socioeconomic status risk, allostatic load, and adjustment: A prospective latent profile analysis with contextual and genetic protective factors. *Developmental Psychology, 49*(5), 913–927.

Carver, C. S., Johnson, S. L., & Joormann, J. (2008). Serotonergic function, two—mode models of self-regulation, and vulnerability to depression: What depression has in common with impulsive aggression. *Psychological Bulletin, 134,* 912–943.

Christensen, A., Atkins, D. C., Baucom, B., & Yi, J. (2010). Marital status and satisfaction five years following a randomized clinical trial comparing traditional versus integrative behavioral couple therapy. *Journal of Consulting and Clinical Psychology, 78,* 225–235. doi:10.1037/a0018132.

Cohen, S., O'Leary, K. D., & Foran, H. (2010). A randomized clinical trial of a brief, problem-focused couple therapy for depression. *Behavior Therapy, 41,* 433–446. doi: 10.1016/j.beth.2009.11.004.

Cummings, E. M., Davies, P. T., & Campbell, S. B. (2000). *Developmental psychopathology and family process: Theory, research, and clinical implications.* New York, NY: Guilford Press.

Cummings, E. M., & Davies, P. T. (2002). Effects of marital conflict on children: Recent advances and emerging themes in process-oriented research. *Journal of Child Psychology and Psychiatry and Allied Disciplines, 43,* 31–63. doi:10.1111/1469-7610.00003.

Davies, P., Sturge-Apple, M., & Cummings, E. (2004). Interdependencies among interparental discord and parenting practices: The role of adult vulnerability and relationship perturbations. *Development and Psychopathology, 16,* 773–797. doi:10.1017/S0954579404004778.

Davila, J., Bradbury, T. N., Cohan, C. L., & Tochluk, S. (1997). Marital functioning and depressive symptoms: Evidence for a stress generation model. *Journal of Personality and Social Psychology, 73,* 849–861. doi:10.1037//0022-3514.73.4.849.

Davila, J., Karney, B. R., Hall, T. W., & Bradbury, T. N. (2003). Depressive symptoms and marital satisfaction: Within-subject associations and the moderating effects of gender and neuroticism. *Journal of Family Psychology, 17,* 557–570. doi:10.1037/0893-3200.17.4.557.

Dessaulles, A., Johnson, S. M., & Denton, W. H. (2003). Emotion-focused therapy for couples in the treatment of depression: A pilot study. *American Journal of Family Therapy, 31,* 345–353. doi:10.1080/01926180390232266.

Duncan, L. E., & Keller, M. C. (2011). A critical review of the first 10 years of candidate gene-by-environment interaction research in psychiatry. *American Journal of Psychiatry, 168,* 1041–1049. doi: 10.1176/appi.ajp.2011.11020191.

Emanuels-Zuurveen, L., & Emmelkamp, P. M. (1996). Individual behavioral-cognitive therapy vs. marital therapy for depression in maritally distressed couples. *British Journal of Psychiatry, 169,* 181–188. doi:10.1192/bjp.169.2.181.

Erel, O., & Burman, B. (1995). Interrelatedness of marital relations and parent-child relations: A meta-analytic review. *Psychological Bulletin, 118,* 108–132. doi:10.1037//0033-2909.118.1.108.

Falzone, T. L., Gelman, D. M., Young, J. I., Grandy, D. K., Low, M. J., & Rubinstein, M. (2002). Absence of dopamine D4 receptors results in enhanced reactivity to unconditioned, but not conditioned, fear. *European Journal of Neuroscience, 15,* 158–164. doi:10.1046/j.0953816x.2001.01842.x.

Fleeson, W. (2004). The quality of American life at the turn of the century. In O. G. Brim, C. D. Ryff, & R. C. Kessler (Eds.), *How healthy are we? A national study of* well-being at midlife (pp. 252–272). Chicago, IL: University of Chicago Press

Foley, S. H., Rounsaville, B. J., Weissman, M. M., Sholomskas, D., & Chevron, E. (1989). Individual versus conjoint interpersonal psychotherapy for depressed patients with marital disputes. *International Journal of Family Psychiatry, 10,* 29–42.

Forehand, R., Wells, K. C., & Griest, D. L. (1980). An examination of the social validity of a parent training program. *Behavior Therapy, 11,* 488–502. doi:10.1016/S0005-7894(80)80065-7.

Gallart, S. C., & Matthey, S. (2005). The effectiveness of group Triple P and the impact of four telephone contacts. *Behaviour Change, 22,* 71–80. doi: 10.1375/bech.2005.22.2.71.

Gelernter, J., Kranzler, H., & Cubells, J. F. (1997). Serotonin transporter protein (SLC6A4) allele and haplotype frequencies and linkage disequilibria in African—and European-American and Japanese populations and in alcohol dependent subjects. *Human Genetics, 101,* 243–246.

Gelfand, D. M., Teti, D. M., Seiner, S. A., & Jameson, P. B. (1996). Helping mother fight depression: Evaluation of a home-based intervention for depressed mothers and their infants. *Journal of Clinical Child Psychology, 24,* 406–422. doi:10.1207/s15374424jccp2504_6.

Gerard, J., Krishnakumar, A., & Beuhler, C. (2006). Marital conflict, parent–child relations, and youth maladjustment: A longitudinal investigation of spillover effects. *Journal of Family Issues, 27,* 951–975. doi:10.1177/0192513X05286020.

Goering, P. N., Lancee, W. J., & Freeman, J. J. (1992). Marital support and recovery from depression. British Journal of Psychiatry, *10,* 29–42. doi:10.1192/bjp.160.1.76.

Gottman, J. M., Murray, J. D., Swanson, C. C., Tyson, R., & Swanson, K. R. (2002). *The mathematics of marriage: Dynamic nonlinear models.* Cambridge, MA: MIT Press.

Greenberg, P. E., Kessler, R. C., Birnbaum, H. G., Leong, S. A., Lowe, S. W., Berglund, P. A., & Corey-Lisle, P. K. (2003). The economic burden of depression in the United States: How did it change between 1990 and 2000? *Journal of Clinical Psychiatry, 64,* 1465–1475. doi:10.4088/JCP.v64n1211.

Goodman, S. H. (2007). Depression in mothers. *Annual Review of Clinical Psychology, 3,* 107–135. doi:10.1146/annurev.clinpsy.3.022806.091401.

Hammen, C. L. (2006). Stress generation in depression: Reflections on origins, research, and future directions. *Journal of Clinical Psychology, 62,* 69–82. doi:10.1002/jclp.20293.

Hooley, J. M. (2007). Expressed emotion and relapse of psychopathology. *Annual Review of Clinical Psychology, 3,* 329–352.

Hutchings, J., Lane, E., & Kelly, J. (2004). Comparison of two treatments for children with severely disruptive behaviors: A four year follow up. *Behavioral and Cognitive Psychotherapy, 32,* 15–30.

Jacobson, N. S., Dobson, K., Fruzzetti, A. E., Schmaling, K. B., & Salusky, S. (1991). Marital therapy as a treatment for depression. *Journal of Consulting and Clinical Psychology, 59,* 547–557. doi:10.1037//0022-006X.59.4.547.

Jones, D. J., Beach, S. R. H., & Forehand, R. (2001). Stress generation in intact community families: Depressive symptoms, perceived family relationship stress, and implications for adolescent adjustment. *Journal of Social and Personal Relationships, 18,* 443–462. doi: 10.1177/0265407501184001.

Kazdin, A. E. (2005). *Parent management training: Treatment for oppositional, aggressive, and antisocial behavior in children and adolescents.* New York, NY: Oxford University Press.

Kessler, R. C., Berglund, P., Demler, O., Jin, R., Koretz, D., Merikangas, K. R.,...Wang, P. S. (2003). The epidemiology of major depressive disorder: Results from the National Comorbidity Survey Replication (NCS-R). *Journal of the American Medical Association, 289,* 3095–3105. doi:10.1001/jama.289.23.3095.

Krishnakumar, A., & Buehler, C. (2000). Interparental conflict and parenting behaviors: A meta-analytic review. *Family Relations, 49,* 25–44. doi:10.1111/j.1741-3729.2000.00025.x.

Kung, W. W., & Elkin, I. (2000). Marital adjustment as a predictor of outcome in individual treatment of depression. *Psychotherapy Research, 10,* 267–278. doi:10.1093/ptr/10.3.267.

Leff, J., Vearnals, S., Brewin, C. R., Wolff, G., Alexander, B., Asen, E.,...Everitt, B. (2000). The London Depression Intervention Trial. *British Journal of Psychiatry, 177,* 95–100. doi:10.1192/bjp.177.2.95.

Lovejoy, M. C., Gracyk, P. A., O'Hare, E., & Neuman, G. (2000). Maternal depression and parenting behavior: A meta-analytic review. *Clinical Psychology Review, 20,* 561–592. doi:10.1016/S0272-7358(98)00100-7.

McClelland, G. H., & Judd, C. M. (1993). Statistical difficulties in detecting interactions and moderator effects. *Psychological Bulletin, 114,* 376–390. doi:10.1037//0033-2909.114.2.376.

McLeod, J. D., & Eckberg, D. A. (1993). Concordance for depressive disorders and marital quality. *Journal of Marriage & Family, 55,* 733–746. doi:10.2307/353353.

Miller, W. R., & Brown, J. M. (1991). Self-regulation as a conceptual basis for the prevention of addictive behaviors. In N. Heather, W. R. Miller, & J. Greely (Eds.), *Self-control and the addictive behaviors* (pp. 3–79). Sydney, Australia: Maxwell MacMillan.

Munafo, M. R., Clark, T. G., & Flint, J. (2004). Are there sex differences in the association between the 5HTT gene and neuroticism? A meta-analysis. *Personality and Individual Differences, 37,* 621–626.

Overbeek, G., Vollebergh, W., de Graaf, R., Scholte, R., de Kemp, R., & Engels, R. (2006). Longitudinal associations of marital quality and marital dissolution with the incidence of *DSM–III–R* disorders. *Journal of Family Psychology, 20,* 284–291. doi:10.1037/0893-3200.20.2.284.

Patterson, G. R., Reid, J. B., & Dishion, T. J. (1992). *Antisocial boys.* Eugene, OR: Castilia.

Propper, C., & Moore, G. A. (2006). The influence of parenting on infant emotionality: A multilevel psychobiological perspective. *Developmental Review, 26,* 427–460. doi:10.1016/j.dr.2006.06.003.

Proulx, C. M., Helms, H. M., & Buehler, C. (2007). Marital quality and personal well-being: A meta-analysis. *Journal of Marriage and Family, 69,* 576–593. doi:10.1111/j.1741-3737.2007.00393.x.

Rounsaville, B. J., Weissman, M. M., Prusoff, B. A., & Herceg-Baron, R. L. (1979). Marital disputes and treatment outcome in depressed women. *Comprehensive Psychiatry, 20,* 483–490. doi:10.1016/0010-440X(79)90035-X.

Rounsaville, B. J., Prusoff, B. A., & Weissman, M. M. (1980). The course of marital disputes in depressed women: A 48-month follow-up study. *Comprehensive Psychiatry, 21,* 111–118. doi:10.1016/0010-440X(80)90087-5.

Rutter, M., Dunn, J., Plomin, R., Simonoff, E., Pickles, A., Maughan, B.,…Eaves, L. (1997). Integrating nature and nurture: Implications of person-environment correlations and interactions for developmental psychopathology. *Development and Psychopathology, 9,* 335–364. doi:10.1017/S0954579497002083.

Sanders, M. R., & McFarland, M. (2000). Treatment of depressed mothers with disruptive children: A controlled evaluation of cognitive behavioral family intervention. *Behavior Therapy, 31,* 89–112. doi:10.1016/S0005-7894(00)80006-4.

Schoots, O., & Van Tol, H. H. (2003). The human dopamine D4 receptor repeat sequences modulate expression. *Pharmacogenomics Journal, 3,* 343–348. doi:10.1038/sj.tpj.6500208.

Snyder, D. K. (1997). *Manual for the Marital Satisfaction Inventory, Revised.* Los Angeles, CA: Western Psychological Services.

Snyder, D. K., Castellani, A. M., & Whisman, M. A. (2006). Current status and future directions in couple therapy. *Annual Review of Psychology, 57,* 317–344. doi:10.1146/annurev.psych.56.091103.070154.

Starrr, L. R., Hammen, C., Brennan, P. A., & Najman, J. M. (2012). Serotonin transporter gene as a predictor of stress generation in depression. *Journal of Abnormal Psychology, 21*(4), 810–818. doi: 10.1037/a0027952.

Taylor, S. E., Repetti, R. L., & Seeman, T. (1997). Health psychology: What is an unhealthy environment and how does it get under the skin? *Annual Review of Psychology, 48,* 411–447. doi:10.1146/annurev.psych.48.1.411.

Teichman, Y., Bar-El, Z., Shor, H., Sirota, P., & Elizur, A. (1995). A comparison of two modalities of cognitive therapy (individual and marital) in treating depression. *Psychiatry, 58,* 136–148.

Wade, T. J., & Pevalin, D. J. (2004). Marital transitions and mental health. *Journal of Health and Social Behavior, 45,* 155–170. doi: 10.1177/002214650404500203.

Waller, N. G., & Meehl, P. E. (1998). *Multivariate taxometric procedures: Distinguishing types from continua.* Thousand Oaks, CA: Sage.

Wang, X., Zhong, P., & Yan, Z. (2002). Dopamine D4 receptors modulate GABAergic signaling in pyramidal neurons of prefrontal cortex. *Journal of Neuroscience, 22,* 9185–9193.

Whiffen, V. E. (2004). Myths and mates in childbearing depression. *Women and Therapy, 27,* 151–163. doi:10.1300/J015v27n03_11.

Whisman, M. A. (2001a). The association between depression and marital dissatisfaction. In S. R. H. Beach (Ed.), *Marital and family processes in depression* (pp. 3–24). Washington, DC: American Psychological Association.

Whisman, M. A. (2001b). Marital adjustment and outcome following treatments for depression. *Journal of Consulting and Clinical Psychology, 69,* 125–129. doi:10.1037//0022-006X.69.1.125.

Whisman, M. A. (2007). Marital distress and DSM-IV psychiatric disorders in a population-based national survey. *Journal of Abnormal Psychology, 116,* 638–643. doi:10.1037/0021-843X.116.3.638.

Whisman, M. A., Beach, S. R. H., & Snyder, D. K. (2008). Is marital discord taxonic and can taxonic status be assessed reliably? Results from a national, representative sample of married couples. *Journal of Consulting and Clinical Psychology, 76,* 745–755. doi:10.1037/0022-006X.76.5.745.

Whisman, M. A., & Bruce, M. L. (1999). Marital distress and incidence of major depressive episode in a community sample. *Journal of Abnormal Psychology, 108,* 674–678. doi:10.1037//0021-843X.108.4.674.

CHAPTER 7

Intimate Partner Violence

A Biopsychosocial, Social Information

Processing Perspective

CHRISTOPHER M. MURPHY, AMBER E. Q. NORWOOD,
AND GINA M. POOLE

The current chapter reviews one of the most direct and troubling associations between relationships and health. We begin by providing an overview of the prevalence and health consequences of intimate partner violence (IPV). By all indications, IPV is a major public health epidemic—one of the primary causes of physically traumatic injuries and a contributing factor to a variety of mental health problems in victims. After reviewing health consequences, this chapter provides a broad conceptual framework for understanding risk and causal mechanisms in IPV perpetration. To date, most theories have been narrow in scope and insufficient to guide prevention and intervention. The field is ripe for a biopsychosocial model that is coherent and integrative. IPV risk factors are present at multiple levels of analysis. Examples include neurocognitive deficits, traumatic stress exposure, alcohol intoxication, and cultural beliefs about gender-appropriate roles and behaviors. We propose the hypothesis that these and many other contributing factors—at biological, psychological, and social levels of analysis—exert their influence on IPV through core aspects of social information processing. More specifically, many IPV risk factors promote hostile biases in interpretation of the partner's behavior and positive valuation of aggressive responses to aversive relationship events. Modern social information processing (SIP) models provide a coherent understanding of risk mechanisms that link both distal and proximal factors to enactment of relationship violence.

Definitions

The US Centers for Disease Control and Prevention (CDC) developed standardized definitions to guide IPV surveillance efforts (Saltzman, Fanslow, McMahon, & Shelley, 1999). Their definitions include 11 categories of intimate partners comprising both current and former relationships between married spouses, cohabiting partners, girlfriend/boyfriends, dating partners, or any couple with a child in common. CDC definitions also include four categories of IPV: (1) physical violence; (2) sexual violence; (3) threat of physical or sexual violence; and (4) psychological/emotional violence. Definitions for each category are quite complex. The following reflects core elements of the CDC definition of physical violence:

> The intentional use of physical force with the potential for causing death, disability, injury, or harm. . . includes, but is not limited to: scratching, pushing, shoving, throwing, grabbing, biting, choking, shaking, poking, hair pulling, slapping, punching, hitting, burning, use of a weapon (gun, knife, or other object), and use of restraints or one's body, size, or strength against another person. (Saltzman et al. 1999, pp. 10–11)

Sexual violence refers to the use of physical acts to force an individual to engage in a sexual act or to engage in such with an individual who has not or is unable to consent. Threat of physical or sexual violence is defined as a communication of intent to cause physical or sexual violence or abusive sexual contact. Psychological/emotional violence refers to acts, threats, or coercive tactics that cause trauma to an individual (e.g., demeaning or degrading statements, stalking, or controlling behaviors) when a history or threat of physical or sexual violence is present.

Prevalence, Morbidity, and Mortality

A 2003 CDC report estimated 5.3 million IPV victimizations annually in the United States, with 2 million total injuries (550,000 requiring medical attention) (National Center for Injury Prevention and Control, 2003). The US Department of Justice National Crime Victimization Survey (NCVS) for 2008 estimated the rates of nonfatal partner violence victimization to be 4.8 per 1,000 for adult women and 0.8 per 1,000 for adult men. In 2007, IPV accounted for 14% of all US homicides, with an annual total of 1,640 female victims and 700 male victims (Catalano, Smith, Snyder, & Rand, 2009).

These high prevalence rates are further reflected in emergency room visits and health costs. Between 1% and 7% of female emergency room patients have acute injuries from IPV, with most estimates in the 2%–4% range (Anglin & Sachs, 2003). Translated to 2012 dollars, CDC estimates place the annual direct health and mental health service costs associated with IPV in the United States at about $5 billion. One ray of hope comes from the fact that US Crime Survey data reveal substantial reductions in IPV across time. From 1993 to 2007, partner homicide rates declined 36% for male victims and 26% for female victims, and nonfatal IPV declined about 50% for both genders (Catalano et al., 2009).

Physical Health Consequences

Adverse physical health outcomes are common consequences of IPV. These include contusions, soft-tissue injuries, sprains, strains, fractures, maxillofacial injuries, and traumatic brain injuries (Mitchell & Anglin, 2009). In contrast to women who have not experienced relationship abuse, IPV victims have more health care visits, more days in bed, and higher rates of serious and chronic illnesses (Campbell, 2002; Campbell & Lewandowski, 1997; Taft, Vogt, Mechanic, & Resick, 2007). Through effects on the endocrine and immune systems, IPV may also contribute to chronic illnesses such as fibromyalgia, irritable bowel syndrome, and cardiovascular disease (Crofford, 2007; Leserman & Drossman, 2007).

Similar to physical assault, psychological aggression also has deleterious health consequences (Taft et al., 2007). For example, after controlling for exposure to physical dating aggression in a sample of female students, psychological aggression was associated with poorer self-reported general and functional health (Straight, Harper, & Arias, 2003). Likewise, women exposed only to psychological aggression have been found to report similar patterns of elevated health symptoms as those experiencing physical aggression and sexual coercion (Coker et al., 2002).

Mental Health Consequences

Negative mental health consequences of IPV exposure have been extensively documented. However, direct causal explanations are complicated by the fact that many IPV victims have prior histories of traumatic stress exposure in childhood or adolescence and live in high-stress environments. In addition, some victims have behavioral or emotional problems, such as substance abuse, that predate exposure to IPV. Efforts to isolate victimization effects on mental health are further complicated by mutual partner engagement in abuse perpetration (Archer, 2000) and the fact that young adults display assortative partnering with respect to antisocial behavior and emotional problems (Kim & Capaldi, 2004).

Bidirectional influences between mental health conditions and IPV are suggested by population studies. For example, in the National Comorbidity Survey, the presence of several premarital mental health conditions, including agoraphobia, social phobia, alcohol dependence, dysthymia, and nonaffective psychosis, conferred significant risk for subsequent IPV victimization in men (Kessler,

Molnar, Feurer, & Applebaum, 2001). However, no consistent associations between premarital mental health problems and IPV victimization were found for women. Predictive associations in the other direction, from IPV to mental health problems, are generally clearer and more robust. For example, using a combined sample of men and women, the National Epidemiological Survey on Alcohol and Related Conditions (NESARC) found that the odds of a new Axis I disorder diagnosis were 2.6 times higher among those with recent IPV exposure (Okuda et al., 2011).

Although explanatory models are complicated by exposure to multiple risk factors and potential bidirectional influences, strong associations between IPV victimization and mental health problems are apparent in research to date. A review by Golding (1999) provided empirical estimates for the prevalence and odds of specific psychological conditions among battered women. The following list contains average empirical prevalence estimates, the number of prevalence studies used to calculate them, and odds ratios associating the disorder with IPV victimization: posttraumatic stress disorder (PTSD), 64% prevalence (N = 11 studies; odds ratio [OR] = 3.7); depression, 48% (N = 18; OR = 3.8); suicidality, 18% (N = 13; OR = 3.6); alcohol abuse or dependence, 18% (N = 10; OR = 5.5); drug abuse or dependence, 9% (N = 4; OR = 5.6). Variation in prevalence was also uncovered, with higher rates found among samples drawn from battered women's shelters than from community or population samples.

More representative samples also display substantial risk for mental health problems in IPV victims. The CDC's 2010 National Intimate Partner and Sexual Violence Survey found that 63% of female IPV victims reported at least one PTSD symptom (Black et al., 2011). The NISVS study found the following odds ratios between new incident diagnoses and recent IPV exposure: any alcohol use disorder (OR = 3.3), any drug use disorder (6.3), any mood disorder (2.6), and any anxiety disorder (2.9) (Black et al., 2011). In summary, among both severely affected service-seeking samples, as well as population samples, IPV victimization is associated with a two- to sixfold increase in the odds of common mental health conditions.

The most prevalent mental health conditions in service-seeking samples of IPV victims appear to be PTSD and major depression. Not surprisingly, PTSD and depression are often comorbid in this population. For example, studies of female IPV victims with PTSD have found rates of comorbid depression ranging from 43% to 64% (Cascardi, O'Leary, & Schlee, 1999; Nixon, Resick, & Nishith, 2004; Stein & Kennedy, 2001). In addition, symptoms of PTSD and depression may persist for many years after an abusive relationship has ended (Campbell & Soeken, 1999; Zlotnick, Johnson, & Kohn, 2006).

Several studies have documented that psychological abuse exposure is also very important in understanding mental health effects of IPV. In the National Violence Against Women Survey, for example, psychological abuse had equally strong associations with PTSD as did physical abuse (Coker, Weston, Creson, Justice, & Blakeney, 2005). In fact, several studies of IPV victim populations have found that psychological abuse is uniquely associated with PTSD symptoms above and beyond the effects of physical assault (e.g., Street & Arias, 2001; Taft, Murphy, King, Dedeyn, & Musser, 2005). One recent study found that this was true even when sexual violence and sexual coercion were included as controls along with physical assault (Norwood & Murphy, 2012).

Summary of Physical and Mental Health Effects

With respect to injuries, the physical health consequences of violent partner assaults are clear, direct, and extensive. Although more challenging to isolate, IPV effects on general health status, health service utilization, and chronic illness presentation are also supported by research to date. Population studies suggest bidirectional influences between mental health conditions and IPV victimization, yet the evidence is more consistent and robust in supporting IPV victimization effects on mental health than mental health effects on IPV victimization. PTSD and depression are the most prevalent conditions among service-involved samples of IPV victims. In addition to physical assaults, psychological abuse has been consistently associated with negative effects on both physical and mental health. A variety of factors, including the type and severity of IPV exposure and previous victimization experiences, appear to influence the onset and continuation of mental health symptoms. Mounting evidence produces an undeniable conclusion that IPV places victims at substantial risk for negative physical and mental health outcomes, and it should receive significant attention in public health research.

PROMINENT THEORIES OF INTIMATE PARTNER VIOLENCE PERPETRATION

To date, the prominent theoretical models in the field have emphasized limited, often singular, causes of IPV. The primary conceptual analyses derive from the 1970s feminist movement in Great Britain and North America and reflect extensive efforts to provide safe houses and support for battered women. Rooted in a feminist analysis of gender and power, IPV is seen as an outgrowth of social dynamics that place men in charge in the domestic sphere (e.g., Dobash & Dobash, 1979; Pence & Paymar, 1993). Relevant research has highlighted cultural variations and social institutions that promote or condone IPV. Associated solutions require social and cultural transformation to promote women's empowerment and equality. A recent synthesis of controlled trial research on interventions for perpetrators and victims of IPV highlighted the scope and influence of feminist models. In 61 published studies located, comprising over 1,000 participants, not one single male victim or female perpetrator was included in any controlled intervention trial (Eckhardt et al., 2013).

While providing trenchant analysis of social, cultural, and historical contributions to IPV, these models have important limitations. First, women's aggressive and violent behavior is either ignored altogether or understood solely as self-defense or violent resistance. Available research indicates a high rate of mutual (bidirectional) aggression (Archer, 2000; Straus, 2011). In addition, women do not invariably see their aggression as self-defense. In fact, women report that they and their male partners are about equally likely to initiate physical aggression (Stets & Straus, 1990). Second, gender-based analyses have difficulty explaining the notable prevalence of IPV in gay and lesbian relationships (Letellier, 1994; Messinger, 2011; Murray, Mobley, Buford, & Searnan-DeJohn, 2007). Finally, the social cognitive emphasis on beliefs about gender and sex roles has not been consistently supported in case-control research on male IPV perpetrators (Eckhardt & Dye, 2000).

Psychopathological models understand IPV as an outgrowth of abusive individuals' trauma histories, personality disorders, and patterns of insecure and disorganized attachment (e.g., Ehrensaft, Moffit, & Caspi, 2004; Ehrensaft, Cohen, & Johnson, 2006; Dutton, 2007). Relevant research has identified numerous personality, emotional, and symptomatic correlates of IPV, and it has produced empirical subtypes of abuse perpetrators in clinical samples of men (e.g., Hamberger & Hastings, 1991; Murphy, Meyer, & O'Leary, 1993). The most prominent subtyping model identifies three groups of IPV perpetrators: (1) generally violent/antisocial; (2) dysphoric/borderline; and (3) family only/nonpathological (Holtzworth-Munroe & Stuart, 1994).

Despite extensive empirical documentation of trauma and personality correlates of IPV, research on psychopathological disorders among IPV perpetrators is complex. Available evidence indicates that only a minority of IPV perpetrators in treatment samples have serious psychopathological conditions such as psychotic disorders, mood disorders, or severe personality disorders (e.g., antisocial or borderline) (Huss & Langhincrichsen-Rohling, 2006), although a much higher proportion report traumatic stress exposure, childhood violence, and attachment problems (Dutton & White, 2012; Theobald & Farrington, 2012). However, the translation to perpetration of IPV is complicated, as many individuals with insecure attachment and traumatic histories do not engage in IPV. The processes and mechanisms linking trauma, personality, and psychopathology to IPV are often murky or ill defined, specifically in explaining how emotional distress translates into violence for some, but not all, individuals with specific personality characteristics, attachment styles, and psychopathological profiles. In addition, these approaches tend to downplay dyadic/interactional, social learning, and sociocultural influences.

Dyadic interactional models, grounded in family systems and behavioral theories of relationships, understand IPV as an outgrowth or expression of relationship distress and dysfunction (e.g., Neidig & Friedman, 1984; Stith, McCollum, Amanor-Boadu, & Smith, 2012). These models emphasize dyadic conflict escalation, poor communication and problem solving, and mutual patterns of abuse. In support of these models, laboratory studies in which couples are asked to discuss and solve an important problem in their relationship have consistently documented aversive patterns of communication and high levels of negative emotion expression and negative reciprocity in couples experiencing IPV (e.g., Cordova, Jacobson, Gottman, Rushe, & Cox, 1993; Margolin, John, & Gleberman, 1988; Murphy & O'Farrell, 1997).

While providing important insights and empirical findings on interactional processes associated with IPV, dyadic and relationship systems models tend to downplay individual risk factors. Unidirectional patterns of abuse and violence, unidirectional escalation of conflict, and individuals who abuse multiple relationship partners across time are not well understood by conflict escalation models. Likewise, the more pernicious forms of abuse, labeled "intimate terrorism" (Johnson & Leone, 2005), may reflect patterns and causal factors that are distinct from common dyadic conflict. Finally, among couples experiencing relationship distress and escalating hostilities, it remains mysterious why some, but clearly not all, escalate their conflicts to physical assault.

BIOPSYCHOSOCIAL DIMENSIONS

Whereas all three approaches highlighted earlier—feminist/gender-based models, psychopathological models, and dyadic process models—provide important insights and research findings on IPV, none seems to sufficiently capture the broad scope of risk and protective factors associated with IPV. In addition, neurobiological factors, which are largely ignored by all prominent conceptual models, may also be important. Several findings are notable in this regard. One is the high rate of head injury found among perpetrators of IPV (Rosenbaum et al., 1994). Detailed analyses have revealed a history of head injury in close to half of partner violent men presenting for treatment, rates that are two to four times higher than nonviolent controls (Cohen, Rosenbaum, Kane, Warnken, & Benjamin, 1999; Cohen et al., 2003). Second, relative to matched controls, IPV perpetrators exhibit poorer average performance on a range of neuropsychological tests measuring executive functions, impulse control, and specific verbal abilities (Cohen et al., 1999, 2003). Third, low brain serotonin levels, which have been associated with generalized aggression in humans and animal models of aggression, also appear to be linked to IPV (Hibbeln et al., 1998). However, serotonin associations with IPV may be moderated by factors such as head injury (Rosenbaum, Abend, Gearan, & Fletcher, 1997) and plasma levels of essential fatty acids (Hibbeln et al., 1998).

In light of emerging neurobiological findings, Rosenbaum, Geffner, and Benjamin (1997) proposed a biopsychosocial model of IPV. Their proposal was motivated by three main considerations: (1) the limited attention paid to biological influences by IPV researchers and practitioners, (2) the heterogeneity of partner violent men as reflected in the proliferation of abuser subtypes and diversity of research findings on this population, and (3) the need for integrative theoretical models to embrace these complex findings.

Expanding upon basic laboratory research on aggression, Rosenbaum and colleagues (1997) proposed a threshold model in which a variety of individual, relational, and contextual factors, including stress and conflict, contribute to the arousal of negative affect. As arousal builds, the individual crosses a threshold, shifting from cognitively controlled behavior to more automatic modes of responding, labeled "behaviors of high habit strength." Disinhibited aggression is one high habit-strength behavior that can emerge after this threshold shift in response tendencies. Whereas contextual and relational factors primarily contribute to arousal, a variety of other factors, including social learning history and cultural constraints on aggression, influence the establishment and enactment of "high habit strength" behaviors. In their model, neurocognitive factors and acute intoxication operate by lowering the threshold for aggressive responding.

Rosenbaum and colleagues' model is integrative, innovative, and linked to basic laboratory investigations of affective arousal and aggression (Zillman, 1983). They also argue that this model is consistent with abusive individuals' subjective experience of a loss of control at the time of aggression, reflecting an apparent threshold shift to more automatic or "primitive" modes of thought and action. However, the ways in which contributing factors influence aggression risk remain complex. For example, the ways in which learning histories establish aggressive response tendencies are not fully articulated. In addition, the specific processes involved in the dramatic cognitive shift to automatic responding remain somewhat elusive and mysterious.

INTIMATE PARTNER VIOLENCE AND SOCIAL INFORMATION PROCESSING

An overlapping, but distinct, approach to integrating biopsychosocial dimensions of IPV derives from research and theory on children's aggression. More specifically, social information processing (SIP) models contextualize peer aggression within a general model of social competence (Crick & Dodge, 1994). Originally, McFall (1982) proposed an information processing model of social competence containing three stages—*decoding* involves the interpretation and understanding of social cues, *decision making* involves the generation and selection of responses, and *enactment* involves the output of behaviors that are judged as socially competent (or problematic) by others. In an early series of case-control studies, Holtzworth-Munroe had excellent success applying McFall's model to IPV perpetrators (Holtzworth-Munroe, 2000). With respect to decoding, when presented with hypothetical relationship scenarios, male IPV perpetrators were more likely than nonviolent controls to display a hostile cognitive bias, attributing more negative intentions to female partners (e.g., Holtzworth-Munroe & Hutchinson, 1993).

With respect to decision making, when asked about how they would respond to hypothetical relationship scenarios involving jealousy, rejection, or wife challenges, male IPV perpetrators generated response options that were judged by third-party raters to be less effective and less socially competent than nonviolent controls (e.g., Holtzworth-Munroe & Anglin, 1991).

The intervening years have witnessed significant developments in both the conceptual models of social information processing and social cognitive research on IPV perpetration. At the conceptual level, Crick and Dodge (1994) proposed a reformulated, six-stage model of SIP designed to explain children's social competence. Unlike the original SIP model, which involved linear steps from input (decoding) to output (response enactment), the reformulated model depicts a circular set of processing stages in which social behaviors can influence subsequent interpretations of social cues and subsequent generation and evaluation of behavioral responses. Notably, at each stage of the process, the reformulated model contains bidirectional influences with a central database of social information in the form of rules, schemas, and accumulated social knowledge. Thus, social information processing does not happen in a vacuum, but in the context of cultural influences, personality, and learning history. Finally, the role of emotion is more fully articulated by conceptualizing internal emotional cues as part of the encoding process and arousal regulation as part of the goal clarification process that precedes response generation and selection. This model has been very fruitful in understanding children's aggression (Crick & Dodge, 1994; Dodge et al., 2002).

Applications to IPV at each step of the reformulated SIP model are presented in Table 7.1. Some of the most robust empirical findings involve the interpretation of partner behavior, as represented in early SIP stages. Persistent and intense attribution of negative intention to the partner is a core cognitive feature shared by the vast majority of IPV perpetrators (Holtzworth-Munroe & Hutchinson, 1993). Hostile attributions work in a reciprocal dynamic with anger arousal, biasing response generation and selection processes toward aggressive options, and creating a need for arousal regulation to inhibit aggressive impulses. As indicated by findings listed in Table 7.1, IPV perpetrators display further problems in subsequent information processing stages as well, including limited verbal/cognitive self-control efforts to downregulate anger arousal, generation of socially incompetent response alternatives in difficult relationship scenarios, and more positive outcome appraisals for aggressive relationship behaviors. The reformulated SIP model provides a powerful heuristic for organizing cognitive-behavioral research findings on IPV perpetration, and it highlights a number of important targets for behavior change interventions.

In another set of important developments, new and innovative strategies have been devised to investigate social cognition in IPV perpetrators. In the articulated thoughts in simulated situations (ATSS) paradigm, individuals listen to audio recordings of hypothetical, anger-inducing relationship scenarios. At regular intervals, the scenario is halted and the individual is asked to articulate ongoing thoughts, which are recorded for subsequent coding. ATSS research has revealed

Table 7.1. STAGES OF SOCIAL INFORMATION PROCESSING (SIP)
FROM CRICK AND DODGE (1994) AND APPLICATIONS TO INTIMATE
PARTNER VIOLENCE (IPV)

SIP Stage	Sample Research Applications to IPV Perpetrators
1. Encoding of cues —External —Internal	External: Low empathic accuracy (decoding of partner's emotions) in review of videotaped couple interaction (Clements, Holtzworth-Munroe, Schweinle, & Ickes, 2007) Internal: High reports of anger in response to a variety of hypothetical partner behaviors (Holtzworth-Munroe & Smutzler, 1996)
2. Interpretation of cues —Causal attributions —Attributions of intent —Evaluations of: Goal attainment Past performance Self and other	Strong and pervasive attribution of negative intention to partner (e.g., Holtzworth-Munroe & Hutchinson, 1993)
3. Clarification of goals —Arousal regulation	Low rates of anger control self-statements in ATSS (although not significantly different from distressed, nonviolent men) (Eckhardt et al., 1998)
4. Response access or construction	Generation of socially incompetent responses to hypothetical relationship scenarios (Holtzworth-Munroe & Anglin, 1991)
5. Response decision	Aggressive behavioral intentions in response to a variety of hypothetical wife behaviors (Holtzworth-Munroe & Smutzler, 1996) More positive outcome appraisals (e.g., win argument) and fewer negative outcome appraisals (e.g., relationship will be interrupted or dissolved) of aggressive relationship behaviors (e.g., Riggs & Caulfield, 1997)
6. Behavioral enactment	Moderate to strong correlations among different forms of abuse, including physical assault, threats, psychological abuse, sexual coercion and violence (e.g., Norwood & Murphy, 2012) Problematic communication, negative reciprocity (e.g., Cordova et al., 1993)
Other considerations	Reciprocal referencing of social knowledge and schemas occurs at each step of the model

that cognitive distortions and irrational beliefs, often not detectable in response to general self-report measures of cognitive style, become highly apparent in response to relationship scenarios that invoke emotional reactions (Eckhardt, Barbour, & Davidson, 1998). Thus, hostile cognitive biases associated with IPV perpetration emerge within specific emotional contexts.

Recent research further suggests that some aspects of social cognition linked to IPV perpetration may be subtle and largely outside of conscious awareness. In the implicit association test (IAT), reaction time differences are used to evaluate implicit schematic processing of information (Greenwald, McGhee, & Schwartz, 1998). Differential response times to different patterns of word pairings reflect accessibility of implicit associations. One example involves response times discriminating associations between violent and nonviolent words as paired with positive and negative emotion words. Using this method in a case-control design, Eckhardt, Samper, Suhr, and Holtzworth-Munroe (2012) found that compared to controls, male IPV perpetrators display a relative bias toward faster reaction times when positive emotion words were paired with violent words, revealing more implicit positive attitudes toward violence. A similar finding emerged for implicit associations between female words and violent words. Thus, automatically accessed implicit associations may fuel biases observed in social information processing studies of IPV.

USING SOCIAL INFORMATION PROCESSING TO UNDERSTAND BIOPSYCHOSOCIAL RISK MECHANISMS FOR INTIMATE PARTNER VIOLENCE

Returning to the need for a biopsychosocial model of IPV, the reformulated SIP model provides a heuristic framework in which a wide array of contributing factors work by influencing core social information processing. Most notably, a variety of factors influence hostile appraisals of the partner's behavior and intentions, arousal regulation in the context of interactional goals, generation and evaluation of response options, and behavioral enactment processes. As highlighted within the reformulated SIP model (Crick & Dodge, 1994), each step in the SIP process is also influenced by, and influences, core social knowledge in the form of social rules and schemas. In this formulation, core SIP mechanisms mediate a wide array of distal and proximal contributing factors, including biological, psychological, and social inputs. In developing prevention and intervention strategies, there may be considerable value in understanding how various contributing factors alter social cognition—that is, to determine the specific mediational processes involved using the SIP model. This integrative hypothesis can be illustrated by examining recent studies of several well-documented risk predictors of IPV. Table 7.2 provides examples of how key biological, psychological, and social factors may influence risk for IPV through SIP processes. The following sections provide more detailed analysis of several examples in which SIP provides a useful mediational framework for a biopsychosocial approach to IPV.

Neurocognitive Abilities and Intimate Partner Violence

In a recent study from our research team, male perpetrators of IPV were administered a series of neuropsychological tests designed to measure executive cognitive functions and impulse control (Persampiere, Poole, & Murphy, in press). Examples include the Wisconsin Card Sort Test, which presents respondents with response

Table 7.2. EXAMPLE INTIMATE PARTNER VIOLENCE (IPV) RISK FACTOR
INFLUENCES ON SOCIAL INFORMATION PROCESSING (SIP)

IPV Risk Factor	IPV-Relevant Effects on SIP
Subtle neurocognitive limitations —Executive functioning —Impulse control	*Hostile bias in cue interpretation:* Enhanced levels of anger reactivity, cognitive distortion, and irrational beliefs during ATSS (Persampiere et al., in press)
Trauma exposure and posttraumatic stress disorder (PTSD) symptoms	*Cue interpretation and response generation:* Predictive effects of PTSD and trauma exposure on IPV mediated by perception of negative partner intentions and socially incompetent response generation to relationship challenges (Taft et al., 2008)
Intergenerational conflict expression	*Response generation and selection:* Predictive effects of witnessed aggression between parents (assessed during childhood) on participation in dating aggression (assessed in young adulthood) are mediated by the tendency to generate and favor aggressive responses to social challenges (assessed in adolescence) (Fite et al., 2008)
Alcohol intoxication	*Cue interpretation:* Heightened perception of negative partner engagement during problem discussions with alcohol administration (Sillars et al., 2002) *Response selection:* Alcohol enhances verbalization of aggressive intentions by IPV perpetrators in ATSS (Eckhardt, 2007)

cards that vary in shape, color, and size and asks the individual to figure out sorting criteria and shift when the task demands (sorting rules) change. This task exerts complex cognitive demands; the individual must retain information about the ongoing task in memory, maintain a mental response set, compare ongoing feedback on each trial to the current hypothesis about sorting rules, generate new hypotheses when needed, shift mental set, and inhibit learned responses that are no longer correct. A number of additional automated neuropsychological tests were also administered, including the continuous performance test, which requires the individual to respond rapidly while inhibiting incorrect responses to simple stimuli (e.g., X's and O's) presented via computer. These individuals also completed the ATSS procedure, providing "talk aloud" data in response to a hypothetical relationship scenario in which they were overhearing a relationship partner say demeaning things about the respondent to a friend.

The findings, although straightforward, were somewhat surprising. IPV perpetrators with relatively poorer performance on "cold" neuropsychological tests assessing executive functions and impulsivity also displayed considerably higher levels of cognitive distortions and irrational beliefs in their articulated thoughts during the ATSS. Whereas some models suggest that neuropsychological deficits may simply lower the response threshold for disinhibition of aggressive outbursts (Rosenbaum et al., 1997), these findings suggest that neurocognitive limitations may influence early stages of SIP, enhancing the shift to distorted and hostile thinking in response to relationship challenges. The broader point here is that neurocognitive contributors to IPV may not operate in a vacuum and may not exert direct disinhibiting effects on aggression, but they may create challenges for core facets of the SIP process, enhancing hostile cognitive biases and perhaps altering one's ability to manage negative affect arousal in light of social and interpersonal goals.

Alcohol Intoxication and Intimate Partner Violence

An extensive body of research has demonstrated that alcohol use is associated with IPV (Foran & O'Leary, 2008), and IPV is highly prevalent in populations suffering from alcohol use disorders (Murphy & O'Farrell, 1996). Important questions arise as to whether elevated rates of IPV in alcohol-dependent samples reflect distal correlated problems versus the proximal effects of acute alcohol intoxication. For example, some individuals have a broad personality-based predisposition to externalizing behavior problems that include both substance abuse and aggression (Krueger & South, 2009). In addition, IPV risk may arise from more general problems with relationship distress, poor problem solving, life stress, and other difficulties correlated with alcohol use disorders (Murphy, O'Farrell, Fals-Stewart, & Feehan, 2001). However, acute effects of alcohol intoxication on IPV risk are also apparent. For example, higher rates of alcohol consumption are present prior to violent versus nonviolent relationship conflicts (Murphy et al., 2005). Experience-sampling research has also documented daily co-occurrence of alcohol use and partner aggression (Moore, Elkins, McNulty, Kivisto, & Handsel, 2011).

The effect of acute alcohol intoxication on risk for IPV provides a second important illustration of the SIP model as an integrative framework. The predominant conceptual model to understand the effects of acute intoxication on social behavior is Steel and Josephs's (1990) alcohol myopia theory. In this model, alcohol influences social behavior indirectly as a function of the interaction of social information processing and elements of the social context. Specifically, alcohol has a direct, dose-dependent effect on speed and depth of cognitive processing. In general terms, the more you drink, the less flexibly and elaborately you think. Reduced information processing capacity produces behavioral effects that depend on the situational context. Specifically, alcohol is thought to bias response selection in situations that combine a strong immediate impulse to act in a specific fashion (i.e., an impulse to aggression) with less obvious reasons to inhibit this impulse (i.e., potential negative consequences of aggression). These situational conditions are labeled "inhibition conflict" by Steele and Josephs (1990).

Using SIP as a framework, one can further decompose the effects of alcohol on aggression. First, it may be possible to determine the extent to which intoxication: (a) enhances problematic initial decoding of social cues (i.e., hostile biases), (b) impairs cognitive regulation of arousal in light of social goals, and/or (c) biases response generation and selection processes. Second, the referencing of social knowledge and schemas that occurs at each step of this process can provide individual-difference components to help understand why aggression is a common behavioral effect of intoxication for some, but clearly not all, individuals.

Relevant studies have used direct manipulation of alcohol (versus placebo) to investigate relevant social cognitive and behavioral processes in perpetrators of IPV. Leonard and Roberts (1998) administered alcohol, placebo, or neither to men with and without a history of IPV prior to a relationship problem-solving communication task. As compared to a baseline communication sample, alcohol administration increased husbands' negative communication behavior independent of IPV status.

Surprisingly, husbands' problem-solving attempts were also increased by alcohol administration and were higher in general among men in the IPV group. It appears that the distorting effect of alcohol on response selection may enhance both the tendency to respond in a hostile fashion and the tendency to proffer solutions to relationship problems. Further analyses (described later) suggest that increased problem solving may reflect a positive (optimistic) shift in appraisals for individuals who have a highly favorable view of their relationship partner. Note, however, that problem-solving attempts as coded in marital interaction research are not uniformly well received by the partner. For some individuals, such attempts may reflect unilateral efforts to impose solutions rather than collaborative efforts to devise solutions. Thus, from the perspective of alcohol myopia theory, alcohol effects on both negative (hostile) relationship exchanges, as well as some problem-solving attempts, may reflect similar alterations in response selection under conditions of inhibitory conflict.

A follow-up analysis of data from the Leonard and Roberts's (1998) study used methodology originally developed by Ickes (1997, 2001) in his study of empathic accuracy in couples to examine social cognition during marital interactions (Sillars, Leonard, Roberts, & Dun, 2002). Immediately after completing the communication task, husbands and wives were brought to separate rooms where they watched a video replay of their discussion. Every 20 seconds, the video was stopped, and the participant was asked to say out loud what he or she was thinking and feeling during the interaction. Their responses were then organized using 50 specific codes encompassing higher order categories that included emotions, appraisals of the issue at hand, person appraisals (of self or partner), and appraisals or descriptions of the interactional process. Dimensions of social cognition could then be examined by contrasting actor and partner's interpretations of events in the interaction, and by comparing thoughts articulated during the video review to behaviors enacted in the interactions.

The effects of alcohol on social cognition during these marital interactions were very different for violent versus nonviolent husbands. One way this was examined was to compare the wife's articulations regarding constructive (versus destructive) engagement in the interaction with the husband's report of the wife's engagement.

Interestingly, in the alcohol condition, nonaggressive husbands displayed a positivity bias in which they attributed more constructive engagement and cooperation to the wife than the wives attributed to themselves. The exact opposite pattern was found for aggressive husbands. In the alcohol condition, aggressive husbands attributed more negative engagement to the partners than the partners attributed to themselves. Thus, alcohol appeared to escalate negative attributions regarding the partner's intentions and behaviors, but only among husbands with a history of relationship aggression. In addition, the associations between articulated negative thoughts (in the video review task) and negative behavior (coded by third-party ratings of the interaction) were stronger among aggressive than nonaggressive husbands, even when controlling for the partner's previous negative behavior, and this linkage was further strengthened by alcohol. Thus, as predicted by alcohol myopia theory, alcohol appears to reduce or prevent any editing process that might otherwise inhibit negative thoughts from being translated directly into negative communication behaviors.

In related work, Eckhardt (2007) administered alcohol or placebo to male IPV perpetrators and controls prior to the ATSS procedure. Participants responded to a neutral ATSS scenario, as well as two anger-invoking relationship scenarios. In examining articulations reflecting aggressive verbalizations and intentions, neither the alcohol manipulation nor the anger-inducing scenarios had a significant impact among nonviolent control subjects; however, IPV perpetrators had higher aggressive verbalizations during the challenging scenarios than the neutral scenario, and this effect was amplified by the administration of alcohol. From the SIP perspective, it is interesting to note that the dependent variable, verbalizations of aggressive thoughts and intentions, reflects later stages of the SIP model involving response generation, selection, and enactment. Interestingly, alcohol myopia theory predicts that alcohol will enhance aggression primarily through response selection processes when aggression is an activated response option. For nonviolent controls, aggressive response options may not be activated by the ATSS scenarios, thus limiting the potential for alcohol to bias the response selection process.

Trauma, Traumatic Stress Symptoms, and Intimate Partner Violence

A final illustration of the integrative value of the SIP model involves trauma, traumatic stress symptoms, and IPV. Extensive research has documented intergenerational patterns of relationship abuse, as well as high rates of childhood trauma exposure in perpetrators of IPV (Ehrensaft et al., 2003, 2004; Fritz, Slep, & O'Leary, 2012). In addition, studies of military veteran samples have documented elevated rates of IPV among veterans with posttraumatic stress disorder (PTSD; Taft, Watkins, Stafford, Street, & Monson, 2011) and indicate that the association between combat exposure and IPV is largely accounted for by PTSD symptoms (Marshall, Panuzio, & Taft, 2005). Conceptual explanations suggest that hyperarousal symptoms contribute to anger dysregulation and enhanced appraisal of threat in response to common social stimuli (Chemtob, Novaco, Hamada, Gross, & Smith, 1997).

Two recent studies have examined SIP variables in mediational models designed to understand intergenerational patterns of abuse and the effects of trauma exposure on IPV perpetration. These studies are described in detail here because they most clearly illustrate the proposed utility of SIP models in understanding IPV risk mechanisms. Fite and colleagues (2008) examined aspects of SIP as mediators of intergeneration patterns of relationship conflict in a large longitudinal study of child development. Interparental conflict was measured by parents' reports of psychological and physical aggression toward one another when the target child was 5 years old. They assessed general SIP variables, which were not specific to intimate relationships, at ages 13 and 16, using socially ambiguous scenarios involving peers or adults that end with some type of provocation. The SIP assessment used a combination of formats to display hypothetical vignettes (e.g., videotapes and line drawings accompanied by narration) and used a combination of closed-ended and open-ended formats to measure encoding of social stimuli, hostile attributions, response generation, and response evaluation. Subsequently, participants reported on their own perpetration and receipt of psychological and physical relationship aggression annually between the ages of 18 and 21 years.

Structural models involving encoding and hostile attributions did not show significant mediational effects. Response generation and evaluation, however, were found to be significant mediators of the longitudinal associations between parental relationship aggression and offspring relationship aggression assessed 13–16 years later. The generation of hostile and aggressive responses to ambiguous social scenarios, in particular, had a strong mediational effect in these models. There was no evidence of significant gender differences in the mediational processes. Fite and colleagues' (2008) findings are noteworthy given the long-term prospective nature of their study; the use of distinct informants and methods to measure parental relationship aggression, SIP, and offspring relationship aggression; and the fact that social information processing was assessed outside the context of intimate relationships.

Another interesting demonstration of SIP as an integrative framework for understanding trauma and IPV examined a community-based sample with high overall rates of IPV perpetration (Taft, Schumm, Marshall, Panuzio, & Holtzworth-Munroe, 2008). Retrospective accounts evaluated physical assault between parental figures, as well as direct experience of parent-to-child physical assault, parental rejection, and exposure to traumatic stress in adulthood. Their model examined the influence of childhood maltreatment on adult IPV perpetration, with PTSD symptoms and SIP variables as mediators. The SIP assessment used hypothetical relationship scenarios to measure attribution of negative intent to partners and competency of responses to challenging relationship scenarios. The SIP variables were thus specific to the relationship domain.

Structural equation analysis provided strong support for a mediational model. Exposure to childhood maltreatment and trauma in adulthood predicted PTSD symptoms. PTSD symptoms predicted social information processing problems, which in turn predicted IPV. Thus, the effects of trauma exposure and PTSD symptoms on IPV were accounted for by the tendency to attribute negative intention to relationship partners and the tendency to generate socially incompetent responses to challenging relationship events.

CONCLUSIONS AND FUTURE DIRECTIONS

Exposure to IPV exerts both direct and indirect effects on health. At a direct level, IPV accounts for about 14% of homicides in the United States, and partner assault is a major cause of physical trauma injuries (Catalano et al., 2009). Effects on general health status and chronic illnesses are also apparent, and negative health impacts are found for exposure to psychological abuse as well as physical violence. With respect to mental health effects, the odds of several common conditions are substantially elevated in IPV victims. Most notably, very high rates of PTSD and depression are consistently found among victims of IPV. The available evidence clearly indicates that IPV is a major public health problem.

Although prominent theories of IPV are limited in scope, empirical research has uncovered a wide array of risk predictors across biological, psychological, and sociocultural domains. Thus, the time is ripe for development of a biopsychosocial approach. To inform policy, practice, and research, new conceptual approaches must be coherent and integrative, not simply a catalogue of predictive factors. Social information processing models, which have been very productive in understanding aggression in children, hold out tremendous promise as an integrating framework for understanding IPV in adults. Early research identified consistent, robust, and direct links to IPV for SIP variables involving the attribution of negative intent to relationship partners, generation of socially incompetent responses to relationship events, and positive appraisal of aggressive responses to interpersonal and relationship problems.

Emerging findings provide exciting new perspectives on IPV risk predictors in light of SIP. Several key contributing factors appear to influence IPV risk through their effects on social cognition. At a neurobiological level, problems with executive cognitive functioning and impulsivity in IPV perpetrators have been linked to highly distorted thinking in response to distressing relationship events. From the SIP perspective, these neurocognitive limitations appear to enhance hostile interpretation of negative relationship events and degrade the ability to regulate emotional arousal in light of interpersonal goals. Although frontal deficits are often loosely thought to disinhibit aggressive behavior directly, these findings suggest that there may also be important effects that occur earlier in the chain of social information processing.

Available evidence suggests that acute alcohol intoxication confers situational risk for IPV by intensifying negative aspects of social information processing. Most notably, consistent with alcohol myopia theory (Steele & Josephs, 1990), alcohol appears to bias response selection processes. Alcohol increases the likelihood that aggressive response options, once cognitively activated, will become aggressive behaviors, and it decreases the likelihood that negative thoughts will be edited in this process. Interestingly, for individuals who are referencing generally positive schemas regarding the partner, alcohol may bias response selection in a favorable direction, enhancing the likelihood that positive emotions and intentions are expressed behaviorally.

Relevant research on intergenerational patterns of relationship aggression, trauma exposure, and PTSD provides a robust example of the potential value of SIP as an integrative framework. Longitudinal research on development from childhood to early adulthood indicates that intergenerational patterns of relationship aggression are mediated by hostile biases in response generation and selection (Fite et al., 2008). Similarly, attributions of negative intention and limitations in the generation of socially competent responses to relationship conflict have been shown to mediate the links between retrospective reports of childhood maltreatment, current PTSD symptoms, and recent expression of IPV (Taft et al., 2008). The use of SIP as a core mediational framework has begun to yield important insights into the ways in which important contributing factors directly influence IPV expression.

Although these findings illustrate the potential value of the SIP approach to understanding IPV, there is a great deal of work to be done. First, it is important to note that the current review is very limited and highly selective in nature. There are dozens of relevant studies examining biological, psychological, and social dimensions of IPV, and many proposed mechanisms of influence.

Despite the limited scope of material presented, our review indicates that more can be done to examine how various risk factors effect IPV through SIP mechanisms. For example, although it seems logical that social and cultural factors would contribute risk for IPV by influencing core aspects of SIP, our review did not uncover direct examinations of SIP as a mediator of social and cultural beliefs on IPV expression. In addition, research on IPV has not been substantially influenced by ongoing developments in SIP research, most notably Crick and Dodge's (1994) reformulated SIP model. This expanded approach includes several features that should promote greater conceptual integration, including the regulation of arousal in light of social (relationship) goals, effects of aggressive responses on subsequent encoding and interpretation of relationship cues, and reciprocal referencing of a central database of social knowledge (e.g., relationship schemas and scripts) at each step of the SIP process. This latter innovation, in particular, highlights the importance of accumulated knowledge of both social and intimate relationships, including roles, rules, and expectancies. This innovation also highlights the potential utility of cognitive assessments, such as the Implicit Association Test (IAT), that access dimensions of social cognition that are largely outside conscious awareness.

Surprisingly, thoroughgoing SIP analyses have not figured prominently in IPV prevention and intervention efforts to date. Although many elements of SIP are touched upon by cognitive-behavioral and relationship systems approaches, more systematic application efforts may be warranted. These include strategies to assess SIP problems associated with IPV as part of individual treatment planning, intervention strategies to alter core aspects of SIP, efforts to evaluate changes in SIP as potential mediators of IPV treatment outcome, and efforts to document whether and how treatments for associated problems, such as substance use disorders and PTSD, may alter ongoing risk for IPV through effects on SIP mechanisms.

REFERENCES

Anglin, D., & Sachs, C. (2003). Preventive care in the emergency department: Screening for domestic violence in the emergency department. *Academic Emergency Medicine, 10,* 1118–1127.

Archer, J. (2000). Sex differences in aggression between heterosexual partners: A meta-analytic review. *Psychological Bulletin, 126,* 651–680.

Black, M. C., Basile, K. C., Breiding, M. J., Smith, S. G., Walters, M. L., Merrick, M. T., ... Stevens, M. R. (2011). *The National Intimate Partner and Sexual Violence Survey (NISVS): 2010 summary report.* Altanta, GA: National Center for Injury Prevention and Control, Centers for Disease Control and Prevention.

Campbell, J. C. (2002). Health consequences of intimate partner violence. *Lancet, 359,* 1331–1336.

Campbell, J. C., & Lewandowski, L. A. (1997). Mental and physical health effects of intimate partner violence on women and children. *Psychiatric Clinics of North America, 20,* 1–23.

Campbell, J., & Soeken, K. L. (1999). Women's responses to battering: A test of the model. *Research in Nursing and Health, 22,* 49–58.

Cascardi, M., O'Leary, K. D., & Schlee, K. A. (1999). Co-occurrence and correlates of post-traumatic stress disorder and major depression in physically abused women. *Journal of Family Violence, 14,* 227–249.

Catalano, S., Smith, E., Snyder, H., & Rand, M. (2009). *Female victims of violence.* Washington, DC: US Department of Justice, Bureau of Justice Statistics.

Chemtob, C. M., Novaco, R. W., Hamada, R. S., Gross, D. M., & Smith, G. (1997). Anger regulation deficits in combat-related posttraumatic stress disorder. *Journal of Traumatic Stress, 10,* 17–36.

Clements, K., Holtzworth-Munroe, A., Schweinle, W., & Ickes, W. (2007). Empathic accuracy of intimate partners in violent versus nonviolent relationships. *Personal Relationships, 14,* 369–388.

Cohen, A. C., Rosenbaum, A. R., Kane, R. L., Warnken, W. J., & Benjamin, S. (1999). Neuropsychological correlates of domestic violence. *Violence and Victims, 14,* 397–410.

Cohen, R. A., Virdette, B., Zawacki, T., Paul, R., Sweet, L., & Rosenbaum, A. (2003). Impulsivity and verbal deficits associated with domestic violent. *Journal of the International Neuropsychological Society, 9,* 760–770.

Coker, A. L., Davis, K. E., Arias, I., Desai, S., Sanderson, M., & Brandt, H. (2002). Physical and mental health effects of intimate partner violence for men and women. *American Journal of Preventative Medicine, 23,* 260–268.

Coker, A. L., Weston, R., Creson, D. L., Justice, B., & Blakeney, P. (2005). PTSD symptoms among men and women survivors of intimate partner violence: The role of risk and protective factors. *Violence and Victims, 20,* 625–643.

Cordova, J. V., Jacobson, N. S., Gottman, J. M., Rushe, R., & Cox, G. (1993). Negative reciprocity and communication in couples with a violent husband. *Journal of Abnormal Psychology, 102,* 559–564.

Crick, N. R., & Dodge, K. A. (1994). A review and reformulation of social information-processing mechanisms in children's social adjustment. *Psychological Bulletin, 115,* 74–101.

Crofford, L. J. (2007). Violence, stress, and somatic syndromes. *Trauma, Violence, and Abuse, 8,* 299–313.

Dobash, R. E., & Dobash, R. (1979). *Violence against wives: A case against the patriarchy.* New York, NY: Free Press.

Dodge, K. A., Laird, R., Lochman, J. E., Zelli, A., & Conduct Problems Prevention Research Group. (2002). Multidimensional latent-construct analysis of children's social information processing patterns: Correlations with aggressive behavior problems. *Psychological Assessment, 14,* 60–73.

Dutton, D. G. (2007) *The abusive personality.* New York, NY: Guilford Press.

Dutton, D. G., & White, K. R. (2012). Attachment insecurity and intimate partner violence. *Aggression and Violent Behavior, 17,* 475–481.

Eckhardt, C. I. (2007). Effects of alcohol intoxication on anger experience and expression among partner assaultive men. *Journal of Consulting and Clinical Psychology, 75,* 61–71.

Eckhardt, C. I., Barbour, K. A., & Davison, G. C. (1998). Articulated thoughts of maritally violent and nonviolent men during anger arousal. *Journal of Consulting and Clinical Psychology, 66,* 259–269.

Eckhardt, C. I., & Dye, M. L. (2000). The cognitive characteristics of maritally violent men. *Cognitive Therapy and Research, 24,* 139–158.

Eckhardt, C. I., Murphy, C. M., Whitaker, D. J., Sprunger, J., Dykstra, R., & Woodard, K. (2013). The effectiveness of intervention programs for perpetrators and victims of intimate partner violence: Findings from the Partner Abuse State of Knowledge Project. *Partner Abuse, 4,* 196–231.

Eckhardt, C. I., Samper, R., Suhr, L., & Holtzworth-Munroe, A. (2012). Implicit attitudes toward violence among male perpetrators of intimate partner violence: A preliminary investigation. *Journal of Interpersonal Violence, 27,* 471–491.

Ehrensaft, M. K., Cohen, P., Brown, J., Smalles, E., Chen, H., & Johnson, J. G. (2003). Intergenerational transmission of partner violence: A 20-year prospective study. *Journal of Consulting and Clinical Psychology, 71,* 741–753.

Ehrensaft, M. K., Cohen, P., & Johnson, J. G. (2006). Development of personality disorder symptoms and the risk for partner violence. *Journal of Abnormal Psychology, 115,* 474–483.

Ehrenshaft, M. K., Moffit, T. E., & Caspi, A. (2004). Clinically abusive relationships in an unselected birth cohort: Men's and women's participation and developmental antecedents. *Journal of Abnormal Psychology, 113,* 258–271

Fite, J. E., Bates, J. E., Holtzworth-Munroe, A., Dodge, K. A., Nay, S. Y., & Pettit, G. S. (2008). Social information processing mediates the intergenerational transmission of aggressiveness in romantic relationships. *Journal of Family Psychology, 22,* 367–376.

Foran, H. M., & O'Leary, K. D. (2008). Alcohol and intimate partner violence: A meta-analytic review. *Clinical Psychology Review, 28,* 1222–1234.

Fritz, P. A. T., Slep, A. M. S., & O'Leary, K. D. (2012). Couple-level analysis of the relation between family-of-origin aggression and intimate partner violence. *Psychology of Violence, 2,* 139–153.

Golding, J. M. (1999). Intimate partner violence as a risk factor for mental disorders: A meta-analysis. *Journal of Family Violence, 14,* 99–132.

Greenwald, A. G., McGhee, D. E., & Schwartz, J. K. L. (1998). Measuring individual differences in implicit cognition: The Implicit Association Test. *Journal of Personality and Social Psychology, 74,* 1464–1480.

Hamberger, L. K., & Hastings, J. E. (1991). Personality correlates of men who batter and nonviolent men: Some continuities and discontinuities. *Journal of Family Violence, 6,* 131–147.

Hibbeln, J. R., Umhau, J. C., Linnoila, M., George, D. T., Ragan, P. W., Shoaf, S. E., . . . Salem, N. (1998). A replication study of violent and nonviolent subjects: Cerebrospinal fluid metabolites of serotonin and dopamine are predicted by plasma essential fatty acids. *Biological Psychiatry, 44,* 243–249.

Holtzworth-Munroe, A. (2000). Social information processing skills deficits in maritally violent men: Summary of a research program. In J. P. Vincent & E. N. Jouriles (Eds.), *Domestic violence: Guidelines for research-informed practice* (pp. 13–36). Philadelphia, PA: Jessica Kingsley.

Holtzworth-Munroe, A., & Anglin, K. (1991). The competency of responses given by maritally violent versus nonviolent men to problematic marital situations. *Violence and Victims, 6,* 257–269.

Holtzworth-Munroe, A., & Hutchinson, G. (1993). Attributing negative intent to wife behavior: The attributions of maritally violent versus nonviolent men. *Journal of Abnormal Psychology, 102,* 206–211.

Holtzworth-Munroe, A., & Smutzler, N. (1996). Comparing the emotional reactions and behavioral intentions of violent and nonviolent husbands to aggressive, distressed, and other wife behaviors. *Violence and Victims, 11,* 319–339.

Holtzworth-Munroe, A., & Stuart, G. L. (1994). Typologies of male batterers: Three subtypes and the differences among them. *Psychological Bulletin, 116,* 476–497.

Huss, M. T., & Langinrichsen-Rohling, J. (2006). Assessing the generalization of psychopathy in a clinical sample of domestic violence perpetrators. *Law and Human Behavior, 30,* 571–586.

Ickes, W. (Ed.). (1997). *Empathic accuracy.* New York, NY: Guilford Press.

Ickes, W. (2001). Measuring empathic accuracy. In J. A. Hall & F. J. Bernieri (Eds.), *Interpersonal sensitivity: Theory and measurement* (pp. 219–241). Mahwah, NJ: Erlbaum.

Johnson, M. P., & Leone, J. M. (2005). The differential effects of intimate terrorism and situational couple violence: Findings from the National Violence Against Women Survey. *Journal of Family Issues, 26,* 322–349.

Kessler, R. C., Molnar, B. E., Feurer, I. D., & Applebaum, M. (2001). Patterns and mental health predictors of domestic violence in the United States: Results from the National Comorbidity Survey. *International Journal of Law and Psychiatry, 24,* 487–508.

Kim, H. K., & Capaldi, D. M. (2004). The association of antisocial behavior and depressive symptoms between partners and risk for aggression in romantic relationships. *Journal of Family Psychology, 18,* 82–96.

Krueger, R. F., & South, S. C. (2009). Externalizing disorders: Cluster 5 of the proposed metastructure for DSM-V and ICD-11. *Psychological Medicine, 39,* 2061–2070.

Leonard, K. E., & Roberts, L. J. (1998). The effects of alcohol on the marital interactions of aggressive and nonaggressive husbands and their wives. *Journal of Abnormal Psychology, 107,* 602–615.

Leserman, J., & Drossman, D. A. (2007). Relationship of abuse history to functional gastrointestinal disorders and symptoms. *Trauma, Violence, and Abuse, 8,* 331–343.

Letellier, P. (1994). Gay and bisexual domestic violence victimization: Challenges to feminist theory and responses to violence. *Violence and Victims, 9,* 95–106.

Margolin, G., John, R. S., & Gleberman, L. (1988). Affective responses to conflictual discussions in violent and nonviolent couples. *Journal of Consulting and Clinical Psychology, 56,* 24–33.

Marshall, A. T., Panuzio, J., & Taft, C. T. (2005). Intimate partner violence among military veterans and active duty servicemen. *Clinical Psychology Review, 25,* 862–876.

McFall, R. M. (1982). A review and reformulation of the concept of social skills. *Behavioral Assessment, 4,* 1–33.

Messinger, P. (2011). Invisible victims: Same-sex IPV in the National Violence Against Women Survey. *Journal of Interpersonal Violence, 26,* 2228–2243.

Mitchell, C., & Anglin, D. (Eds.) (2009). *Intimate partner violence: A health-based perspective.* New York, NY: Oxford University Press.

Moore, T. M., Elkins, S. R., McNulty, J. K., Kivisto, A. J., & Handsel, V. A. (2011). Alcohol use and intimate partner violence perpetration among college students: Assessing the temporal association using electronic diary technology. *Psychology of Violence, 1,* 315–328.

Murray, C. E., Mobley, A. K., Buford, A. P., & Seaman-DeJohn, M. M. (2007). Same-sex intimate partner violence: Dynamics, social context, and counseling implications. *Journal of LGBT Issues in Counseling, 1,* 7–30.

Murphy, C. M., Meyer, S. L., & O'Leary, K. D. (1993). Family of origin violence and MCMI-II psychopathology among partner assaultive men. *Violence and Victims, 8,* 165–176.

Murphy, C. M., & O'Farrell, T. J. (1996). Marital violence among alcoholics. *Current Directions in Psychological Science, 5,* 183–186.

Murphy, C. M., & O'Farrell, T. J. (1997). Couple communication patterns of maritally aggressive and nonaggressive male alcoholics. *Journal of Studies on Alcohol, 58,* 83–90.

Murphy, C. M., O'Farrell, T. J., Fals-Stewart, W., & Feehan, M. (2001). Correlates of intimate partner violence among male alcoholic patients. *Journal of Consulting and Clinical Psychology, 69,* 528 540.

Murphy, C. M., Winters, J., O'Farrell, T. J., Fals-Stewart, W., & Murphy, M. (2005). Alcohol consumption and intimate partner violence by alcoholic men: Comparing violent and non-violent conflicts. *Psychology of Addictive Behaviors, 19,* 35–42.

National Center for Injury Prevention and Control. (2003). *Costs of intimate partner violence against women in the United States.* Atlanta, GA: Centers for Disease Control and Prevention.

Neidig, P. H., & Friedman, D. H. (1984). *Spouse abuse: A treatment program for couples.* Champaign, IL: Research Press.

Nixon, R. D., Resick, P. A., & Nishith, P. (2004). An exploration of comorbid depression among female victims of intimate partner violence with posttraumatic stress disorder. *Journal of Affective Disorders, 82,* 315–320.

Norwood, A., & Murphy, C. (2012). What forms of abuse correlate with PTSD symptoms in partners of men being treated for intimate partner violence? *Psychological Trauma: Theory, Research, Practice, and Policy, 6,* 596–604.

Okuda, M., Olfson, M., Hasin, D., Grant, B. F., Lin, K., & Blanco, C. (2011). Mental health of victims of intimate partner violence: Results from a national epidemiologic survey. *Psychiatric Services, 62,* 959–962.

Pence, E., & Paymar, M. (1993). *Education groups for men who batter: The Duluth Model.* New York, NY: Springer.

Persampiere, J., Poole, G. M, & Murphy, C. M. (in press). Neuropsychological correlates of anger, hostility, and relationship-relevant distortions in thinking among partner violent men. *Journal of Family Violence*

Riggs, D. A., & Caulfield, M. B. (1997). Expected consequences of male violence against their female dating partners. *Journal of Interpersonal Violence, 12,* 229–240.

Rosenbaum, A., Abend, S. S., Gearan, P. J., & Fletcher, K. E. (1997). Serotonergic functioning in partner violent men. In A. Raine, P. A. Brennan, D. P. Farrington, & S. A. Mednick (Eds.), *Biosocial bases of violence* (pp. 329–332). New York, NY: Plenum Press.

Rosenbaum, A., Geffner, R., & Benjamin, M. (1997). A biopsychosocial model for understanding relationship aggression. *Journal of Aggression, Maltreatment, and Trauma, 1,* 57–79.

Rosenbaum, A., Hoge, S., Adelman, S., Warnken, W., Fletcher, K., & Kane, R. (1994). Head injury in partner abusive men. *Journal of Consulting and Clinical Psychology, 62,* 1187–1193.

Saltzman, L. E. Fanslow, J. L., McMahaon, P. M., & Shelley, G. A. (1999). *Intimate partner violence surveillance: Uniform definitions and recommended data elements.* Atlanta, GA: Centers for Disease Control and Prevention.

Sillars, A., Leonard, K. E., Roberts, L. J., & Dun, T. (2002). Cognition and communication during marital conflict: How alcohol affects subjective coding of interaction in aggressive and nonaggressive couples. In P. Noller & J. A. Feeney (Eds.), *Understanding marriage: Developments in the study of couple interaction* (pp. 85–112). New York, NY: Cambridge University Press.

Steele, C. M., & Josephs, R. A. (1990). Alcohol myopia: Its prized and dangerous effects. *American Psychologist, 45,* 921–933.

Stein, M. B., & Kennedy, C. (2001). Major depressive and posttraumatic stress disorder comorbidity in female victims of intimate partner violence. *Journal of Affective Disorders, 66,* 133–138.

Stets, J. E., & Straus, M. A. (1990). Gender differences in reporting marital violence and its medical and social consequences. In M. A. Straus & R. J. Gelles (Eds.), *Physical violence in American families* (pp. 151–165). New Brunswick, NJ: Transaction.

Straight, E. S., Harper, F. W. K., & Arias, I. (2003). The impact of partner psychological abuse on health behaviors and health status in college women. *Journal of Interpersonal Violence, 18,* 1035–1054.

Stith, S. M., McCollum, E. E., Amanor-Boadu, Y., & Smith, D. (2012). Systemic perspectives on intimate partner violence treatment. *Journal of Marital and Family Therapy, 38,* 220–240.

Straus, M. A. (2011). Gender symmetry and mutuality in perpetration of clinical-level partner violence: Empirical evidence and implications for prevention and treatment. *Aggression and Violent Behavior, 16,* 279–288.

Street, A. E., & Arias, I. (2001). Psychological abuse and posttraumatic stress disorder in battered women: Examining the roles of shame and guilt. *Violence and Victims, 16,* 65–78.

Taft, C. T., Murphy, C. M., King, L. A., DeDeyn, J. M., & Musser, P. H. (2005). Posttraumatic stress disorder symptomatology among partners of men in treatment for relationship abuse. *Journal of Abnormal Psychology, 114,* 259–268.

Taft, C. T., Schumm, J. A., Marshall, A. D., Panuzio, J., & Holtzworth-Munroe, A. (2008). Family-of-origin maltreatment, posttraumatic stress disorder symptoms, social information processing deficits, and relationship abuse perpetration. *Journal of Abnormal Psychology, 117,* 637–646.

Taft, C., Vogt, D. S., Mechanic, M. B., & Resick, P. A. (2007). Posttraumatic stress disorder and physical health symptoms among women seeking help for relationship aggression. *Journal of Family Psychology, 21,* 354–362.

Taft, C. T., Watkins, L. E., Stafford, J., Street, A. E., & Monson, C. M. (2011). Posttraumatic stress disorder and intimate relationship problems: A meta-analysis. *Journal of Consulting and Clinical Psychology, 79,* 22–33.

Theobald, D., & Farrington, D. (2012). Child and adolescent predictors of male intimate partner violence. *Journal of Child Psychology and Psychiatry, 53,* 1242–1249.

Zillman, D. (1983). Arousal and aggression. In R. G. Geen & E. I. Donnerstein (Eds.), *Aggression: Theoretical and empirical reviews* (Vol. 1, pp. 75–101). New York, NY: Academic Press.

Zlotnick, C., Johnson, D. M., & Kohn, R. (2006). Intimate partner violence and long-term psychosocial functioning in a national sample of American women. *Journal of Interpersonal Violence, 21,* 262–275.

CHAPTER 8

Interparental Conflict and Children's Mental Health

Emerging Directions in Emotional Security Theory

E. MARK CUMMINGS, KALSEA J. KOSS, AND
REBECCA Y. M. CHEUNG

Conflict is inevitable in personal relationships and carries important implications for mental and physical health. Conflict present in the marital relationship not only impacts members of the marital union but also plays an important role for children in the family. The way in which parents manage conflict in the marital relationship is critically pertinent for children's mental health and well-being (Cummings, 1998). Destructive conflict, conflict that is characterized by anger, aggression, and hostility in the marital relationship, has negative implications for the family. Children exposed to destructive marital conflict are at risk for developing a host of negative outcomes, including internalizing and externalizing behaviors, disrupted sleep patterns, lower social competence, problematic peer relationships, and lower school performance (e.g., Cummings, Goeke-Morey, & Papp, 2004; Cummings, Schermerhorn, Davies, Goeke-Morey, & Cummings, 2006; El-Sheikh, Buckhalt, Keller, Cummings, & Acebo, 2007; Stocker, &Youngblade, 1999). Murphy and colleagues (Chapter 7, this volume) call attention to the widespread negative effects of intimate partner violence on biological and psychosocial functioning. Conflict that is constructive in nature, characterized by the use of problem-solving techniques, compromise, and resolution, is linked with better outcomes for children, including increased prosocial behavior and decreased aggression (e.g., Cummings, Goeke-Morey, & Papp, 2004; Goeke-Morey, Cummings, Harold, & Shelton, 2003; Goeke-Morey, Cummings, & Papp, 2007; McCoy, Cummings, & Davies, 2009; for a review, see Cummings & Davies, 2010).

Given the long-established relations between marital conflict and child adjust-ment (e.g., Emery, 1982; Grych & Fincham, 1990), process-oriented investigations of the causal mechanisms accounting for this relationship have been a focus for research for the past two decades (Cummings & Davies, 1994a; Fincham, 1994), including the development of empirically supported theoretical models (Davies & Cummings, 1994; Grych & Fincham, 1990). In this regard, emotional security theory (EST; Davies & Cummings, 1994) has emerged as a promising theoretical model for understanding associations between marital conflict and children's health and well-being. EST has been the subject of increasing investigation as a conceptual model for understanding the impact of interparental conflict on children (Cummings & Davies, 2010) and to account for the impact of broader contexts of discord and violence, including community violence, on children (Cummings et al., 2011).

The focus of the present chapter is on a series of recent studies that further extends the investigation of EST as a theoretical model. We will consider both empirical support for EST as an explanatory mechanism and also evidence that physiological as well as psychological processes merit inclusion in the conceptual-ization and assessment of emotional security in the context of family stress. After an introduction to the key tenets of EST, we will examine a series of studies reflecting recent advances in the study of children's health and well-being from this theoreti-cal perspective, including (a) longitudinal research supporting emotional insecu-rity as an explanatory mechanisms for children's adjustment between childhood and adolescence, (b) studies that advance the conceptualization of EST as a mul-tidimensional regulatory system by examining relations between physiological and psychological indicators of EST (Cummings & Davies, 1996), (c) a recent prospec-tive study of EST as a mediating process in relations between parental depressive symptoms and child adjustment, and (d) findings supporting emotional insecurity as a mediating process in the context of a social ecological investigation of relations between political and sectarian community violence and children's adjustment.

EMOTIONAL SECURITY THEORY AS A THEORETICAL FRAMEWORK

EST provides a theoretical framework to understand and guide the study of child development in contexts of family risk, including marital conflict. Using a process-oriented approach that relies on careful assessment of specific regulatory processes, EST is conceptualized from a developmental psychopathology framework to eluci-date the processes (the "why" and "how") and conditions (for "whom" and "when") underlying the relations between marital conflict and child adjustment and malad-justment (Davies & Cummings, 2006). EST posits that children have a set goal to feel safe and secure within the family. Children's goal of security results in the moti-vation to preserve and promote their sense of security when family events threaten this sense of security. In other words, children's views and expectations about the family settings, including the context of the marital relationship, are related to their sense of security, safety, and protection, which are among the most salient in the hierarchy of human goals (Bowlby, 1973; Waters & Cummings, 2000).

With origins in attachment theory (Bowlby, 1969, 1973), EST extends notions of emotional security to reflect a broader family-wide perspective, postulating that children's emotional security is an explanatory mechanism in the relations between marital conflict and child adjustment. Moving beyond the importance of the parent–child dyad, EST posits that children also derive their sense of security from other important family relationships. In particular, the marital dyad carries important implications for the stability and safety of the family unit; for example, problems in the marital relationship have the possibility of undermining the quality of parenting or over time contributing to the dissolution of the family, making the marital relationship a particularly salient family relationship for children's security (see also Chapter 6, this volume).

Notably, a substantial body of theory and research has accumulated to support that children's emotional security about parent–child and marital/family relationships matters to their well-being, emotional and social functioning, and adjustment in the context of developmental processes from infancy through adolescence (Cummings & Davies, 2010). EST has recently been extended to contribute to understanding the effects of community conflict and violence on children's well-being and adjustment (Cummings et al., 2009). According to EST, children's emotional security about community is related to their sense of protection, safety, and security, with implications for their optimal socioemotional regulation.

A useful analogy is to think about emotional security as a bridge between the child and the world. When family and community relationships are functioning well, they serve as a secure base, supporting the child's exploration and relationships with others. When destructive family and community relations erode the bridge, children may become hesitant to move forward, lack confidence, or may move forward in an uncertain way, unable to find appropriate footing within themselves or in interaction with others.

Although the child evaluates interpersonal contexts in relation to multiple goals, EST postulates that safety and security are among the most salient in the hierarchy of human goals throughout development, from infancy through adolescence, and across the life span (Waters & Cummings, 2000). Thus, although research has traditionally focused on parent–child emotional security within the tradition of attachment theory (Cassidy & Shaver, 2008), there is also a long-standing literature that has posited that emotional security is a family-wide construct (e.g., Bowlby, 1949). Moreover, the purview of EST has been extended to children's sense of security about other environmental contexts (Cummings, Goeke-Morey, Schermerhorn, Merrilees, & Cairns, 2009), with recent empirical research demonstrating that emotional security about community also mediates child adjustment (Cummings et al., 2011).

With regard to emotional security about family as a mechanism affecting child well-being and adjustment, distressing family events motivate children to regain their sense of security. For example, in the context of destructive conflict between parents, children may experience a prolonged defense system through which their actions and reactions function to safeguard their felt security. EST posits that threats to children's security are manifested in various responses, which are thought to reflect their appraisals of emotional insecurity and may also serve to motivate additional behavioral actions necessary to maintain or restore security. Insecurity may manifest through a variety of emotional responses, including anger, fear, and sadness. Additionally, insecurity may be evident by children's efforts to mediate their parents' conflicts as well as in their cognitions about the safety and security of the family in the short and long term.

The emotional security system is involved in the appraisal, organization, and the motivation of responses to violations of children's "set goals" for emotional security (Bowlby, 1969; Davies & Cummings, 1994). In a further extension beyond traditional attachment theory conceptualizations, social defense is also posited as a salient element of the evaluation of emotional security, relevant to children's evaluation of their own well-being and that of their family (Davies & Sturge-Apple, 2007; Davies & Woitach, 2008). Regulatory strategies for regaining security include emotional, behavioral, and cognitive responses (e.g., Davies, Forman, Rasi, & Stevens, 2002; Harold, Shelton, Goeke-Morey, & Cummings, 2004). Children's behavioral response strategies, driven by their insecurity, may also serve to regulate their exposure to marital conflict. For example, children's avoidance or involvement in conflict may serve to alleviate the threat of conflict. Past experiences with conflict may also shape children's expectations about the implications of conflict on the family. Internal representations of the family may impact how they interpret subsequent conflicts' threatening nature. Children consistently exposed to destructive conflict may perceive subsequent conflict as more threatening to their security given their past experiences with conflict. Current research and theory further posit that neurobiological and attentional responses may also serve as regulatory processes to promote and restore security (Davies, Sturge-Apple, Cicchetti, & Cummings, 2007, 2008; Davies, Woitach, Winter, & Cummings, 2008; Sturge-Apple, Davies, Cicchetti & Cummings, 2009; see Cummings & Davies, 1996).

A strong point of EST is that the manifestation of insecurity is hypothesized to be measurable in terms of multiple regulatory processes which are observable and/or amenable to objective assessment across multiple domains of functioning, including emotional, behavioral, cognitive, and physiological responses. As we have indicated, multiple dimensions of measurable responses to family stress can serve as indicators of children's emotional security. Moreover, emotional security is posited as a higher order organizational construct, with multiple dimensions of responding expected to provide the most valuable and reliable indices of emotional security (Davies & Cummings, 2006). Accordingly, a goal of assessment of emotional security as a mediating or moderating process is to assess emotional security as a latent construct, based on children's responding across two or more domains (e.g., emotional, behavioral, cognitive).

A LONG-TERM TEST OF EMOTIONAL SECURITY AS A
MEDIATOR OF CHILDREN'S MENTAL HEALTH

The mediating role of emotional security has now been demonstrated in multiple empirical studies. Over time, children are hypothesized to be at risk for developing poorer mental and physical outcomes due to a lack security about the family. Specifically, exposure to destructive conflict has been associated with child maladjustment in a variety of domains with emotional security serving as an explanatory mechanism in these relations. Consistent with this hypothesis, children's insecurity has been found to serve as an explanatory mechanism through which marital discord influences their outcomes. In a cross-sectional study, Davies and Cummings (1998) found that emotional insecurity mediated the association between marital conflict and children's internalizing and externalizing symptoms (see also El-Shiekh, Cummings, Kouros, Elmore-Staton, & Buckhalt, 2008; El-Sheikh et al., 2007). Further supporting the cogency of emotional security as a mediating variable, this study was followed by several short-term longitudinal studies providing support for emotional security as a mediator between destructive marital conflict and child adjustment (e.g., Harold et al., 2004; Schacht, Cummings, & Davies, 2009). Similarly, Cummings, Schermerhorn, Davies, Goeke-Morey, and Cummings (2006) found in two independent short-term prospective studies that destructive conflict predicted maladjustment among children and adolescents through a greater sense of emotional insecurity. In another short-term prospective study that explored the longitudinal impact of constructive versus destructive interparental conflict on children's adjustment, McCoy, Cummings, and Davies (2009) reported that constructive conflict behavior, as indicated by self-report and observational measures of support, including verbal and physical affection, and problem-solving behavior, was associated with children's subsequently greater level of helping behavior through emotional security. Conversely, destructive conflict behavior, as indicated by various measures of verbal aggression, nonverbal anger, stonewalling, and withdrawal, was related to children's subsequently lower levels of helping behavior through decreased emotional security. This line of research has thus demonstrated both concurrently and longitudinally that children's felt security and interpretations of marital conflict have a striking impact on their social and psychological outcomes.

However, until recently, evaluation of the pertinence of EST for understanding child adjustment was limited to short-term longitudinal studies. Thus, questions remained about whether emotional security was pertinent to predicting child adjustment over extended periods of time or across major periods of and transitions in development. That is, there was no evidence concerning whether emotional security had implications for children's long-term health and well-being, despite the fact that both attachment theory and EST supported predictions of relatively long-lasting implications of early experiences for children's well-being and adjustment (e.g., Waters, Weinfield, & Hamilton, 2000). Specifically, according to EST, children's response processes, including their representations of family relationships and their emotional and physiological response processes based on experiences with interparental conflict, were expected to be relatively long-lasting (Cummings & Davies, 2010). Addressing this gap, in a study spanning across childhood into adolescence, Cummings, George, McCoy, and Davies (2012) examined relations between interparental conflict in kindergarten, children's emotional insecurity in the early school years, and subsequent adolescent internalizing and externalizing problems. This research was groundbreaking in examining the long-term effects of early marital conflict and emotional insecurity on children's long-term adjustment. This study was based on a representative community sample, multimethod and multireporter assessments, and structural equation modeling tests of the hypothesized model that included stringent autoregressive controls for prior level of functioning of both mediating (i.e., emotional insecurity) and outcome variables (i.e., internalizing problems, externalizing problems, and adjustment). The findings provided support for emotional insecurity in early childhood as an explanatory mechanism for long-term implications of marital conflict for child adjustment. In particular, kindergarten children's exposure to marital conflict and subsequent insecurity predicted increased levels of internalizing and externalizing problems in adolescence.

The findings from this study indicate that the influence of emotional security is robust and long lasting, and the significance of early experiential histories with interparental conflict to children's later health and well-being was indicated. Notably, consistent with the notion of emotional security as an organizational construct based on multiple, measurable dimensions of regulatory functioning, emotional security was assessed as a robust latent construct based on multiple theoretically driven components (i.e., emotional reactivity, behavioral dysregulation, avoidance, and involvement). One implication is that prior psychological organizations and experiences with interparental conflict have influence over long periods of development. A complementary hypothesis is that early experiences with family adversity prime children to be reactive to interparental conflict throughout childhood and adolescence. These results are also suggestive of the possibility of long-term cascade effects reflecting family systems processes that may further solidify these trajectories (Masten & Cicchetti, 2010). The many transactions and interactions over time among interparental conflict, child emotional insecurity in the context of marital conflict, and child adjustment problems may serve both to solidify these interrelations and also result in more widespread difficulties (Kouros, Cummings, & Davies, 2010). Thus, many avenues toward further understanding the bases for the long-term effects of interparental conflict on children's mental health in the context of EST are suggested.

ADVANCES IN THE CONCEPTUALIZATION OF EMOTIONAL SECURITY AS A REGULATORY CONSTRUCT

In addition to behavioral, affective, and cognitive responses to conflict exposure, physiological responses may also reflect regulatory processes pertinent to assessments of emotional insecurity. From an evolutionary perspective, there are advantages to appropriate physiological responses to family stresses over time, in concert with the organization and motivation of psychological responses (Davies, Sturge-Apple, & Cicchetti, 2011). Thus, physiological responses may be relevant to an organizational perspective on emotional insecurity that reflects a more complete understanding of emotional security as a response to stressful events, including distressing family environments (Cummings & Davies, 1996). These notions are consistent with broader notions regarding associations between relationship disruptions and psychophysiological functioning (see Chapter 4, this volume).

At a biological level, acute stress responses ready the body to respond with the necessary resources to cope with threatening or distressing events. Both physical and psychological threats can trigger the stress response system. Given the threatening nature of marital conflict and violence and the role of the emotional security system in children's social defense (Davies & Sturge-Apple, 2007), these events likely cause a mounting biological response in children. Multiple biological systems are sensitive to environmental influences and may be activated in the context of conflict, including the parasympathetic nervous system, the sympathetic nervous system, and the adrenocortical axis (e.g., Davies, Sturge-Apple, Cicchetti, & Cummings, 2007; El-Sheikh, 2005; El-Sheikh et al., 2009). More specifically, as a second wave of autonomic response to stress, neuroendocrine functioning is activated in times of stress. The hypothalamic-pituitary-adrenal axis (HPA) is responsible for assembling and activating the resources necessary to cope with stress (see Chapter 3, this volume). The HPA axis response consists of a cascade of events resulting in the release of its end product hormone, cortisol. An efficient, adaptive HPA response includes effective activation, regulation, and termination of this system. Long-term activation of these responses can lead to dysregulation of the stress response system; dysregulation in the stress response system has been found in both subsequent reactivity and alterations in steady resting states.

Two forms of altered HPA responses have been related to children's exposure to marital conflict. A sensitization hypothesis posits an amplified HPA response to witnessing conflict. This type of pattern suggests elevated cortisol levels as well as heightened reactivity and a lengthier return to prestressor hormone levels. On the other hand, an attenuation hypothesis posits that over time stress serves to decrease the sensitivity of the HPA response exhibiting lower levels and blunted, flattened reactivity patterns. Both forms of altered cortisol responses have been linked with children's exposure to marital conflict and violence. For example, research finds elevated cortisol levels have been associated with poor marital functioning and violence (e.g., Davies, Sturge-Apple, Cicchetti, Manning, & Zale, 2009; Pendry & Adam, 2007; Saltzman, Holden, & Holahan, 2005), and elevated levels of temperamental inhibition and vigilance (Davies et al., 2011). Similarly, lower cortisol levels have also been related to destructive marital conflict (e.g., Davies, Sturge-Apple, Cicchetti, & Cummings, 2007; Sturge-Apple, Davies, Cicchetti, & Manning, 2012) and aggressive temperamental characteristics (Davies et al., 2011).

Physiological responses to family risk are an important dimension of regulation and these responses may have important implications for children's emotional security (Cummings & Davies, 1996). Moreover, recent research on family stress and children's cortisol stress reactivity suggests that children's cortisol reactivity demonstrates specificity, such that relations with family stress are specific to the construct (e.g., interparental conflict) the task is eliciting and not broad dimensions of family functioning. This suggests that biological responses to conflict may be an additional indicator of the manifestation of emotional insecurity (Sturge-Apple, Davies, Cicchetti, & Manning, 2012). Recent work has begun to explore the ways in which children's neuroendocrine responses in the context of marital conflict relate to other known indicators of children's emotional security. For example, Davies, Sturge-Apple, Cicchetti, and Cummings (2008) found that children's behavioral distress to witnessing conflict was related to higher cortisol activity. Relatedly, in toddlers, angry emotional reactivity has been found to mediate links between interparental aggression and neuroendocrine and parasympathetic nervous system functioning (Davies, Sturge-Apple, Cicchetti, Manning, & Zale, 2009). Children's cortisol reactivity has also been found to moderate the relations between emotional reactivity and behavioral regulation in the context of interparental conflict, reflecting the interactive nature of multiple domains of children's emotional insecurity (Koss et al., 2011). Moreover, feeling threatened by the presence of conflict, children displaying decreasing cortisol levels after exposure to marital conflict (indicative of recovery) utilized more active forms of behavioral involvement to manage their exposure to discord. Children unable to downregulate their adrenocortical reactivity after the cessation of marital conflict were more likely to display vigilant behavioral responses regardless of feelings of fear. Taken together, these results suggest that children's emotional and physiological responses to conflict may impact their ability to enact effective behavioral regulation to manage their exposure to conflict.

Recent work suggests pathways of risk through both forms of dysregulation of reactivity patterns may be associated with marital conflict and children's emotional security (Davies, Sturge-Apple, & Cicchetti, 2011; Koss et al., 2012). In a study of first-grade children witnessing a simulated phone anger and resolution task, children's cortisol responses revealed distinct patterns of responses (Koss et al., 2012). Two subsets of children displayed altered cortisol patterns. Indicative of an attenuation hypothesis, one group of children exhibited low, unchanging cortisol levels in response to witnessing the marital dispute and resolution. Parents of these children displayed higher rates of observable destructive marital conflict in the laboratory setting, suggesting these children may be exposed to more destructive conflict in everyday life which may result in the emergence of an altered form of reactivity to family stress. A second group of children, indicative of a sensitization hypothesis, exhibited rising cortisol levels in response to witnessing the phone anger and phone resolution task. These children reported the highest levels of perceived threat and child-related disagreement exposure suggesting that these children find marital conflict to be a particularly salient and stressful event. The children also had higher rates of child maladjustment and emotional insecurity, indexed by increased emotional reactivity, behavioral dysregulation, and involvement in marital conflict. This recent study provides support for associations between children's emotional security in response to conflict and altered physiological response patterns, supporting the potential for these responses to be included in higher order multidimensional assessments of emotional security as an additional regulatory process.

Moving beyond investigating single systems of physiological responsivity in isolation, children's physiological response may be even better understood from a multisystem perspective (e.g., Bauer, Quas, & Boyce, 2002) that investigates the interactive nature of multiple systems simultaneously. This approach may shed light on the role of physiological responses in children's ability to maintain and restore their sense of security in the face of distressing events. The autonomic nervous system (ANS) is also activated in response to stressful events. Salivary alpha amylase is an enzyme secreted in saliva that has been linked to ANS activity. Both the ANS and HPA axis respond to stress; however, less is known about how associations or disassociations in the activation of these systems at the same time relate to an adaptive stress response in children.

Along these lines, our recent work has begun to explore the interactive nature of the ANS in conjunction with children's neuroendocrine responses to witnessing marital conflict (Koss et al., 2012). Second-grade children's cortisol (e.g., neuroendocrine responses) and salivary alpha amylase (e.g., autonomic nervous system responses) were assessed in response to viewing videotaped marital conflict vignettes. In this study, asymmetry among cortisol and salivary alpha amylase responses was linked with children's emotional security and mental health. Moreover, responses were moderated by the level of conflict exposure a child experienced in the home in the prediction of behavioral and emotional indices of children's emotional security. In particular, low cortisol and high alpha amylase levels were associated with increased internalizing problems and emotional insecurity (e.g., emotional reactivity, behavioral dysregulation, and involvement). These results thus supported a complex relation among multiple regulation systems associated with emotional security, providing further support for the notion that children's strategies for managing family stress reflect higher order organizations of systems in the response to conflict exposure.

In summary, children's physiological responding was supported by this series of studies as an additional dimension of the regulatory processes children utilize to restore and maintain their sense of security when faced with the threatening context of destructive interparental conflict. Furthermore, a suggestion of these results is that the strategies children use to regulate and maintain security may emerge from their history of exposure to marital conflict and aggression in the family, highlighting the role of individual differences in responses.

EMOTIONAL SECURITY THEORY IN BROADER FAMILY CONTEXT: PARENTAL DEPRESSIVE SYMPTOMS AND CHILD ADJUSTMENT

EST posits that children have a goal of security both in the family as a whole as well as in different relationships within the family (Cummings & Davies, 1996). Research investigating the explanatory role of emotional security in children's development has typically focused on the role of the marital relationship or the parent–child relationship. While the parent–child and marital relationships may be particularly salient contexts for children's derived sense of security, it is likely that other family relationships and processes have implications for children's security and warrant further investigation. The construct of emotional security, and associated regulatory systems for responding to threats to security, are inherently applicable to other family processes and processes beyond the family (Waters & Cummings, 2000), for example, threats of sectarian community violence to children's security about the community (Cummings et al., 2011). Family processes may impact children's security in multiple ways, including direct effects of exposure to family stressors or indirect effects by altering other family processes (e.g., parenting, Cummings & Davies, 2010). For example, family risk, such as parental depression or parental alcohol use, may function similar to the role of marital conflict and may serve to directly affect children's assessments of their sense of security by exposure to behaviors indicative of these problems, or indirectly by changing parenting or other family processes (e.g., Keller, Cummings, Davies, & Mitchell, 2008). Research on depression in adults highlights the interrelations between depression and marital conflict (Chapter 6, this volume). These additional family risk factors may thus undermine children's sense of security by creating family contexts that threaten the stability of the family unit.

In addition to family processes that may serve to directly affect children's sense of security, family processes may also serve to moderate the relationship between marital conflict and children's security and subsequent adjustment. Children's adjustment and health outcomes develop in the context of a multitude of risk and protective factors that interact with one another. Research on cumulative risk shows that the presence of multiple risk factors is detrimental to children's development (e.g., Appleyard, Egeland, van Dulmen, & Sroufe, 2005). The presence of additional family risk factors may exacerbate the effects of marital conflict on children's security by creating a family context in which marital conflict is particularly threatening. Conflict occurring in an already compromised family system may carry additional implications for children's security.

On the other hand, protective family processes may serve to promote adaptive functioning and buffer against negative outcomes despite the presence of risk. Conflict occurring in the context of family protective factors, such as a cohesive, warm family, may carry fewer implications for children's security. Children in these family contexts may feel secure within the family unit and conflict may not be seen as a threat to the stability of the family unit. Understanding how family risk and protective factors interact may help to shed light on the processes that prevent some children from the detrimental effects of destructive conflict. The broader family context has been found to alter the effects of conflict on children's sense of security. For example, parental alcohol use and marital aggression has been shown to interactively impact children's responses to marital conflict (Keller, Gilbert, Koss, Cummings, & Davies, 2011).

One particularly salient family context with implications for children's sense of security is parental depression. Children of depressed parents are two to five times more likely to develop various disorders than children of nondepressed parents (e.g., Beardslee, Bemporad, Keller, & Klerman, 1983; Goodman, 2007). Of note, both fathers' and mothers' depressive symptoms may affect child adjustment and maladjustment (e.g., Downey & Coyne, 1990; Du Rocher Schudlich & Cummings, 2003, 2007; Ramchandani et al., 2008; Shelton & Harold, 2008). However, there is a paucity of research that incorporates *both* parents in our research on relations between family processes and children's mental health and well-being, leaving many questions about the relative effects of paternal depressive symptoms (Cummings, Merrilees, & George, 2010).

Amid other mechanisms posited to link parental depressive symptoms and child maladjustment (e.g., Lewis, Rice, Harold, Collishaw, & Thapar, 2011; Rutter, 2007), family-wide research plays a major role in understanding the heterogeneity of pathways between parental dysphoria and child development (Cummings, Davies, & Campbell, 2000). Since the home setting brings about a shared environment, processes occurring in the family might be particularly salient in affecting parental and children's well-being. Of all the family correlates linked to spousal depression, marital discord has emerged as one of the major variables (for a review, see Chapter 6, this volume). As to child adjustment, both parental depressive symptoms and marital conflict have emerged as predictors (e.g., Downey & Coyne, 1990; Du Rocher Schudlich & Cummings, 2003; Fendrich, Warner, & Weissman, 1990).

To further account for why marital conflict affects child adjustment in relation to parental depressive symptoms, recent studies have begun to use an EST framework. In general, findings indicate that both parental depressive symptomatology and destructive marital conflict threaten children's goals of security (e.g., Cummings, Cheung, & Davies, 2013; Du Rocher Schudlich & Cummings, 2007; Kouros, Merrilees, & Cummings, 2008). Further tests of mediating and moderating effects of parental depression and children's insecurity have delineated specific processes associated with adjustment outcomes. For example, Kouros, Merrilees, and Cummings (2008) found that parental depressive symptomatology interacted with marital conflict, such that marital conflict predicted emotion insecurity more strongly in children whose fathers reported high levels of depression, compared to those whose fathers reported lower levels of depression. In testing alternative hypotheses, findings also supported a mediating effect of emotional insecurity between maternal depressive symptoms and children's externalizing problems, when paternal depressive symptoms were controlled. This study implicated the effects of both maternal and paternal psychopathology on the developing child, and also unfolded the intricate moderating and mediating roles of parental depressive symptoms and emotional insecurity on children's well-being.

In exploring the question of which conflict styles are most saliently affected by parental depressive symptoms in predicting emotional insecurity, Du Rocher Schudlich and Cummings (2007) examined three conflict tactics (i.e., depressive, destructive, and constructive) and found that both maternal and paternal depressive symptoms predicted greater levels of depressive conflict tactics (e.g., negative affect and withdrawal) and lower levels of constructive conflict tactics (e.g., affection and use of problem-solving techniques). Also, paternal depressive symptoms predicted greater levels of destructive marital conflict tactics (e.g., hostility and pursuit). Consistent with previous research, children's emotional insecurity mediated relations between depressive marital conflict tactics and child maladjustment. In addition to advancing our understanding of relations between parental dysphoria and marital conflict (e.g., Kouros & Cummings, 2011), this research has demonstrated the differential impact of mothers' and fathers' symptomatology on conflict styles. Emotional insecurity is supported in this research as bridging relations among parental and family processes and child adjustment.

To further examine the differential impact of parental depression on children's emotional insecurity, we have begun to explore the possible explanatory role of emotional expressiveness. Previous research has indicated that compared to nondepressed parents, depressed parents express more negative affect, are more critical, less warm, and less supportive (Cummings & Davies, 1994b; Downey & Coyne, 1990; Oyserman, Mowbray, Meares, & Firminger, 2000). Thus, parental depression might undermine children's felt security and well-being by setting in motion dysfunctional self and familial emotional expressions. Negative expressivity might, in turn, account for the effects of dysphoria on family processes and, subsequently, child development.

In our recent study (Cummings, Cheung, & Davies, 2013), we longitudinally examined the roles of parental negative expressiveness and emotional security as mediators between parental depressive symptoms and child adjustment. Building on the conceptual framework of EST, this study longitudinally examined multiple factors linking parental depressive symptoms and child internalizing symptoms. Assessments included mothers' and fathers' depressive symptoms when children were in kindergarten, parents' negative expressiveness when children were in first grade, children's emotional insecurity 1 year later, and children's internalizing symptoms in kindergarten and second grade, with the former assessment providing autoregressive controls over initial levels of functioning to allow for assessment of change over time.

Findings revealed both mothers' and fathers' depressive symptoms were related to their own negative expressiveness (interestingly, not to their partners'). Mothers' and fathers' negative expressiveness were each associated with children's emotional insecurity, which, in turn, was related to their internalizing symptoms. In addition to these similar pathways, distinctive pathways as a function of parental gender were identified. That is, paternal depressive symptoms were also directly related to children's emotional insecurity. One possible explanation is that depressive symptoms in fathers may be perceived as less acceptable or normative, so that children's emotional insecurity is directly threatened. Moreover, maternal negative emotional expressiveness was directly associated with children's internalizing symptoms. One hypothesis is mothers' negative emotional expressiveness impacts parenting and other aspects of family functioning that directly affect children's adjustment, without regard to children's emotional security. That is, as the parent who often assumes the primary caregiving role, mothers' depressive symptoms may have a greater impact on parenting and other variables not assessed in this study that affect children's adjustment. Thus, when both mothers' and fathers' depressive symptoms were included, both similarities and differences were found in pathways to children's internalizing symptoms.

In addition to supporting the role of depressive symptoms on children's emotional security, these findings lend support to the role of negative emotional expressiveness as an additional family process affecting children's insecurity and their subsequent risk for maladjustment. Negative emotional expressiveness by the parents has been related to the impact of parental depressive symptoms on children's appraisals of the security and safety of family environments and children's risk for adjustment problems (e.g., Lee & Gotlib, 1991). These behaviors may constitute a significant pathway through which parental depressive symptoms affect family and child functioning (see Cummings et al., 2000), supporting the utility of the construct of parental emotional expressiveness for understanding children's development in families (Halberstadt, 1983, Halberstadt, Crisp, & Eaton, 1999).

These findings have implications for prevention and intervention measures in families with parents who exhibit depressive symptomatology. The importance of the parents' emotional behaviors associated with depressive symptoms was underscored (Restifo & Bögels, 2009). *Both* parents should be made aware of the impact of their expressions of emotions in the family on children's appraisals of safety and security. Parents may be able to reduce children's risk for emotional insecurity and internalizing problems by altering their pattern of emotional expression toward others in the family (e.g., Dix & Meunier, 2009; Shelton & Harold, 2008). Psychological interventions geared toward improving emotional communications in the family by parents with depressive symptoms merit investigation, in regard to possibly improving children's functioning.

CHILDREN'S SECURITY IN BROADER SOCIOCULTURAL SETTINGS

Findings from the past decade conducted in the United States have indicated the significance of emotional security on adjustment among American children. However, validation studies are essential to enable tests of EST in other cultures.

The concept of emotional security has been recently examined in an Eastern culture. In this study, with a sample from Mideast China, the authors validated the Security in the Interparental Subsystem Scales (SIS; Davies et al., 2002), an emotional security measure, and found that overt and covert marital conflict predicted emotional insecurity among adolescents who reported a high level of social harmony. That is, compared to individuals who are more individualistic, adolescents who place a higher value on social harmony reported greater felt insecurity in the face of marital conflict. Thus, even race or country may serve as a proxy for culture, with specific cultural values such as social harmony strengthening or weakening the marital conflict–emotional insecurity relationship in Eastern societies.

Moving beyond establishing the importance of children's sense of security in additional cultural contexts, it is also important to consider the role of extrafamilial contexts. Political conflict and violence may have important implications for understanding family conflict on children; these broader sociocultural factors provide the setting in which families live. Recent work by our group has been concerned with testing a social ecological model for links between political violence and child adjustment in Northern Ireland (Cummings et al., 2009).

The negative effects of political violence on children's mental health, including the implications of intergenerational transmission of sectarian hostilities and animosities for lasting peace processes in areas of sectarian conflict and war, are matters of international concern. Political violence has long been related to child adjustment problems, including aggressive behavior, depressive symptoms, posttraumatic stress symptoms, poor academic performance, and engagement by youth in political violence. However, the mechanisms through which political violence impacts children's well-being are not well understood (Cairns & Dawes, 1996). Relatively few tests of explanatory models have been undertaken, with longitudinal tests of theoretical models remaining rare to this point (Dubow et al., 2010).

Cummings et al. (2009) proposed a social ecological framework for conceptualizing relations between political violence and children's adjustment, positing that historical political violence, sectarian and nonsectarian community violence, and family and child psychological processes relate to children's maladjustment in these contexts. Cross-sectional tests have supported the promise of this approach for advances in understanding of mechanisms and contexts underlying relations between political violence and child adjustment (Cummings, Merrilees, et al., 2010; Cummings, Schermerhorn, et al., 2010). However, although cross-sectional studies are informative about explanatory processes, causal models of pathways of influence from a developmental perspective are further explicated by longitudinal model testing.

Our prospective research on relations between political violence and child adjustment in Belfast, Northern Ireland, began in 2005. To examine longitudinal pathways involving the larger social context, interparental conflict, emotional security about family, and child adjustment, Cummings and colleagues (2012) assessed mothers and their adolescent children from two-parent families in Catholic and Protestant working-class neighborhoods in Belfast, Northern Ireland (N = 1,015 mother–child dyads). Both parents and children completed measures assessing multiple levels of a social ecological model over 3 consecutive years. Families were surveyed across 24 wards in Belfast, all among the most socially deprived. In order to test a social ecological model, associations were examined among political violence (i.e., historical death rates in communities), sectarian and nonsectarian community violence (T1), family conflict and emotional security about family conflict (T2), and child internalizing and externalizing problems (T3), with autoregressive controls over adjustment at T1. This three-wave longitudinal model test supported a specific pathway linking sectarian community violence, family conflict, children's insecurity about family relationships, and adjustment problems, with historical death rates due to political violence predicting both sectarian and nonsectarian community violence (see Fig. 8.1). That is, historical levels of political violence were associated with reports of violence in the community, and in turn sectarian community violence was related to family conflict 1 year later. Children who experienced family conflict evidenced negative emotional and behavioral reactions indicative of emotional insecurity. Emotional insecurity, in turn, was related to more mental health symptoms and conduct problems over time.

Concerns have long been raised about the negative effects of political violence on children's adjustment and the intergenerational transmission of political violence (e.g., Sagi-Schwartz, 2008). The results of our study suggest that these effects may be explained, in part, by community and family factors and child psychological processes. Emotional insecurity about family relationships was again identified as an explanatory variable for adjustment problems associated with family conflict, including both internalizing and externalizing problems (Cummings & Davies, 2010), with the unique contribution that the broader social ecology associated with political violence was related to greater family conflict and violence.

The implications for peace processes warrant note. Agreements between leaders are only one step toward lasting peace, that is, "reaching a peace deal is not the same as reaching peace" (MacGinty et al., 2007, p. 1). The impact of political discord on communities, families, and children needs to be understood and addressed successfully for greater promise of sustained peace. Although policy makers have long recognized the negative impact of political violence on children (United Nations, 1997), limited recommendations have often been the result, such as "blandly accepting the truism that mothers can act as buffers for children exposed to political violence" (Cairns & Dawes, 1996, p. 131). The present research begins to support intervention strategies toward more holistic preventative approaches for communities. For example, one approach that is indicated is that community interventions should be broadly directed toward ameliorating children's emotional insecurity, including emotional insecurity about community and the family, in contexts of political violence.

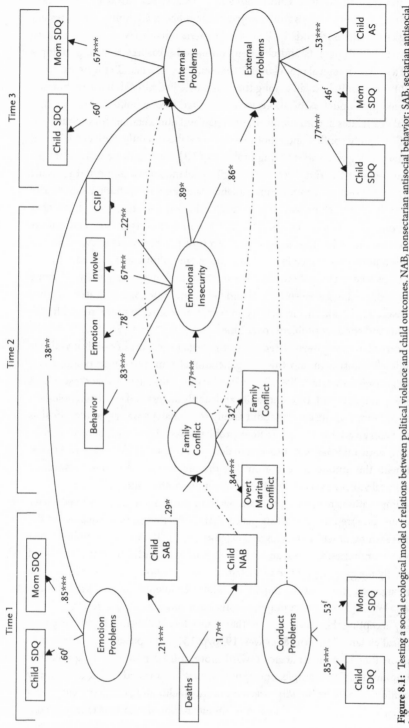

Figure 8.1: Testing a social ecological model of relations between political violence and child outcomes. NAB, nonsectarian antisocial behavior; SDQ, Strengths and Difficulties Questionnaire. Standardized path coefficients reported. f superscripts denote fixed factor loadings. Solid lines denote significant paths; dashed lines indicate nonsignificant paths. *p < .05; **p < .01; ***p < .001. Model fit: χ^2 (144) = 254.90, p < .001; χ^2/df = 1.77; NFI = .79; CFI = .89; RMSEA = .051 (90% CI: .04–.06). (Reprinted from Cummings, E. M., Merrilees, C. E., Schermerhorn, A. C., Goeke-Morey, M. C., Shirlow, P், & Cairns, E. [2012]. Political violence and child adjustment: Longitudinal tests of sectarian antisocial behavior, family conflict and insecurity as explanatory pathways. *Child Development, 83*, 461–468.)

SUMMARY AND FUTURE DIRECTIONS

Children's emotional security based on EST is further supported in the research reviewed in this chapter as a robust mediator of children's social functioning and adjustment from childhood to adolescence. Multiple processes were found to be related to children's regulation of emotional insecurity and adjustment, including dimensions of biological functioning. Moreover, children's emotional security played a role in multiple social ecological contexts, including parents' psychological symptoms and broader social ecologies of community and political violence. Emotional security was thus identified as a psychological mechanism related to child mental health and well-being in multiple social and family contexts. Support was also found for children's physiological responses to conflict as an additional regulatory system related to the functioning of the emotional security system.

These findings are consistent with a wider literature demonstrating the interplay between relationship functioning and mental health (see Introduction and Chapter 12, this volume). An important future direction is the development of intervention and prevention programs to take advantage of the accumulating knowledge to increase children's emotional security as an avenue toward better mental health and adjustment. Moreover, significant associations between dimensions of emotional insecurity and dimensions of physiological functioning call attention to the importance of being aware of possible implications for physical health of relationship processes that threaten emotional security (see Chapter 3, this volume). Notably, the research of El-Sheikh and colleagues (2009) supports the promise of examining relationships between improved marital and family conflict and cardiovascular functioning, consistent with advanced studies of these issues among adults (see Chapter 2, this volume). Thus, future programs should both target and assess possible benefits for dimensions of physical as well as psychological functioning. Various directions are ongoing (see Cummings & Davies, 2010), but much more needs to be done, including the development and rigorous testing of programs in multiple pertinent social ecological contexts. For example, in addition to programs being developed and tested for children and adolescents in two-parent families (Cummings & Schatz, 2012), programs are needed to increase children's emotional security in single-parent families, families faced with high levels of family stress (e.g., divorcing or custody disputing families), and families challenged by community and political violence. As reviewed by Beach (Chapter 6, this volume), considerable evidence suggests that interventions for marital conflict may serve to ameliorate depression in adults, with the implication that interventions for conflict behaviors in families may be a promising direction to ameliorate both adult and adolescent mental health (see also Restifo & Bögels, 2009).

In addition, given that emotional security is a construct pertinent to mental health and well-being across the life span (Cassidy & Shaver, 2008), extending EST to additional developmental periods is an important goal. With over a decade of research supporting emotional security about family relationships as a major process for child and adolescent development (Cummings & Davies, 2010; Waters & Cummings, 2000), advancing the understanding of its long-term significance across the life span is an important goal for future research. For example, emerging adults, who have not been systematically studied in relation to EST, are grappling with a new set of stage-salient challenges and tasks, such as establishing autonomy and occupational identity, managing risky behaviors such as substance use and unprotected sex, and forming new friendships and romantic relationships. Successful coping with all of these stage-salient challenges might be fostered by emerging adults achieving a positive sense of emotional security about family and other significant relationships. Along the same lines, future research is needed to examine how past (i.e., childhood) and present emotional security among young adults when they become parents is associated with felt security of their own children.

In conclusion, this chapter reviews recent evidence and theory supporting the significance of interparental conflict for children's mental health. Moreover, these findings suggest that the impact of interparental conflict on adjustment relates to broader processes pertinent to children's well-being, specifically, emotional security. This construct provides bases both for rigorous empirical model testing of family-wide constructs and ways to conceptually and empirically integrate interparental conflict with other sources of support and stress during child, adolescent, and young adult development, such as relations between interparental conflict and dimensions of parenting (Cummings & Davies, 2010). Further, given the implications for adults and children, and normal development as well as the development of psychopathology, there are strong bases for supporting connections between social, developmental, and clinical psychological approaches in future research on EST and interpersonal relationships and health (see Introduction and Chapter 12, this volume). Finally, EST also yields bases for conceptually including family factors with influences from a broader social ecological perspective, thereby making family more clearly amenable to inclusion in models for multiple real-world influences on children's development, including contexts of war, political violence, and variations across other cultural contexts.

REFERENCES

Appleyard, K., Egeland, B., van Dulmen, M. H. M., & Sroufe, L. A. (2005). When more is not better: The role of cumulative risk in child behavior outcomes. *Journal of Child Psychology and Psychiatry, 46*, 235–245. doi:10.1111/j.1469-7610.2004.00351.x.

Bauer, A. M., Quas, J. A., & Boyce, W. T. (2002). Associations between physiological reactivity and children's behavior: Advantages of a multisystem approach. *Developmental and Behavioral Pediatrics, 23*, 102–113. doi:10.1097/00004703-200204000-00007.

Beardslee, W. R., Bemporad, J., Keller, M. B., & Klerman, G. L. (1983). Children of parents with major affective disorder: A review. *The American Journal of Psychiatry, 140*, 825–832.

Bowlby, J. (1949). The study and reduction of group tensions in the family. *Human Relations, 2*, 123–128. doi: 10.1177/001872674900200203.

Bowlby, J. (1969). *Attachment and loss, Vol. 1. Attachment.* New York, NY: Basic Books.

Bowlby, J. (1973). *Attachment and loss, Vol. 2. Separation.* New York, NY: Basic Books.

Cairns, E., & Dawes, A. (1996). Children: Ethnic and political violence—A commentary. *Child Development, 67,* 129–139. doi:10.2307/1131691.

Cassidy, J., & Shaver, P. R. (2008). *Handbook of attachment: Theory, research, and clinical applications* (2nd ed.). New York, NY: Guilford Press.

Cummings, E. M. (1998). Stress and coping approaches and research: The impact of marital conflict on children. *Journal of Aggression, Maltreatment and Trauma, 2,* 31–50. doi:10.1300/J146v02n01_03.

Cummings, E. M., Cheung, R. Y. M., & Davies, P. T. (2013). Prospective relations between parental depression, negative expressiveness, emotional insecurity, and children's internalizing symptoms. *Child Psychiatry and Human Development, 44,* 698–708.

Cummings, E. M., & Davies, P. T. (1994a). *Children and marital conflict: The impact of family dispute and resolution.* New York, NY: The Guilford Press.

Cummings, E. M., & Davies, P. T. (1994b). Maternal depression and child development. *Journal of Child Psychology and Psychiatry, 35,* 73–112. doi:10.1111/j.1469-7610.1994.tb01133.x.

Cummings, E. M., & Davies, P. T. (1996). Emotional security as a regulator process in normal development and the development of psychopathology. *Development and Psychopathology, 8,* 123–139. doi: 10.1017/S0954579400007008.

Cummings, E. M., & Davies, P. T. (2010). *Marital conflict and children: An emotional security perspective.* New York, NY: Guilford Press.

Cummings, E. M., Davies, P. T., & Campbell, S. B. (2000). *Developmental psychopathology and family process: Theory, research, and clinical implications.* New York, NY: Guilford Press.

Cummings, E. M., DeArth-Pendley, G., Du Rocher Schudlich, T., & Smith, D. (2000). Parental depression and family functioning: Towards a process-oriented model of children's adjustment. In S. R. H. Beach (Ed.), *Marital and family processes in depression* (pp. 89– 110). Washington, DC: American Psychological Association.

Cummings. E. M., George, M. W., McCoy, K., & Davies, P. T. (2012). Interparental conflict in kindergarten and adolescent adjustment: Prospective investigation of emotional security as an explanatory mechanism. *Child Development, 83,* 1703–1715. doi: 10.1111/j.1467-8624.2012.01807.x.

Cummings, E. M., Goeke-Morey, M. C., & Papp, L. M. (2004). Everyday marital conflict and child aggression. *Journal of Abnormal Child Psychology, 32,* 191–202. doi:10.1023/B:JACP.0000019770.13216.be.

Cummings, E. M., Goeke-Morey, M. C., Schermerhorn, A. C., Merrilees, C. E., & Cairns, E. (2009). Children and political violence from a social ecological perspective: Implications for research on children and families in Northern Ireland. *Clinical Child and Family Psychology Review, 12,* 16–38. doi: 10.1007/s10567-009-0041-8.

Cummings, E. M., Merrilees, C. E., & George, M. (2010). Fathers, marriages and families: Revisiting and updating the framework for fathering in family context. In M. Lamb (Ed.), *The role of the father in child development* (5th ed., pp. 154–176). New York, NY: Wiley.

Cummings. E. M., Merrilees, C. M., Schermerhorn, A. C., Goeke-Morey, M. C., Shirlow, P., & Cairns, E. (2010). Testing a social ecological model for relations between political violence and child adjustment in Northern Ireland. *Development and Psychopathology, 22,* 405–418. doi: 10.1017/S0954579410000143.

Cummings, E. M., Merrilees, C. E., Schermerhorn, A. C., Goeke-Morey, M., Shirlow, P., & Cairns, E. (2011). Longitudinal pathways between political violence and child adjustment: The role of emotional security about the community in Northern Ireland. *Journal of Abnormal Child Psychology, 39,* 213–224. doi:10.1007/s10802-010-9457-3.

Cummings, E. M., Merrilees, C. E., Schermerhorn, A. C., Goeke-Morey, M. C., Shirlow, P., & Cairns, E. (2012). Political violence and child adjustment: Longitudinal tests of sectarian antisocial behavior, family conflict and insecurity as explanatory pathways. *Child Development*, *83*, 461–468. doi: 10.1111/j.1467-8624.2011.01720.x.

Cummings, E. M., & Schatz, J. N. (2012). Family conflict, emotional security, and child development: Translating research findings into a prevention program for community families. *Clinical Child and Family Psychology Review*, *15*, 14–27. doi:10.1007/s10567-012-0112-0.

Cummings, E. M., Schermerhorn, A. C., Davies, P. T., Goeke-Morey, M., & Cummings, J. S. (2006). Interparental discord and child adjustment: Prospective investigations of emotional security as an explanatory mechanism. *Child Development*, *77*, 132–152. doi:10.1111/j.1467-8624.2006.00861.x.

Cummings, E. M., Schermerhorn, A. C., Merrilees, C. M., Goeke-Morey, M. C., & Cairns, E. (2010). Political violence and child adjustment in Northern Ireland: Testing pathways in a social ecological model including single—and two-parent families. *Developmental Psychology*, *46*, 827–841. doi: 10.1037/a0019668.

Davies, P. T., & Cummings, E. M. (1994). Marital conflict and child adjustment: An emotional security hypothesis. *Psychological Bulletin*, *116*, 387–411. doi: 10.1037/0033-2909.116.3.387.

Davies, P. T., & Cummings, E. M. (1998). Exploring children's emotional security as a mediator of the link between marital relations and child adjustment. *Child Development*, *69*, 124–139. doi:10.2307/1132075.

Davies, P. T., & Cummings, E. M. (2006). Interparental discord, family process, and developmental psychopathology. In D. Cicchetti & D. Cohen (Eds.), *Developmental psychopathology, Vol. 3. Risk, disorder, and adaptation* (2nd ed., pp. 86–128). New York, NY: Wiley.

Davies, P. T., Forman, E. M., Rasi, J. A., & Stevens, K. I. (2002). Assessing children's emotional security in the interparental relationship: The security in the interparental subsystem (SIS) scales. *Child Development*, *73*, 544–562. doi: 10.1111/1467-8624.00423.

Davies, P. T., & Sturge-Apple, M. L. (2007). Advances in the formulation of emotional security theory: An ethologically based perspective. *Advances in Child Development and Behavior*, *35*, 87–137. doi: 10.1016/B978-0-12-009735-7.50008-6.

Davies, P. T., Sturge-Apple, M. L., & Cicchetti, D. (2011). Interparental aggression and children's adrenocortical reactivity: Testing an evolutionary model of allostatic load. *Development and Psychopathology*, *23*, 801–814. doi:10.1017/S0954579411000319.

Davies, P. T., Sturge-Apple, M. L., Cicchetti, D., & Cummings E. M. (2007). The role of child adrenocortical functioning in pathways between interparental conflict and child maladjustment. *Developmental Psychology*, *43*, 918–930. doi: 10.1037/0012-1649.43.4.918.

Davies, P. T., Sturge-Apple, M. L., Cicchetti, D., & Cummings, E. M. (2008). Adrenocortical underpinnings of children's psychological reactivity to interparental conflict. *Child Development*, *79*, 1693–1706. doi: 10.1111/j.1467-8624.2008.01219.x.

Davies, P. T., Sturge-Apple, M. L., Cicchetti, D., Manning, L. G., & Zale, E. (2009). Children's patterns of emotional reactivity to conflict as explanatory mechanisms in links between interpartner aggression and child physiological functioning. *Journal of Child Psychology and Psychiatry*, *50*, 1384–1391. doi: 10.1111/j.1469-7610.2009.02154.x.

Davies, P. T., & Woitach, M. J. (2008). Children's emotional security in the interparental relationship. *Current Directions in Psychological Science*, *17*, 269–274. doi:10.1111/j.1467-8721.2008.00588.x.

Davies, P. T., Woitach, M. J., Winter, M. A., & Cummings, E. M. (2008). Children's insecure representations of the interparental relationship and their school adjustment: The mediating role of attention difficulties. *Child Development*, *79*, 1570–1582. doi: 10.1111/j.1467-8624.2008.01206.x.

Dix, T., & Meunier, L. N. (2009). Depressive symptoms and parenting competence: An analysis of 13 regulatory processes. *Developmental Review, 29*, 45–68. doi: 10.1016/j. dr.2008.11.002.

Downey, G., & Coyne, J. C. (1990). Children of depressed parents: An integrative review. *Psychological Bulletin, 108*, 50–76. doi: 10.1037/0033-2909.108.1.50.

Dubow, E. F., Boxer, P., Huesmann, L. R., Shikaki, K., Landau, S., Gvirsman, S. D., & Ginges, J. (2010). Exposure to conflict and violence across contexts: Relations to adjustment among Palestinian children. *Journal of Clinical Child and Adolescent Psychology, 39*, 103–116. doi: 10.1080/15374410903401153.

Du Rocher Schudlich, T., & Cummings, E. M. (2003). Parental dysphoria and children's internalizing symptoms: Marital conflict styles as mediators of risk. *Child Development, 74*, 1663–1681. doi:10.1046/j.1467-8624.2003.00630.x.

Du Rocher Schudlich, T., & Cummings, E. M. (2007). Parental dysphoria and children's adjustment: Marital conflict styles, children's emotional security, and parenting as mediators of risk. *Journal of Abnormal Child Psychology, 35*, 627–639. doi:10.1007/s10802-007-9118-3.

El-Sheikh, M. (2005). The role of emotional responses and physiological reactivity in the marital conflict-child functioning link. *Journal of Child Psychology and Psychiatry, 46*, 1191–1199. doi: 10.1111/j.1469-7610.2005.00418.x.

El-Sheikh, M., Buckhalt, J. A., Keller, P. S., Cummings, E. M., & Acebo, C. (2007). Child emotional insecurity and academic achievement: The role of sleep disruptions. *Journal of Family Psychology, 21*, 29–38. doi:10.1037/0893-3200.21.1.29.

El-Sheikh, M., Cummings, E. M., Kouros, C. D., Elmore-Staton, L., & Buckhalt, J. A. (2008). Marital psychological and physical aggression and children's mental and physical health: Direct, mediated, and moderated effects. *Journal of Consulting and Clinical Psychology, 76*, 138–148. doi:10.1037/0022-006X.76.1.138.

El-Sheikh, M., Kouros, C. D., Erath, S., Cummings, E. M., Keller, P., & Staton, L. (2009). Marital conflict and children's externalizing behavior: Interactions between parasympathetic and sympathetic nervous system activity. *Monographs of the Society for Research in Child Development, 74*, 1–79.

Emery, R. E. (1982). Interparental conflict and the children of discord and divorce. *Psychological Bulletin, 92*, 310–330. doi:10.1037/0033-2909.92.2.310.

Fendrich, M., Warner, V., & Weissman, M. M. (1990). Family risk factors, parental depression, and psychopathology in offspring. *Developmental Psychology, 26*, 40–50. doi: 10.1037/0012-1649.26.1.40.

Fincham, F. D. (1994). Understanding the association between marital conflict and child adjustment: Overview. *Journal of Family Psychology 8*, 123–127. doi:10.1037/0893-3200.8.2.123.

Goeke-Morey, M. C., Cummings, E. M., Harold, G. T., & Shelton, K. H. (2003). Categories and continua of destructive and constructive marital conflict tactics from the perspective of US and Welsh children. *Journal of Family Psychology, 17*, 327–338. doi: 10.1037/0893-3200.17.3.327.

Goeke-Morey, M. C., Cummings, E. M., & Papp, L. M. (2007). Children and marital conflict resolution: Implications for emotional security and adjustment. *Journal of Family Psychology, 21*, 744–753. doi:10.1037/0893-3200.21.4.744.

Goodman, S. H. (2007). Depression in mothers. *Annual Review of Clinical Psychology, 3*, 107–135. doi: 10.1146/annurev.clinpsy.3.022806.091401.

Grych, J. H., & Fincham, F. D. (1990). Marital conflict and children's adjustment: A cognitive-contextual framework. *Psychological Bulletin, 108*, 267–290. doi:10.1037/0033-2909.108.2.267.

Halberstadt, A. G. (1983). Family expressiveness styles and nonverbal communication skills. *Journal of Nonverbal Behavior, 8*, 14–26. doi:10.1007/BF00986327.

Halberstadt, A. G., Crisp, V. W., & Eaton, K. L. (1999). Family expressiveness: A retrospective and new directions for research. In P. Philippot, R. S. Feldman, & E. J. Coats (Eds.), *The social context of nonverbal behavior* (pp. 109–155). New York, NY: Cambridge University Press.

Harold, G. T., Shelton, K. H., Goeke-Morey, M., & Cummings, E. M. (2004). Marital conflict, child emotional security about family relationships and child adjustment. *Social Development, 13*, 350–376. doi:10.1111/j.1467-9507.2004.00272.x.

Keller, P. S., Cummings, E. M., Davies, P. T., & Mitchell, P. M. (2008). Longitudinal relations between parental drinking problems, family functioning, and child adjustment. *Development and Psychopathology, 20*, 195–212. doi:10.1017/S0954579408000096.

Keller, P. S., Gilbert, L. R., Koss, K. J., Cummings, E. M., & Davies, P. T. (2011). Parental problem drinking, marital aggression, and child emotional insecurity: A longitudinal investigation. *Journal of Studies on Alcohol and Drugs, 75*, 711–722.

Koss, K. J., George, M. R. W., Bergman, K. N., Cummings, E. M., Davies, P. T., & Cicchetti, D. (2011). Understanding children's emotional processes and behavioral strategies in the context of marital conflict. *Journal of Experimental Child Psychology, 109*, 336–352. doi: 10.1016/j.jecp.2011.02.007.

Koss, K. J., George, M. R. W., Davies, P. T., Cicchetti, D., Cummings, E. M., & Sturge-Apple (2012). Patterns of children's adrenocortical reactivity to interparental conflict and associations with child adjustment: A growth mixture modeling approach. *Developmental Psychology, 49*(2), 317–326. doi: 10.1037/a0028246.

Kouros, C. D., & Cummings, E. M. (2011). Transactional relations between marital functioning and spouses' depressive symptoms. *American Journal of Orthopsychiatry, 81*, 128–138. doi: 10.1111/j.1939-0025.2010.01080.x.

Kouros, C. D., Cummings, E. M., & Davies, P. T. (2010). Early trajectories of interparental conflict and externalizing problems as predictors of social competence in preadolescence. *Development and Psychopathology, 22*, 527–537. doi:10.1017/S0954579410000258.

Kouros, C. D., Merriless, C. E., & Cummings, E. M. (2008). Marital conflict and children's emotional security in the context of parental depression. *Journal of Marriage and Family, 70*, 684–697. doi:10.1111/j.1741-3737.2008.00514.x.

Lee, C. M., & Gotlib, I. H. (1991). Adjustment of children of depressed mothers: A 10-month follow-up. *Journal of Abnormal Psychology, 100*, 473–477. doi:10.1037/0021-843X.100.4.473.

Lewis, G., Rice, F., Harold, G. T., Collishaw, S., & Thapar, A. (2011). Investigating environmental links between parent depression and child depressive/anxiety symptoms: Using an assisted conception design. *Journal of the American Academy of Child and Adolescent Psychiatry, 50*, 451–459. doi:10.1016/j.jaac.2011.01.015.

MacGinty, R., Muldoon, O. T., & Ferguson, N. (2007). No war, no peace: Northern Ireland after the agreement. *Political Psychology, 28*, 1–11. doi: 10.1111/j.1467-9221.2007.00548.x.

Masten, A. S., & Cicchetti, D. (2010). Developmental cascades. *Development and Psychopathology, 22*, 491–495. doi:10.1017/S0954579410000222.

McCoy, K., Cummings, E. M., & Davies, P. T. (2009). Constructive and destructive marital conflict, emotional security and children's prosocial behavior. *Journal of Child Psychology and Psychiatry, 50*, 270–279. doi:10.1111/j.1469-7610.2008.01945.x.

Oyserman, D., Mowbray, C., Allen-Meares, P., & Firminger, K. (2000). Parenting among mothers with serious mental illness. *American Journal of Orthopsychiatry, 70*, 296–315. doi:10.1037/h0087733.

Pendry, P., & Adam, E. K. (2007). Associations between parents' marital functioning, maternal parenting quality, maternal emotion and child cortisol levels. *International Journal of Behavioral Development, 31*, 218–231. doi: 10.1177/0165025407074634.

Ramchandani, P. G., O'Connor, T. G., Evans, J., Heron, J., Murray, L., & Stein, A. (2008). The effects of pre—and postnatal depression in fathers: A natural experiment comparing the effects of exposure to depression on offspring. *Journal of Child Psychology and Psychiatry, 49*, 1069–1078. doi:10.1111/j.1469-7610.2008.02000.x.

Restifo, K., & Bögels, S. (2009). Family processes in the development of youth depression: Translating the evidence to treatment. *Clinical Psychology Review, 29*, 294–316. doi: 10.1016/j.cpr.2009.02.005.

Rutter, M. (2007). Gene-environment interdependence. *Developmental Science, 10*, 12–18. doi:10.1111/j.1467-7687.2007.00557.x.

Sagi-Schwartz, A. (2008). The well being of children living in chronic war zones: The Palestinian-Israeli case. *International Journal of Behavioral Development, 32*, 322–336. doi:10.1177/0165025408090974.

Saltzman, K. M., Holden, G. W., & Holahan, C. J. (2005). The psychobiology of children exposed to marital violence. *Journal of Clinical Child and Adolescent Psychology, 34*, 129– 139. doi:10.1207/s15374424jccp3401_12.

Schacht, P. M., Cummings, E. M., & Davies, P. T. (2009). Fathering in family context and child adjustment: A longitudinal analysis. *Journal of Family Psychology, 23*, 790–807. doi: 10.1037/a0016741.

Shelton, K. H., & Harold, G. T. (2008). Interparental conflict, negative parenting, and children's adjustment: Bridging links between parents' depression and children's psychological distress. *Journal of Family Psychology, 22*, 712–724. doi:10.1037/a0013515.

Stocker, C. M., & Youngblade, L. (1999). Marital conflict and parental hostility: Links with children's sibling and peer relationships. *Journal of Family Psychology, 13*, 598–609. doi:10.1037/0893-3200.13.4.598.

Sturge-Apple, M. L., Davies, P. T., Cicchetti, D., & Cummings, E. M. (2009). The role of mothers' and fathers' adrenocortical reactivity in spillover between interparental conflict and parenting practices. *Journal of Family Psychology, 23*, 215–225. doi: 10.1037/a0014198.

Sturge-Apple, M. L., Davies, P. T., Cicchetti, D., & Manning, L. G. (2012). Interparental violence, maternal emotional unavailability, and children's cortisol functioning in family contexts. *Developmental Psychology, 48*, 237–249. doi:10.1037/a0025419.

United Nations. (1997). *United Nations convention on the rights of the child.* Geneva, Switzerland: Office of the United Nations High Commissioner for Human Rights.

Waters, E., & Cummings, E. M. (2000). A secure base from which to explore close relationships. *Child Development, 49*, 164–172. doi:10.1111/1467-8624.00130.

Waters, E., Weinfield, N. S., & Hamilton, C. E. (2000). The stability of attachment security from infancy to adolescence and early adulthood: General discussion. *Child Development, 71*, 703–706. doi:10.1111/1467-8624.00179.

CHAPTER 9
Social Connectedness at Older Ages and Implications for Health and Well-Being

LINDA J. WAITE, JAMES IVENIUK,
AND EDWARD O. LAUMANN

Social connections are closely linked to health, so that, for example, married people tend to live longer, healthier lives than those who are not married (Holt-Lunstad & Birmingham, 2008; Waite & Gallagher, 2000). Social connections have been theorized to reduce exposure to stress, to moderate the negative effects of stress, and to aid recovery from stress, leading to better mental and physical health (Thoits, 2011). Lonely people—those who view their social relationships as inadequate—tend to sleep more poorly (Cacioppo et al., 2002), get inadequate exercise (Hawkley, Thisted, & Cacioppo, 2009), are more likely to face increases in depressive symptoms over time, and are more likely to die, than those who feel socially connected (Luo, Hawkley, Waite, & Cacioppo, 2012).

One of the major challenges to developing a scientific understanding of the link between social connectedness and health during aging is obtaining good data. Many datasets used to study health are convenience samples involving clinical populations, which do not represent the population at large; are recruited through connections to a health care provider; and select on the outcome of interest. Where datasets are large and nationally representative, biological measures of health are expensive and difficult to incorporate into surveys, and detailed information about respondents' social lives can be costly to obtain in terms of time spent in an interview. Finally, it is rare to find all of these features (national representation, biological and psychological measures, fine-grained information on social context) together in the same dataset, making it hard to establish how it is that these factors come together to produce good or ill health.

In this chapter, we synthesize major findings from the National Social Life, Health and Aging Project (NSHAP), a nationally representative survey that fulfills all these criteria. NSHAP provides us with the first opportunity to see, in great detail, how social, emotional, cognitive, and physical well-being intersect and depend upon one another. NSHAP also contains a large number of questions about sexuality at older ages—another topic which has been hampered by a lack of good data. As such, we will use this chapter to provide the reader with a condensed account of some major findings from NSHAP, specifically findings that we believe provide windows into how social, psychological, and biological factors operate together at older ages. We show that connectedness leads to better psychological and physical health, but only when connections carry resources, such as information or social support. Furthermore, the majority of older adults appear to have relatively large networks of people they are close to, and they are sexually active with their partners—another aspect of their social life that may be important for their overall well-being. In short, we will demonstrate that a plurality of older Americans have social lives that are conducive to good health.

CONCEPTUAL FRAMEWORK

The theoretical framework we will employ here conceptualizes health as produced in social and cultural contexts that provide people with resources through other individuals, family, and social environments.[1] Figure 9.1 illustrates this overarching framework, which we call the interactive biopsychosocial model (IBM). The model comprises (1) an orientation toward health rather than illness; (2) analytic capacity for outcomes of health or illness; (3) parity among the three domains of capital (biophysical, psychocognitive, and social) as factors in an individual's health endowment; (4) consideration of causality and feedback between various types of capital and health; (5) conceptualization of individual health or illness embedded in intimate dyads, the family, or other social networks; (6) interdependency of social and life course dynamics; and (7) the potential of capital inputs to act as assets or liabilities (Lindau, Laumann, Levinson, & Waite, 2003). Biophysical, psychocognitive, and social capital make up an individual's health endowment. Biophysical capital includes genetic composition, physiology, physique, sensory function, nutrition, strength, and appearance, all of which affect an individual's physical and physiological capacity for health. Psychocognitive capital includes intelligence, personality, emotional well-being, happiness, attitudes, perceptions, and evaluations. Social capital refers to the networks of relationships with others (kin, friends, neighbors, physicians), some of whom may be connected to each other, and to the quality of those relationships. Sociocultural context is the broader environment of social locations (ethnic, religious, regional, gendered, political, or economic class), which carry social expectations, norms, and differential access to scarce resources that influence health. The health endowment of the individual is inextricably linked to socially relevant others (partner, kin, friends) with whom the

1. This section was adapted from Waite, L., & Das, A. (2010). Families, social life, and well-being at older ages. *Demography, 47*, S87–S109.

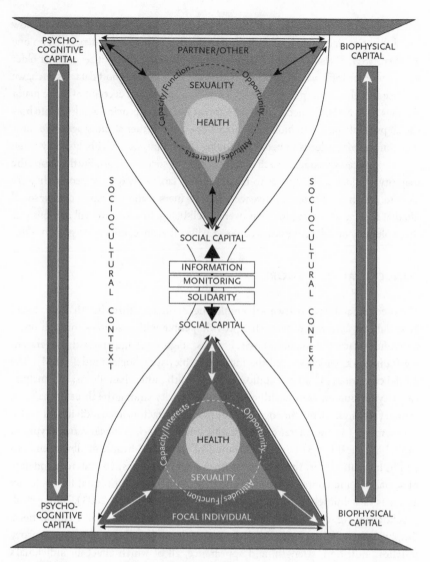

Figure 9.1: The Interactive Biopsychosocial Model (IBM).
Source: Lindau et al., 2003.

individual may pool resources, exchange services, and provide advice and support. In our model, this interdependency allows two healthy individuals acting jointly to generate better health than each would generate alone. The interdependency occurs through repeated small exchanges and specialization of roles within the relationship and serves to maximize efficiency and efficacy, as well as perpetuating their interdependency (Lindau et al., 2003).

According to the IBM, health at older ages develops and changes within a social context and within a family and/or intimate partnership that also changes in both form and function. We will use research from the NSHAP survey to describe empirical links between social connections, families, and well-being among older adults. These results illustrate the utility of the IBM for thinking about interrelationships between social, psychological, and biological well-being at older ages.

NSHAP

All findings reported here use data from the first wave of NSHAP, a nationally representative, population-based study funded by the National Institutes of Health and conducted by NORC at the University of Chicago. The first wave of the study consists of interviews with 3,005 community-dwelling older adults, conducted between autumn 2005 and spring 2006. The sample was selected from a multistage area probability design screened by the Institute for Social Research (ISR) for the Health and Retirement Study (HRS). From the HRS sample surplus, NSHAP selected 4,400 potential respondents, ages 57–85 years. The original HRS design oversampled Blacks and Hispanics. NSHAP retained this design and also oversampled by age and gender to produce approximately equal cell sizes by gender across three age categories. The final response rate for Wave 1 is 75.5%. NSHAP fielded Wave 2 in 2010, and 2,261 of the original 3,005 Wave 1 respondents were reinterviewed (75.2%). Among those not reinterviewed, 318 were deceased and 115 were in too poor health for inclusion. During Wave 2, NSHAP added the spouses and cohabiting partners of 955 respondents to its sample. Complete interviews were conducted with all spouses and cohabiting partners, providing detailed information on the social connections and health of both members of these dyads.

Social Networks

NSHAP collected extensive information about respondents' egocentric social networks and community involvement, as well as partnership history, sexual activity, physical and mental health, health-related behaviors, medication use, and biomeasures. Interviewers asked older adults to list people with whom they discuss "things that are important to you." This question elicits names of strong, frequently accessed, long-term contacts (Marin, 2004; Ruan, 1998). Such contacts are also more able to influence individual behaviors and apply normative pressure (Burt, 1984). Respondents could name up to five people; however, if the spouse was not listed among the first five, the interviewer prompted the respondent to add his or her spouse to the list, in order to ensure NSHAP collected data on intimate partnerships. NSHAP maintained a cap on the number of people that the respondent could list, in order to ensure that those individuals contained in the roster were more likely to be members of the respondents' core discussion network; while this truncates the distribution of network size, it allowed respondents to more easily map the structure of relations among their confidants, and thus provide data that develop our understanding of the implications of network structure for health. These data provide the basis for NSHAP's measures of older adults' egocentric network size, volume of contact with network members, emotional closeness to network members, network composition, and network density (Cornwell, Laumann, & Schumm, 2008).

Sexuality

NSHAP focused on respondents' sexual relationships during the past 5 years. This included the current spouse, cohabiting partner, or romantic/intimate partner and either one or two of the next most recent spouses or cohabiting partners within the past 5 years, for a maximum of two partners overall. NSHAP also included a suite of measures dedicated to sexual behavior and function, sexual satisfaction, coital frequency, and sexual attitudes and practices. Overall, 2% to 7% of respondents declined to answer any given question about sexual activities and problems.

Biomeasures

The range of biomeasures collected in NSHAP represents a balance between the scientific value of the data, minimally invasive techniques accepted by respondents, practical considerations of implementation, and budget constraints. A total of 13 biomeasures were collected for Wave 1 of the study, including measured weight, height, blood pressure, heart rate, pulse, mobility, and sensory function. Biological samples of saliva, blood spots, and vaginal swabs were also obtained. During the in-person interview, all respondents were administered measures of quality of life, cognition, and psychological health. These include anxiety, stress, depression, loneliness, emotional health, happiness, cognitive function, and self-esteem (Shiovitz-Ezra, Leitsch, Graber, & Karraker, 2009).

THE FINDINGS

Social Connectedness and Aging—Descriptive Statistics

According to one set of theories, old age is not only a time of potential physical and psychological decline but also of social decline and social isolation.[2,3] Modernization

---

2. All analyses and descriptive statistics employ survey weighting, clustering by primary sampling unit, and variance adjusted for stratification and sampling design.

3. This section was adapted from Cornwell, B., Laumann E. O., & Schumm, L. P. (2008). The social connectedness of older adults: A national profile. *American Sociological Review, 73,* 185–203, as well as Cornwell, B., Schumm, L. P., Laumann, E. O., & Graber, J. (2009). Social networks in the NSHAP Study: Rationale, measurement, and preliminary findings. *Journals of Gerontology Series B: Psychological Sciences and Social Sciences, 64B,* i47–i55.

theories describe the breakdown of traditional extended families, precipitating a loss of social standing for older adults (Burgess, 1960; Cowgill, 1986). One classic social-psychological model developed from a modernization framework is social disengagement theory (Cumming & Henry, 1961), which argues that older adults' isolation results from a gradual and irreversible abandonment of social roles, narrowing role sets, and the weakening of existing social ties. The proposed mechanism behind this change was that as older adults approach the end of their lives, they withdraw their expectations of social connectedness at the same time as their confidants withdraw from the older adult.

In response to these accounts, some researchers have turned to a life course perspective (Elder, 1985; George, 1993) in order to underscore later life challenges for older adults' social integration. This line of research portrays older adults as preserving their social connections and staving off isolation in the face of potentially isolating life-course events like retirement and bereavement. Activity theory notes that some older adults adjust to later life transitions by remaining socially active, which helps them to remain relatively happy and healthy (Cavan, Burgess, Havinghurst, & Goldhammer, 1949; Lemon, Bengtson, & Peterson, 1972). Similarly, continuity theory argues that people attempt to maintain social roles and activities through life course transitions, in part by remaining socially engaged in voluntary organizations and leisure activities that they enjoyed earlier in life (Atchley, 1989; Rowe & Kahn, 1998; Thoits, 1992).

Many of the samples that have been used to make statements about the makeup and structure of older adults' social networks have been small and non–nationally representative, meaning it is hard to state what the expected baseline of social interaction should be for this age group. By some accounts, social networks at older ages should be quite small with weak ties, while others would suggest that they would be filled with close confidants (Marsden, 1987; McPherson, Smith-Lovin, & Brashears, 2006; Shaw, Krause, Liang, & Bennett, 2007). Therefore, we begin by providing descriptive statistics about what older adults' networks look like, according to the measures employed in NSHAP, and how these measures' scores vary by key sociodemographic characteristics. Note that in line with terminological conventions in social network analysis, we will refer to the focal respondent as *ego* in the analyses herein, and their confidants as *alters*. All descriptive statistics come from Table 9.1.

Network Size

The most basic measure one can derive from NSHAP's social network roster is network size, which may provide more opportunity for the transmission and accumulation of social capital. Few respondents reported having no confidants. In fact, the modal number of alters reported by NSHAP respondents was five, with over one third of the sample reporting that they have five or more confidants. These are relatively large networks compared to the average network sizes reported for adults of all ages in other studies (McPherson et al., 2006), and they contrast with the expected picture from modernization/isolation theories mentioned earlier. As shown in Table 9.1, women, Whites, higher educated people, and healthier respondents also reported having larger networks.

Network Composition

Network composition can be defined in various ways, such as the prevalence of specific types of tie (e.g., friends) in the network or the overall diversity of ties within it. Many researchers in medical sociology and social gerontology focus on proportion kin because kin relations are the most likely to provide unconditional support in the face of health crises (Antonucci & Akiyama, 1995; Hurlbert, Haines, & Beggs, 2000).

To make it possible to identify a wider variety of relationship types in older adults' networks, NSHAP asked respondents to characterize their relationship with each alter as one of the following 18 types: spouse; ex-spouse; romantic/sexual partner; parent; parent-in-law; child; stepchild; sibling; other relative; other in-law; friend; neighbor; coworker or boss; minister/priest/other clergy; psychiatrist/ psychologist/counselor/therapist; caseworker/social worker; housekeeper/home health care provider; or other. As seen from Table 9.1, older adults' networks are mainly kin centered; however, there are some differences in network composition across demographic groups. Latinos tended to report more kin-centered networks than Whites. About two thirds of Whites' and Blacks' networks comprised kin compared with nearly 80% of Latinos' networks. People with less formal education also reported networks with a higher proportion of kin. With respect to other aspects of network composition, men reported fewer alters than did women, as did Whites (compared with Blacks) and less highly educated people. About one fourth of alters lived with ego (e.g., about 80% of coresident network members were the respondent's spouse or current partner). Older respondents, women, and Whites (compared with Latinos) reported fewer coresident confidants.

Emotional Closeness to Network Members

The subjective, emotional quality of relationships has been linked to well-being (Wellman & Wortley, 1990) and may moderate the effect of other network features on well-being (Fiori, Antonucci, & Cortina, 2006; Luo & Waite, 2011). Unlike studies that conceptualize emotional closeness in terms of relationship type (e.g., automatically assuming that kin ties are closer), NSHAP measured relationship quality directly by asking respondents: "How close do you feel is your relationship with [name]?" Possible responses included "not very close," " somewhat close," "very close," or "extremely close" (in that order). Emotional closeness is summarized in

Table 9.1. SOCIODEMOGRAPHIC DISTRIBUTIONS AND SUMMARY STATISTICS OF KEY SOCIAL NETWORK MEASURES

Attribute	Network Size	Proportion Kin	Proportion Female	Proportion Cohabit	Closeness to Alters	Volume of Contact	Network Density	Bridging Potential[a]
Age								
57–64	3.54	0.66	0.63	0.27	3.21	727.24	0.86	0.08
65–74	3.46	0.67	0.63	0.24	3.13	661.16	0.84	0.10
75–85	3.40	0.69	0.64	0.18	3.10	639.80	0.85	0.11
Trend test	p = 0.09	p = 0.19	p = 0.58	p = 0.00	p = 0.00	p = 0.00	p = 0.30	p = 0.10
Gender								
Female	3.69	0.66	0.71	0.16	3.19	734.24	0.83	0.12
Male	3.26	0.68	0.54	0.32	3.12	629.39	0.87	0.07
Trend test	p = 0.00	p = 0.20	p = 0.00	p = 0.00	p = 0.00	p = 0.00	p = 0.00	p = 0.01
Race/ethnicity								
White	3.59	0.66	0.62	0.23	3.15	684.52	0.85	0.10
Black	3.10	0.67	0.68	0.20	3.22	691.18	0.84	0.11
Hispanic, non-Black	2.86	0.79	0.66	0.34	3.16	670.95	0.90	0.07
Other	3.26	0.72	0.60	0.27	3.12	666.74	0.93	0.03
Trend test	p = 0.00	p = 0.00	p = 0.03	p = 0.00	p = 0.19	p = 0.94	p = 0.00	p = 0.02
Education								
< High school	2.97	0.72	0.66	0.25	3.15	653.69	0.89	0.08
High school	3.34	0.71	0.64	0.22	3.18	685.64	0.88	0.10
Some college	3.62	0.64	0.63	0.22	3.15	697.38	0.83	0.11
≥BA	3.85	0.63	0.59	0.26	3.14	686.34	0.82	0.09
Trend test	p = 0.00	p = 0.00	p = 0.01	p = 0.53	p = 0.56	p = 0.22	p = 0.00	p = 0.59
Self-rated health								
Poor/fair	3.29	0.68	0.63	0.22	3.09	681.34	0.86	0.10
Good	3.37	0.69	0.63	0.25	3.16	675.56	0.85	0.11
Very good/excellent	3.66	0.66	0.63	0.24	3.19	689.09	0.85	0.09
Trend test	p = 0.00	p = 0.17	p = 0.98	p = 0.15	p = 0.01	p = 0.60	p = 0.51	p = 0.21
Overall weighted mean	3.48	0.67	0.63	0.24	3.16	683.42	0.85	0.10
Standard deviation	1.49	0.34	0.30	0.28	0.54	363.85	0.25	0.30
Skewness	-0.44	-0.67	-0.42	1.51	-0.32	0.53	-1.74	2.62

Note. Estimates refer to network members in respondents' top five only.
[a]Bridging scores relevant only to those with two or more network members (*n* = 2,589).
Source: Cornwell et al, 2009.

Table 9.1 using the average closeness rating (coded 1–4) across alters. Most older adults are close to those in their networks. However, the oldest old, men, and those who are in poorer health reported being less close with their confidants.

Volume of Contact With Network Members

All else equal, many researchers hold that more contact with confidants means more access to resources and social support (Lin, Woelfel, & Light, 1985; Munch, McPherson, & Smith-Lovin, 1997). Frequent contact therefore affects the potential impact of networks on health (Seeman & Berkman, 1988, Terhell, Broese van Groenou, & van Tilburg, 2007). NSHAP respondents reported how often they talk to each alter on an 8-point scale, ranging from "every day" to "less than once per year." One can score these responses according to the approximate number of times per year ego interacts with alter (e.g., "once a month" = 12; "every day" = 365) and sum these scores across respondents' top five confidants to obtain a measure of overall volume of contact with alters. This measure depends both on average frequency of interaction with each network member and on network size, so it is closely related to both. The findings presented in Table 9.1 show that, on average, older adults report nearly two contacts per day with a close confidant. The oldest adults in the sample and men reported fewer contacts per year than younger adults and women, respectively.

Network Density

While many existing studies of social connectedness focus on network composition and closeness, few consider the importance of network structure, that is, the presence and nature of relationships among alters. One way to address this is through the concept of network density, defined as the proportion of all possible pairs among the alters in which the two individuals know each other. High-density networks constitute close-knit social contexts in which alters can share and compare information, coordinate caregiving duties, and pool resources. Thus, high network density is associated with more reliable and more frequent activation of informal support (Haines, Hurlbert, & Beggs, 1996). We can see that more educated people have networks that are less dense, which could be an indicator of greater geographic mobility for keeping in contact with unconnected confidants.

Network Bridging Potential

Network bridging occurs when a respondent maintains connections with at least two alters who are not connected to each other except through the respondent. Serving as a bridge can be useful for a variety of reasons. For example, those who occupy bridging positions can coordinate the transfer of resources and information between unconnected parties (Burt, 1992, 2005). An individual who occupies a bridging position can also access information that a closed, highly interconnected network might unknowingly shut out (Granovetter, 1973). Density may also sometimes be a disadvantage, if it leads to insulation from valuable resources or information that could be helpful. Like network density, bridging potential is evaluated using information on the presence or absence of relationships among alters. A person has bridging potential whenever two confidants are unconnected to each other. Therefore, a person's bridging potential could be quantified as the number of pairs of alters in his or her network who are not directly connected to each other—the number that reportedly "have never spoken to each other." However, it is important to recognize that some other individual apart from the respondent could serve as an indirect link between the unconnected pair. This is not likely to be the case for confidants who have had no contact with any of the respondent's other alters. Therefore, we operationalize bridging potential as a dichotomous indicator of whether there is any confidant in the respondent's network who is unconnected to all other confidants (Cornwell, 2009a, 2009b). In such cases, ego constitutes the sole bridge between this alter and others within his or her egocentric network (other bridges may exist which involve individuals outside the respondent' s egocentric network). All else equal, those who have low network density will have the most bridging potential. Therefore, it is not surprising that men, Latinos, and those in the "other" racial/ethnic category exhibited significantly less bridging potential.

Social Connectedness and Aging—Analyses

We now turn to the question of how social connectedness varies by age in the population of older Americans.[4] Figure 9.2 shows the predicted probability of having three, four, or five or more alters in one's network. These predicted probabilities were computed using a generalized ordered logit model, controlling for gender, ethnicity, retirement, widowhood, and self-rated physical health. The association between age and network size was negative and significant at $p < 0.005$, even when controlling for covariates. Models showed that older adults are about 86% as likely as those 10 years younger than them (e.g., 85-year-olds versus 75-year-olds) to have larger networks. The probability that a 57-year-old has more than four network members is 0.60, compared to 0.49 among 85-year-olds. These results are consistent with disengagement theory, which predicts a decline in interpersonal connectedness in later life. Widowhood, retirement, and health factors do not significantly alter the association between age and network size, meaning neither of these fully accounts for the association with age.

4. This section was adapted from Cornwell, B., Laumann, E. O., & Schumm, L. P. (2008). The social connectedness of older adults: A national profile. *American Sociological Review, 73*, 185–203.

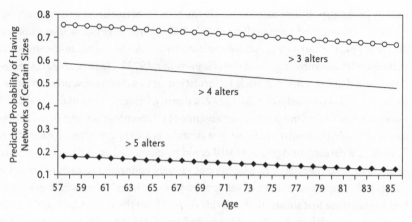

Figure 9.2: Predicted network sizes of older adults, by age.
Source: Cornwell et al., 2008.

Figure 9.3 presents findings from separate ordered logit models, predicting three forms of community involvement—religious services, neighborly socializing, and volunteering. All results control for marital status, ethnicity, education, number of children, self-rated health, functional health (problems with activities of daily living), network size, and religion. Lines displaying religious service participation and volunteer participation also control for retirement and widowhood ("life course factors"). A key finding here is that the oldest adults are the most connected to the community. A 10-year increment in age is associated with a 29% increment in the odds of socializing with neighbors on a weekly basis, but this relationship is no longer significant after controlling for covariates. Figure 9.3 also shows the association between age and the predicted probability of weekly socializing with neighbors before and after controlling for life course factors. The results show that transitioning to retirement is associated with an increase of .225 in the log odds of socializing more frequently with neighbors (odds ratio, 1.25). Older adults are consistently more involved in religious services as well. A 10-year increment in age is associated with a 40% increment in the odds of attending religious services at least once a week. The predicted probability of weekly religious services attendance is 0.42 among the youngest respondents, and 0.65 among the oldest. The oldest adults in this sample are also more likely to volunteer frequently. A 10-year increment in age is associated with a 20% increment in the odds of weekly volunteering. The predicted probability of an 85-year-old volunteering at least once a week is 0.29, compared to a 0.20 probability for a 57-year-old.

Our analyses suggest that old age is indeed related to several aspects of social network connectedness. The oldest-old have smaller social networks, but age is positively correlated with frequency of socializing with neighbors, attending religious services, and volunteering in this age category. We therefore find that older adults' social lives are more complicated than many existing perspectives would have predicted. This finding is reconcilable with work that emphasizes adaptation to changes accompanying

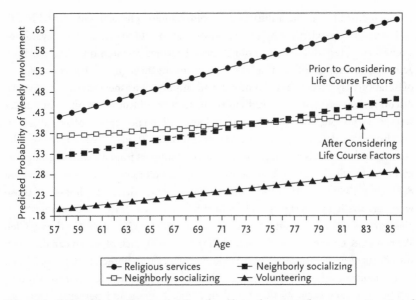

Figure 9.3: Older adults' predicted probability of weekly involvement in three community-oriented social activities by age.
Source: Cornwell et al., 2008.

the aging process (e.g., Utz, Carr, Nesse, & Wortman, 2002). Interpersonal network ties are difficult to control and predict, since they are a product of both one's own and one's network members' behaviors and experiences. Older adults often contend with sudden and irreversible changes to their interpersonal networks. Close confidants or intimate partners who die are not necessarily replaced quickly or easily. In this light, the greater involvement of the oldest adults in our sample in social organizations could be understood as an effort to regain control over their social environment (Baltes & Carstensen, 1996). If this is the case, then it is fair to say that older adults are not simply reacting to increasing age and infirmity passively; rather, they are actively involved in constructing their social world in a way that could build social capital and create opportunities for receiving social support in times of need.

Connectedness, Isolation, and Health

While these findings suggest that earlier theories have overstated the level of social isolation at older ages, they also show that isolation might be a problem for some nontrivial portion of older adults.[5] We are also interested in knowing whether social

5. This section was adapted from York Cornwell, E., & Waite, L. J. (2009). Social disconnectedness, perceived isolation, and health among older adults. *Journal of Health and Social Behavior, 50*, 31–48, as well as York Cornwell, E., & Waite, L. J. (2012). Social network resources and management of hypertension: Evidence from a national sample of older adults. *Journal Health and Social Behavior, 52*, 215–231.

connectedness can make a difference to older adults' physical and mental health and, accordingly, whether it is worth investing in interventions that develop or strengthen older adults' social connections. Previous research on social isolation across age groups points to a variety of mechanisms through which various aspects of isolation may affect health. Some mechanisms link two aspects of isolation, social disconnectedness and perceived isolation, to worse health outcomes in similar ways. For example, both social connectedness and the perception of available support buffer the deleterious effects of stress exposure (Thoits, 1992, 2011). Socially connected individuals may receive instrumental support from network members or coresidents, which may assist in active coping and ultimately reduce stress (Waite & Hughes, 1999). Similarly, individuals who rarely experience loneliness and those who perceive high levels of social support tend to have more active coping strategies, greater self-esteem, and greater sense of control (Cornman, Goldman, Glei, Weinstein, & Chang, 2003; Ernst & Cacioppo, 1999), each of which can diminish the effects of stress (Pearlin, 1989; Steptoe, Owen, Kunz-Ebrect, & Brydon, 2004).

Evidence of other mechanisms that link one or the other form of isolation to health outcomes suggests that social disconnectedness and perceived isolation may separately affect health. For example, social connectedness, indicated by one's social network and level of social participation, can provide access to material resources such as information, transportation, financial loans, or emotional support (Ellison & George, 1994; Haines & Hurlbert, 1992; Lin, 2001). Aspects of perceived isolation are often linked to health outcomes through different mechanisms. The modification of health-related behaviors has not been found to account for the link between loneliness or the perception of a lack of social support and worse health outcomes (Hawkley et al., 2003; Seeman, 2000; Steptoe et al., 2004). However, a large body of research suggests a potentially strong correlation between perceived isolation and mental health problems, especially depression (Weeks, Michela, Peplau, & Bragg, 1980). Loneliness is a key predictor of depression among older adults, in particular (Cacioppo, Hughes, Waite, Hawkley, & Thisted, 2006; Heikkinen & Kauppinen, 2004). Similarly, perceived social support is more important for mental health outcomes than indicators of social connectedness, such as received support (Krause, 1987) and network size (Brummett, Barefoot, Siegler, & Clapp-Channing, 2001). To the extent that mental health problems put individuals at risk for physical health problems (Mehta, Yaffe, & Covinsky, 2002; Sorkin, Rook, & Lu, 2002), perceived isolation may affect physical health through its impact on mental health.

Previous research has employed indicators of numerous aspects of isolation, but no single indicator captures the complex nature of social isolation. One of the strengths of the NSHAP data is its variety of social connectedness measures. We construct a *social disconnectedness scale* based on eight items assessing respondents' lack of connectedness to other individuals and social groups. The scale has acceptable internal consistency, with an alpha of .73 and moderate to strong item-rest correlations. Social network characteristics comprise four of the scale items: (1) social network size indicates the number of network members identified by the respondent; (2) the proportion of social network members who live in the household, with a high proportion of network members in the home resulting in relatively fewer connections with individuals outside the home; (3) social network range indicates the extent to which the respondent is connected to a variety of types of individuals (e.g., spouse, friend, coworker); and (4) frequency of contact with network members indicates an individual's exposure to his or her network members. The social disconnectedness scale also incorporates the number of friends reported by each respondent and lack of participation in social activities outside of the home (e.g., how often they volunteer, attend meetings of an organized group, and socialize with friends and family). The eight variables are standardized, their values are averaged, and the computed scores are reversed so that they indicate disconnectedness rather than connectedness.

We measured perceived isolation using a scale combining nine items that assess loneliness and perceived (lack of) social support. The *perceived isolation scale* has acceptable internal consistency ($\alpha = .70$) and moderate to strong item-rest correlations. The nine items in the scale are as follows: how often the respondent feels he or she can open up to his or her family; how often the respondent feels he or she can rely on his or her family; the same two questions again, asked about friends and the respondent's spouse; and the three items comprising the loneliness scale developed by Hughes et al. (2004). The *perceived isolation scale* is constructed by standardizing each of these items and then averaging the scores. Scores on the scale range from -0.98 to 3.63, with a weighted mean of -0.01 and a standard deviation of 0.59. Higher scores indicate greater perceived isolation.

Our dependent variables include self-rated measures of physical and mental health status, as well as an indicator of depressive symptoms. *Self-rated physical health* was assessed using a standard question: "Would you say your health is excellent, very good, good, fair, or poor?" This question is widely used in epidemiological and population-based survey research. Although it does not directly define health, individuals' self-ratings of their overall health have been shown in numerous studies to be predictive of mortality (Idler & Benyamini, 1997). The effectiveness of the self-rated health measure may stem, in part, from the fact that it reflects physical health status, symptoms, function, and health behaviors (Fayers & Sprangers, 2002), as well as emotional, spiritual, or psychological characteristics that may be important health trajectories (Idler, Hudson, & Leventhal, 1999; Molarius & Janson, 2002). The measure is reliable across age, gender, and racial and ethnic groups (Finch, Hummer, Reindl, & Vega, 2002; Johnson & Wolinsky, 1994).

We also use a single item capturing *self-rated mental health*. Following the self-rated physical health question, respondents were asked, "What about your emotional or mental health? Is it excellent, very good, good, fair, or poor?" This measure has not been validated against clinical assessments of mental health disorders, but the distribution of NSHAP responses mirrors that found in recent research

(Mulvaney-Day, Alegria, & Sribney, 2007). Both self-rated physical health and self-rated mental health are coded so that higher values indicate better health.

A lack of social connectedness is not always accompanied by feelings of loneliness and isolation. In fact, the correlation between social disconnectedness and perceived isolation is only weak to moderate in strength ($r = .25$, $p <.001$) within this population-based sample of older adults. Since objective and subjective isolation are conceptually distinct and are not strongly correlated, it is possible that they are independently associated with health.

Figures 9.4 and 9.5 consider both social disconnectedness and perceived isolation simultaneously, using ordinal logit models controlling for age, gender, ethnicity, education, and marital status. Results show that both disconnectedness and perceived isolation are independently associated with poorer self-rated health. An increment of one standard deviation in social disconnectedness is associated with about 30% lower odds of rating one's health above a given category. Similarly, older adults whose perceived isolation score is one standard deviation above average face 30% lower odds of being above any category of self-rated health. Older adults who are socially connected or perceive high levels of support and companionship from others have a nearly 70% chance of reporting very good or excellent health. However, those who report extreme social disconnectedness or perceived isolation have only a 40% chance of reporting very good or excellent health.

Figure 9.5 presents results from ordered logistic regression analyses predicting self-rated mental health. Net of a number of sociodemographic covariates, social disconnectedness and perceived isolation, are each negatively related to self-rated mental health. Perceived isolation, however, has a decidedly stronger association than social disconnectedness with mental health. The strong relationship between

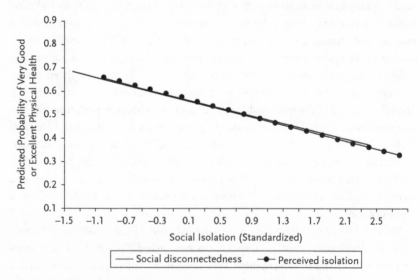

Figure 9.4: Self-rated physical health, social connectedness and perceived isolation.
Source: Cornwell et al., 2008.

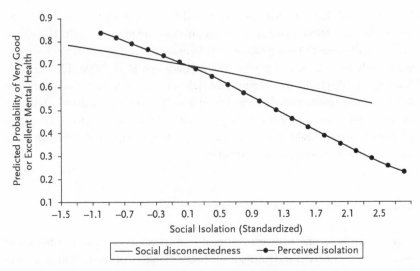

Figure 9.5: Self-rated mental health, social connectedness and perceived isolation.
Source: York Cornwell & Waite, 2009.

perceived isolation and mental health is in line with previous research suggesting that loneliness is particularly deleterious for mental health (Cacioppo et al., 2006; Heikkinen & Kauppinen, 2004). An increase of one standard deviation on the perceived isolation scale is associated with about a one-half reduction in the odds of having better mental health. However, the health risks of disconnectedness appear to operate through the strong, negative association between perceived isolation and mental health. When we control for perceived isolation, social disconnectedness has only a slight association with the probability of having very good or excellent mental health. Individuals who do not perceive themselves to be isolated have a nearly 85% chance of having very good or excellent mental health. But those who feel extremely isolated have only about a 25% chance of claiming very good or excellent mental health.

Our findings that two distinct forms of social isolation are both associated with worse physical and mental health should not come as a surprise. The variety of operationalizations of social isolation in previous research has made it difficult to determine whether particular aspects of isolation are more or less consequential for health. Our findings demonstrate that social disconnectedness and perceived isolation are not interchangeable indicators. Instead, they have separate and distinct associations with physical and mental health. Social disconnectedness is associated with worse physical health, regardless of whether it prompts feelings of loneliness or a perceived lack of social support. On the other hand, at all levels of social disconnectedness (or connectedness), the perception that one lacks social resources may take a toll on physical health.

With respect to physical health outcomes, then, both situational and perceived isolation matter. This is not the case with respect to mental health. The relationship between social disconnectedness and mental health appears to operate through the strong association between perceived isolation and mental health. These findings support research noting robust links between aspects of subjective isolation, particularly loneliness, and mental health (Cacioppo et al., 2006; Heikkinen & Kauppinen, 2004). The role of perceived isolation as a mediator in the association between social disconnectedness and mental health has not been demonstrated so clearly in prior work. Our results suggest that socially disconnected older adults have worse mental health only to the extent that they feel isolated. This is an interesting finding that deserves more attention.

Social Networks and Disease Management

This picture is in line with conventional understandings of connectedness and health: More connected, less isolated individuals should be better off than those who lack connections or perceive themselves as alone.[6] NSHAP data can also be used to address a long-standing but seldom examined question about social networks: When do social networks help the person to achieve better health, and when do they harm? According to the IBM model, network connectedness does not generate returns to health by itself, but only under particular conditions, when social connections conduct forms of capital to the focal person. Presently, it is an established topic to investigate contagion of poor health through social networks (e.g., Christakis & Fowler, 2007); it is also possible, however, to imagine burdensome or stressful networks. Some studies have found negative associations between network size and disease management (e.g., Kaplan & Hartwell, 1987), which may reflect social obligations and responsibilities that take time away from self-care. We now probe this area of poor health arising from social networks, using biomeasured and self-reported hypertension.

We focus on hypertension for two reasons. First, about two thirds of older adults have hypertension, yet rates of management are relatively low. Roughly a quarter of those with hypertension are unaware of their condition, and more than half are uncontrolled. Rates of uncontrolled hypertension are even higher among African American older adults (Ostchega Dillon, Hughes, Carroll, & Yoon, 2007). Second, there are reasons to believe that social context may play a particularly important role in the diagnosis and control of hypertension. Because hypertension is commonly asymptomatic, individuals are unlikely to seek treatment because of discomfort or declining function. Therefore, social capital factors that encourage individuals to undergo preventive screenings are critical. Once diagnosed, management of hypertension involves substantial daily effort, including multiple antihypertensive medications, weight reduction, and changes in physical activity, diet, and alcohol and tobacco use

---

6. This section was adapted from York Cornwell, E., & Waite, L. J. (2012). Social network resources and management of hypertension: Evidence from a national sample of older adults. *Journal Health and Social Behavior, 52*, 215–231

(National Heart, Lung and Blood Institute, 2003). Social network ties and network-based resources such as support may promote or impede these behaviors.

Interactions with network members that involve discussions about health may be particularly efficacious for disease diagnosis and management. Network ties can serve as a conduit for information (Berkman, Glass, Rissette, & Seeman, 2000), particularly regarding health-related issues (e.g., see Kinney, Bloor, Martin, & Sandler, 2005; Perry & Pescosolido, 2010). Research on health communication, for example, indicates that "storytelling" about health experiences increases health knowledge within local networks (Kim, Moran, Wilkin, & Ball-Rokeach, 2011) and families (Warren-Findlow, Seymour, & Shenk, 2010). Pecchioni and Sparks (2007) found that many patients with cancer turn first to family members and close friends for information following diagnosis, and they report greatest satisfaction with the health information obtained through these sources, perhaps because their relationships tend to be imbued with trust and intimacy. These types of health-related discussions may also constitute key mechanisms through which family and friends attempt to control health behaviors

We combine self-reported and biological measures to assess hypertension diagnosis and control. Respondents reported whether medical doctors had ever told them that they had high blood pressure or hypertension. In addition, each respondent underwent two seated blood pressure measurements. If the two readings differed by more than 20 mm Hg systolic or 14 mm Hg diastolic, interviewers collected a third blood pressure reading. Respondents whose mean blood pressures (on the basis of all readings taken) exceeded either 140 mm Hg systolic or 90 mm Hg diastolic were considered hypertensive. We use lower cutoffs of either 130 mm Hg systolic or 90 mm Hg diastolic for respondents who reported that they had been diagnosed with diabetes (National Heart, Lung, and Blood Institute, 2003).

On the basis of self-reported hypertension and blood pressure, we place each respondent into one of four categories: *Nonhypertensive* ($n = 687$, 25.9%) have normal blood pressure and did not self-report hypertension; *undiagnosed hypertensive* ($n = 445$, 16.7%) did not report that they had hypertension but had elevated blood pressure; *controlled hypertensive* ($n = 614$, 23.1%) reported that they had hypertension, but blood pressure was normal; and finally *uncontrolled hypertensive* ($n = 912$, 34.3%), who said they had hypertension and who indeed had elevated blood pressure. Note that the modal category is uncontrolled hypertension, and about half of the older adults in our sample had undiagnosed or uncontrolled hypertension.

We found that social networks were particularly beneficial for disease management when they provide access to health-relevant information. Using a multinomial logit model, we predicted membership in the aforementioned four categories, using network size, frequency of interaction with confidants, discussing health with confidants, and instrumental and emotional support as independent variables. We also included an interaction between network size and heath communication. There was a significant interaction term crossing network size with network-based health communication, indicating that the association between network size and undiagnosed hypertension varies according to the level of health communication. A similar pattern was observed with respect to uncontrolled hypertension. Figure 9.6 depicts this pattern by showing predicted probabilities of uncontrolled hypertension calculated from model 1. We allow network size to vary from one to seven and use values for network-based health discussions that correspond with the original question: 1 indicates that the respondent is "not likely" to discuss health with his or her network members, 2 indicates that he or she is "somewhat likely" to discuss health, and 3 indicates that he or she is "very likely" to discuss health. The predicted probabilities illustrate that those who have larger networks have lower risk for uncontrolled hypertension, provided that they are very likely to discuss health problems with their network members. For those who are less likely to talk about health problems with their family and friends, the risk for unmanaged hypertension increases as network size increases. Note that individuals with small networks, who do not talk to their confidants about their health, are less likely to have undiagnosed hypertension. One reason for this may be that stress is associated with those individuals in one's network to whom one is not particularly open, so the absence of such persons may actually be a health benefit.

Older adults who have larger social networks, and are likely to talk with their network members about health problems, have lower risks for undiagnosed and uncontrolled hypertension. These individuals may benefit from others' advice, experiences, and expertise regarding health care and disease management (Perry & Pescosolido, 2010; Warren-Findlow et al., 2010). But for those who are unlikely

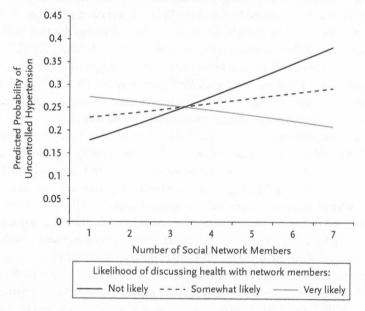

Figure 9.6: Uncontrolled hypertension by social network size, for varying levels of discussing health with social network members.
Source: York Cornwell & Waite, 2012.

to communicate about health, the risk for undiagnosed and uncontrolled hypertension increases with network size. This contradicts a general assumption that having more social relationships is always beneficial. Our results suggest that when lines of communication about health are closed, relationships may present more costs than benefits. In the final section of this chapter, we present another example of relationships creating health problems, instead of good health, using NSHAP's rich information about sexuality at older ages.

Sexual Function and Relationships

Sexuality represents an essential nexus for the interaction among social life, culturally determined beliefs and practices, psychological processes, and the biological mechanisms of aging, health, and disease.[7] Sexual activity and functioning are determined by the interaction of each partner's sexual capacity, motivation, conduct, and attitudes. They are further shaped by the quality and condition of the dyadic relationship itself. For older adults in the generations represented in NSHAP, marriage provides the social and emotional context for the vast majority of all sexual activity. Marriage also provides opportunity for intimacy and improves sexual satisfaction (Waite & Joyner, 2001).

Thus, the IBM conceptualizes partnered sexual behavior as a key feature of the overall relational context within which health is jointly produced. In turn, both physical and mental health have a strong impact on the capacity and motivation for sex (Das, Laumann, & Waite, 2012; Laumann, Das, & Waite, 2008; Lindau et al., 2007); sexual well-being is not only a key component of healthy aging but also has a mutually constitutive relationship with health. As with other relational factors, this important asset also disappears with the loss of a partner.

We will begin by providing a basic description of sexual function at older ages. Figure 9.7 shows the probability of having had sex with a partner in the past year, by gender and levels of self-rated physical health. The probability of being sexually active declines steadily with age and is uniformly lower among women than among men. In addition, the likelihood of being sexually active is positively associated with self-reported health. The odds ratio for being sexually active among those who reported their health to be "poor" or "fair" as compared with those reporting "very good" or "excellent" health was 0.21 (95% confidence interval [CI], 0.14 to 0.32) for men and 0.36 (95% CI, 0.25 to 0.51) for women. At any given age, women are less likely than men to be in a marital or other intimate relationship. This results from the

---

7. This section was adapted from Waite, L. J., Laumann, E. O., Das, A., & Schumm, L. P. (2009). Sexuality: Measures of partnerships, practices, attitudes, and problems in the National Social Life, Health, and Aging Study. *Journals of Gerontology Series B: Psychological Sciences and Social Sciences, 64B,* i56–i66, as well as Cornwell, B., & Laumann, E. O. (2011). Network position and sexual dysfunction: Implications of partner betweenness for men. *American Journal of Sociology, 117,* 172–208.

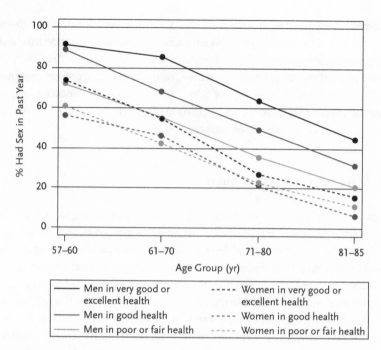

Figure 9.7: Sex in the past year over gender and age group.
Source: Lindau et al., 2007.

tendency of women to marry or partner with men who are somewhat older, combined with the longer life expectancy of women (Lindau et al., 2007). Thus, women are much more likely than men to experience the death of their spouse or partner and less likely to repartner if this happens. Of the 1,198 men and 815 women in a relationship, only 3 men and 5 women reported that the relationship was with someone of the same sex. Among those who were not in a relationship, 22% of men and 4% of women reported being sexually active in the previous year.

Among men and women of the same age, men with a spousal or other intimate relationship were more likely to be sexually active than women with such a relationship. The difference in the rates of sexual activity between men and women was considerably smaller among those with a spousal or intimate relationship; this difference reflects, in part, the disparity in ages between men and women within current relationships. Among all current marital and intimate relationships in the sample, the mean (± SD) difference in age between male and female partners was 3.2 years (SD = 5.7).

Among respondents who were sexually active, the frequency of sex was lower among those who were 75 to 85 years of age than among younger persons. Even in this oldest age group, 54% of sexually active persons reported having sex at least two to three times per month, and 23% reported having sex once a week or more. Fifty-eight percent of sexually active respondents in the youngest age group reported engaging in oral sex, as compared with 31% in the oldest age group.

Table 9.2 lists the prevalence of sexual problems among respondents who were sexually active and the associations of these problems with the respondents' age. Approximately half of all respondents (both men and women) reported having at least one bothersome sexual problem, and almost one third of men and women reported having at least two bothersome sexual problems. Among men, the most prevalent sexual problems and the corresponding percentages of those who were bothered by them were difficulty in achieving or maintaining an erection (37% and 90%, respectively), lack of interest in sex (28% and 65%), climaxing too quickly (28% and 71%), anxiety about performance (27% and 75%), and inability to climax (20% and 73%). For women, the most common sexual problems and the percentages of those who were bothered by them were lack of interest in sex (43% and 61%, respectively), difficulty with lubrication (39% and 68%), inability to climax (34% and 59%), finding sex not pleasurable (23% and 64%), and pain (most commonly felt at the vagina during entry) (17% and 97%). As compared with respondents who rated their health as being excellent, very good, or good, respondents who rated their health as being fair or poor had a higher prevalence of several problems, including difficulty with erection or lubrication, pain, and lack of pleasure.

Our findings indicate that the majority of older adults are engaged in spousal or other intimate relationships and regard sexuality as an important part of life. The

Table 9.2. PERCENT OF RESPONDENTS WITH SEXUAL DYSFUNCTIONS AMONG OLDER MEN AND WOMEN, ACROSS AGE GROUPS

	Age Group		
Dysfunction	Aged 57–64	Aged 65–74	Aged 75–85
Lack of interest in sex			
Men	28.2%	28.5%	24.2%
Women	44.2%	38.4%	49.3%
Erectile dysfunction			
Men	30.7%	44.6%	43.5%
Difficulty with lubrication			
Women	35.9%	43.2%	43.6%
Climaxing too quickly			
Men	29.5%	28.1%	21.3%
Inability to climax			
Men	16.2%	22.7%	33.2%
Women	34.0%	32.8%	38.2%
Anxiety about performance			
Men	25.1%	28.9%	29.3%
Women	10.4%	12.5%	9.9%

Note. All cells show percent of persons within each age category with the specific sexual dysfunction indicated in the rows.
Source: Lindau et al., 2007.

prevalence of sexual activity declines with age, yet a substantial number of men and women engage in vaginal intercourse, oral sex, and masturbation even in the eighth and ninth decades of life. The findings can be thought of as putting forth the same sort of argument as in our studies on social networks: Far from a narrative of universal decline, NSHAP's data show that sexual life, like social life, often does carry on, even for many of the oldest old. Thus, if sexual life and social life are still active at older ages, there is reason to believe that social factors could still be active in shaping older adults' sexual lives.

Consider the following network. A husband and a wife live together; there is a third alter in this network as well, and this third alter is a confidant to both the husband and the wife. Where ego is the husband, one can imagine a situation where the husband has less contact with his confidant than his wife does. Furthermore, the wife has more access to both parties than they have to each other. Drawing on social network approaches, we refer to this circumstance as *partner betweenness*. In network terms, ego's partner can inadvertently constrain his bridging potential in the joint network and is in a position to act as a mediator in the ego–confidant relationship.

Situations of betweenness could result from a number of different circumstances, ranging from an ill ego who has a very helpful partner who facilitates communication between ego and his confidants, to a domineering female partner who insists on acting as a gatekeeper, to an ego who is poorly connected in the first place and whose main source of social contact is his spouse's confidants. Regardless of its cause, given what we know from relational perspectives on gender, it is plausible that partner betweenness has important implications for men. Egos in this position no longer have exclusive access to resources from this confidant. Also, it implies that ego is dependent on their partner to some extent for continued contact with their confidant, and accordingly that ego lacks control over information in this part of his network. This may create a lack of privacy, since information that passes through this confidant is less likely to be confidential, especially if ego wishes to discuss his partner. In sum, partner betweenness proxies a number of circumstances that can block men from expressing or demonstrating key components of traditional masculinity. These results persist regardless of whether the nonspousal alter is male or female, kin or nonkin.

One study of young couples found that men who perceive that they and their partners are too dependent on their relationship have lower self-esteem, whereas perceived dependence does not trouble women in the same way (Galliher, Rotosky, Welsh, & Kawaguchi, 1999). To the extent that partner betweenness indexes lack of involvement with other social contacts, this could lower men's self-esteem, sense of control, and autonomy and, more directly, their sense of masculinity (e.g., Avison & Cairney, 2003). This could also have negative consequences for the quality of men's relationships with their female partners by engendering feelings of resentment toward them, and accordingly it could put strain on the relationship (see Foreman & Dallos, 1992).

If partner betweenness has the potential to compromise older men's gender identity and sense of autonomy, it bears investigating, since having a sense of masculinity is tied to men's sexual function (Hale & Strassberg, 1990; Laumann, Paik, & Rosen, 1999; Laumann et al., 2006; Sand, Fisher, Rosen, Heiman, & Eardley, 2008). For men, reduced autonomy, sense of control, and self-efficacy are associated with sexual function, in part because masculine identity is inextricably tied to the penis (Martino & Pallotta-Chiarolli, 2003; Zilbergeld, 1992). In the context of sexual relationships, masculinity is expressed through "erection, penetration, and climax," so it is possible that threats to masculine autonomy can physically manifest themselves in sexual problems, including erectile dysfunction (Oliffe, 2005; also see Lee & Owens, 2002). In fact, erectile dysfunction has been theorized as a loss of manhood and masculinity that is closely linked to feelings of inadequacy and weakness (Edgar, 1997; Kimmel, 1987; Lee & Owens, 2002; Leiblum & Rosen, 1991; Oliffe, 2005; Sand et al., 2008; Zilbergeld, 1992). Network autonomy may be a kind of social resource for bolstering masculine identity, and so where network autonomy is compromised by partner betweenness, older adults may experience a loss of masculine identity. Thus, in the analysis that follows, we consider implications of partner betweenness for erectile dysfunction, a key health outcome tied to masculinity.

We found that partner betweenness is a significant predictor of erectile dysfunction in logit regressions controlling for age, retirement, marriage, network proportion kin, network proportion female, coital frequency, marital quality, prostate trouble, diabetes, and self-rated health. A man whose female partner has greater contact with some of his confidants than he does is about 92% more likely to have had trouble getting or maintaining an erection than a man who has greater access than his partner does to all of his confidants (odds ratio, 1.916; 95% confidence interval, 1.274–2.881). The significance of partner betweenness is neither explained nor appreciably reduced by the inclusion of control measures.

Our main models suggested that age is positively associated with erectile dysfunction, whereas retirement is not. To push this further, a related question is whether the challenges of later life reduce or amplify the impact of partner betweenness on erectile dysfunction. To test this idea, we considered interactions between age and partner betweenness. The results of this analysis are shown in Figure 9.8. It shows that the positive association between partner betweenness and erectile dysfunction is smaller among the older age groups as compared to the youngest age group—significantly so among men between 65 and 74 years of age. Therefore, partner betweenness is more closely related to erectile dysfunction among the youngest men in the NSHAP sample. It could be that the interaction shown in Figure 9.8 is driven by a combination of factors that change throughout later life, including unmeasured facets of health, new social activities, and bereavement. This significant interaction with age may exist because age proxies this broader complex of factors. Thus, network resources may have different benefits not only for different kinds of network structure but also at different stages in the life course, reinforcing

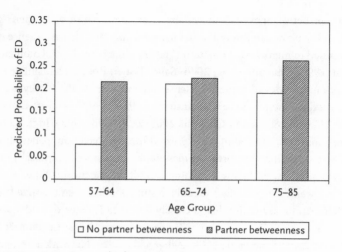

Figure 9.8: Erectile Dysfunction (ED) and partner betweenness, over age groups.
Source: Cornwell & Laumann, 2011.

the interdependency of social-structural and life course factors for generating good or ill health.

CONCLUSION

None of the findings reported earlier, unfortunately, make any use of longitudinal data, making causality almost impossible to determine. This problem is addressed by NSHAP's Wave 2 of data collection, which occurred in 2010; 2,261 respondents out of the original 3,005 were reinterviewed, meaning the first and second waves of NSHAP are able to provide researchers with some ability to separate out the effect of individual aging from chronological age. It could be that increased participation in social organization is not a result of getting older, but simply a characteristic of the cohort of older adults in our present sample. It may also be that if we were able to observe people over time, we might see that partner betweenness actually follows upon erectile dysfunction rather than preceding it.

In addition to this, NSHAP is currently limited in how well it can test the IBM, because while the IBM holds that health is jointly produced in relationships, for the most important relationship for older adults, their spouse, we only have information on one half of the marital dyad at Wave 1. Wave 2 addressed this limitation by conducting interviews with all available spouses and cohabiting partners of the Wave 1 respondents. These 955 individuals, all members of intimate dyads, were added to the Wave 2 sample.

Understanding health is not only a matter of understanding what goes on under the skin or in the mind. Health may ultimately reside within the person, but the precipitants of good health are also environmental. Human beings are often deeply embedded in networks of support, such as families, households and neighborhoods, or organizations with different functions; sometimes these bring conflict, demands, and burdens that threaten the well-being of older adults. We would therefore contend that understanding the role of social relationships and the social environment is essential for understanding the dynamic processes through which health is produced.

REFERENCES

Antonucci, T. C., & Akiyama, H. (1995). Convoys of social relations: Family and friendships within a life span context. In R. Blieszner & V. H. Bedford (Eds.), *Handbook of aging and the family* (pp. 355–371). Westport, CT: Greenwood.

Atchley, R. C. (1989). The continuity theory of normal aging. *Gerontologist, 29*, 183–190.

Avison, W. R., & Cairney, J. (2003). Social structure, stress and personal control. In S. H. Zarit, L. I. Pearlin, & K. W. Schaie (Eds.), *Personal control in social and life contexts* (pp. 127–164). New York, NY: Springer.

Baltes, M. M., & Carstensen, L. L. (1996). The process of successful ageing. *Ageing and Society, 16*, 397–422.

Berkman, L. F., Glass, T., Rissette, I., & Seeman, T. E. (2000). From social integration to health: Durkheim in the new millenium. *Social Science and Medicine, 51*, 843–857.

Brummett, B. H., Barefoot, J. C., Siegler, I. C., & Clapp-Channing, N. E. (2001). Characteristics of socially-isolated patients with coronary artery disease who are at elevated risk for mortality. *Psychosomatic Medicine, 63*, 267–272.

Burgess, E. W. (1960). *Ageing in western societies.* Chicago, IL: University of Chicago Press.

Burt, R. (1984). Network items and the general social survey. *Social Networks, 6*, 293–340.

Burt, R. (1992). *Structural holes: The social structure of competition.* Cambridge, MA: Harvard University Press.

Burt, R. (2005). *Brokerage and closure: An introduction of social capital.* Oxford, UK: Oxford University Press.

Cacioppo, J. T., Hawkley, L. C., Berntson, G. G., Ernst, J. M., Gibbs, A. C., Stickgold, R., & Hobson, J. A. (2002). Do lonely days invade the nights? Potential social modulation of sleep efficiency. *Psychological Science, 13*, 384–387.

Cacioppo, J. T., Hughes, M. E., Waite, L. J., Hawkley, L. C., & Thisted, R. A. (2006). Loneliness as a specific risk factor for depressive symptoms: Cross-sectional and longitudinal analyses. *Psychology and Aging, 21*, 140–151.

Cavan, R. S., Burgess, E. W., Havinghurst, R. J., & Goldhammer, H. (1949). *Personal adjustment in old age.* Chicago, IL: Science Research Associates.

Christakis, N. A., & Fowler, J. H. (2007). The spread of obesity in a large social network over 32 years. *New England Journal of Medicine, 357*, 370–379.

Cornman, J. C., Goldman, N., Glei, D. A., Weinstein, M., & Chang, M-C. (2003). Social ties and perceived support: Two dimensions of social relationships and health among the elderly in Taiwan. *Journal of Aging and Health, 15*, 616–644.

Cornwell, B. (2009a). Good health and the bridging of structural holes. *Social Networks, 31*, 92–103.

Cornwell, B. (2009b). Network bridging potential in later life: Life-course experiences and social network position. *Journal of Aging and Health, 21*, 129–154.

Cornwell, B., & Laumann, E. O. (2011). Network position and sexual dysfunction: Implications of partner betweenness for men. *American Journal of Sociology, 117*, 172–208

Cornwell, B., Laumann, E. O., & Schumm, L. P. (2008). The social connectedness of older adults: A national profile. *American Sociological Review, 73*, 185–203.

Cornwell, B., Schumm, L. P., Laumann, E. O., & Graber, J. (2009). Social networks in the NSHAP study: Rationale, measurement, and preliminary findings. *Journals of Gerontology Series B: Psychological Sciences and Social Sciences, 64B*(Suppl. 1), i47–i55.

Cowgill, D. O. (1986). *Aging around the world*. Belmont, CA: Wadsworth.

Cumming, E., & Henry, W. E. (1961). *Growing old: The process of disengagement*. New York, NY: Basic Books.

Das, A., Laumann, E. O., & Waite, L. J. (2012). Sexual expression over the life course: Results from three landmark surveys. In J. Delamater & L. Carpenter (Eds.), *Sexualities over the life course: Emerging perspectives* (pp. 236–259). New York, NY: New York University Press.

Edgar, D. (1997). *Men, mateship, marriage*. Sydney, Australia: Harper Collins.

Elder, G. H., Jr. (1985). *Life course dynamics*. Ithaca, NY: Cornell University Press.

Ellison, C. G., & George, L. K. (1994). Religious involvement, social ties and social support in a Southeastern community. *Journal for the Scientific Study of Religion, 33*, 46–61.

Ernst, J. M., & Cacioppo, J. T. (1999). Lonely hearts: Psychological perspectives on loneliness. *Applied and Preventative Psychology, 8*, 1–22.

Fayers, P. M., & Sprangers, M. A. G. (2002). Understanding self-rated health. *Lancet, 359*, 187–188.

Finch, B. K., Hummer, R. A., Reindl, M., & Vega, W. A. (2002). Validity of self-rated health among Latino(a)s. *Journal of Epidemiology, 155*, 755–759.

Fiori, K. L., Antonucci, T. C., & Cortina, K. S. (2006). Social network typologies and mental health among older adults. *Journals of Gerontology Series B: Psychological Sciences and Social Sciences, 61*, P25–P32.

Foreman, S., & Dallos, R. (1992). Inequalities of power and sexual problems. *Journal of Family Therapy, 14*, 349–369.

Galliher, R. V., Rotosky, S. S., Welsh, D. P., & Kawaguchi, M. C. (1999). Power and psychological well-being in late adolescent romantic relationships. *Sex Roles, 40*, 689–710.

George, L. K. (1993). Sociological perspectives on life transitions. *Annual Review of Sociology, 19*, 353–373.

Granovetter, M. S. (1973). The strength of weak ties. *American Journal of Sociology, 78*, 1360–1380.

Haines, V. A., & Hurlbert, J. S. (1992). Network range and health. *Journal of Health and Social Behavior, 33*, 254–266.

Haines, V. A., Hurlbert, J. S., & Beggs, J. J. (1996). Exploring the determinants of support provision: Provider characteristics, personal networks, community contexts and support following life events. *Journal of Health and Social Behavior, 37*, 252–264.

Hale, V. E., & Strassberg, D. S. (1990). The role of anxiety on sexual arousal. *Archives of Sexual Behavior, 19*, 569–658.

Hawkley, L. C., Burleson, M. H., Berntson, G. G., & Cacioppo, J. T. (2003). Loneliness in everyday life: Cardiovascular activity, psychosocial context and health behaviors. *Journal of Personality and Social Psychology, 85*, 105–120.

Hawkley, L. C., Thisted, R. A., & Cacioppo, J. T. (2009). Loneliness predicts reduced physical activity: Cross-sectional and longitudinal analyses. *Health Psychology, 28*, 354–363.

Heikkinen, R-L., & Kauppinen, M. (2004). Depressive symptoms in late life: A 10-year follow-up. *Archives of Gerontology and Geriatrics, 38*, 239–250.

Holt-Lunstad, J., & Birmingham, W. (2008). Is there something unique about marriage? The relative impact of marital status, relationship quality and network social support on ambulatory blood pressure and mental health. *Annals of Behavioral Medicine, 35*, 239–244.

Hughes, M. E., Waite, L. J., Hawkley, L. C., & Cacioppo, J. T. (2004). A short scale for measuring loneliness in large surveys: Results from two population-based studies. *Reseach on Aging, 26*, 655–672.

Hurlbert, J. S., Haines, V. A., & Beggs, J. J. (2000). Core networks and tie activation: What kinds of routine networks allocate resources in nonroutine situations? *American Sociological Review, 65*, 598–618.

Idler, E., & Benyamini, Y. (1997). Self-rated health and mortality: A review of twenty-seven community studies. *Journal of Health and Social Behavior, 38*, 21–37.

Idler, E. L., Hudson, S. V., & Leventhal, H. (1999). The meanings of self-rated health: A qualitative and quantitative approach. *Reseach on Aging, 21*, 458–476.

Johnson, R. J., & Wolinsky, F. D. (1994). Gender, race and health: The structure of health status among older adults. *Gerontologist, 34*, 24–35.

Kaplan, R. M., & Hartwell, S. L. (1987). Differential effects of social support and social networks on physiological and social outcomes in men and women with type II diabetes mellitus. *Health Psychology, 6*, 387–398.

Kim, Y-C., Moran, M. B., Wilkin, H. A., & Ball-Rokeach, S. J. (2011). Integrated connection to neighborhood storytelling network, education and chronic disease knowledge among African Americans and Latinos in Los Angeles. *Journal of Health Communication, 16*, 393–415.

Kimmel, M. S. (1987). *Changing men: New directions in research on men and masculinity.* Newbury Park, CA: Sage.

Kinney, A. Y., Bloor, L. E., Martin, C., & Sandler, R. S. (2005). Social ties and colorectal cancer screening among blacks and whites in North Carolina. *Cancer Epidemiology, Biomarkers and Prevention, 14*, 182–189.

Krause, N. (1987). Satisfaction with social support and self-rated health in older adults. *Gerontologist, 27*, 301–308.

Laumann, E. O., Das, A., & Waite, L. J. (2008). Sexual dysfunction among older adults: Prevalence and risk factors from a nationally representative U.S. probability sample of men and women 57–85 years of age prevalence. *Journal of Sexual Medicine, 5*, 2300–2311.

Laumann, E. O., Paik, A., Glasser, D. B., Kang, J.-H., Wang, T., Levinson, B.,...Gingell, C. (2006). A cross-national study of subjective sexual well-being among older women and men: Findings from the Global Study of Sexual Attitudes and Behaviors. *Archives of Sexual Behavior, 35*, 143–159.

Laumann, E. O., Paik, A., & Rosen, R. C. (1999). Sexual dysfunction in the U.S.: Prevalence and predictors. *Journal of the American Medical Association, 281*, 537–544.

Lee, C., & Owens, R. G. (2002). *The psychology of men's health.* Philadelphia, PA: Open University Press.

Leiblum, S. R., & Rosen, R. C. (1991). Couples therapy for erectile disorder: Conceptual and clinical considerations. *Journal of Sex and Marital Therapy, 17*, 147–159.

Lemon, B. W., Bengtson, V. L., & Peterson, J. A. (1972). An exploration of the activity theory of aging: Activity types and life satisfaction among in-movers to a retirement community. *Journal of Gerontology, 27*, 511–523.

Lin, N. (2001). *Social capital: A theory of social structure and action.* Cambridge, UK: Cambridge University Press.

Lin, N., Woelfel, M. W., & Light, S. C. (1985). The buffering effect of social support subsequent to an important life event. *Journal of Health and Social Behavior, 26*, 247–263.

Lindau, S., Schumm, L. P., Laumann, E., Levinsion, W., O'Muircheartaigh, C., & Waite, L. (2007). A study of sexuality and health among older adults in the United States. *New England Journal of Medicine, 357*, 762–774.

Lindau, S. T., Laumann, E. O., Levinson, W., & Waite, L. J. (2003). Synthesis of scientific disciplines in pursuit of health: The interactive biopsychosocial model. *Perspectives in Biology and Medicine, 46*(3 Suppl.), S74–S86.

Luo, Y., Hawkley, L. C., Waite, L. J., & Cacioppo, J. T. (2012). Loneliness, health and mortality in old age: A national longitudinal study. *Social Science and Medicine, 74*, 907–914.

Luo, Y., & Waite, L. J. (2011). Mistreatment and psychological well-being among older adults: Exploring the role of psychosocial resources and deficits. *Journals of Gerontology Series B: Psychological Sciences and Social Sciences, 66*, 217–229.

Marsden, P. V. (1987). Core discussion networks of Americans. *American Sociological Review, 52*, 122–131.

Marin, A. (2004). Are respondents more likely to list alters with certain characteristics? Implications for name generator data. *Social Networks, 26*, 289–307.

Martino, W., & Pallotta-Chiarolli, M. (2003). *"So what's a boy?" Addressing issues of malculinity in schooling.* London, UK: Open University Press.

McPherson, J. M., Smith-Lovin, L., & Brashears, M. E. (2006). Social isolation in America: Changes in core discussion networks over two decades. *American Sociological Review, 71*, 353–375.

Mehta, K. M., Yaffe, K., & Covinsky, K. E. (2002). Cognitive impairment, depressive symptoms and functional decline in older people. *Journal of the American Geriatrics Society, 50*, 1045–1050.

Molarius, A., & Janson, S. (2002). Self-rated health, chronic diseases and symptoms among middle-aged and elderly men and women. *Journal of Clinical Epidemiology, 55*, 364–370.

Mulvaney-Day, N. E., Alegria, M., & Sribney, W. (2007). Social cohesion, social support and health among Latinos in the United States. *Social Science and Medicine, 64*, 477–495.

Munch, A., McPherson, J. M., & Smith-Lovin, L. (1997). Gender, chidren and social contact: The effects of childrearing for men and women. *American Sociological Review, 62*, 509–520.

National Heart, Lung, and Blood Institute. (2003). *The seventh report of the Joint National Committee on Prevention, Detection, Evaluation and Treatment of High Blood Pressure.* Bethesda, MD: US Department of Health and Human Services.

Oliffe, J. (2005). Constructions of masculinity following prostatectomy-induced impotence. *Social Science and Medicine, 60*, 2249–2259.

Ostchega, Y., Dillon, C. F., Hughes, J. P., Carroll, M., & Yoon, S. (2007). Trends in hypertension prevalence, awareness, treatment and control in older U.S. adults: Data from the National Health and Nutrition Examination Survey 1988 to 2004. *Journal of the American Geriatrics Society, 55*, 1056–1065.

Pearlin, L. I. (1989). The sociological study of stress. *Journal of Health and Social Behavior, 20*, 241–256.

Pecchioni, L. L., & Sparks, L. (2007). Health information sources of individuals with cancer and their family members. *Health Communication, 21*, 143–151.

Perry, B. L., & Pescosolido, B. A. (2010). Functional specificity in discussion networks: The influence of general and problem-specific networks on health outcomes. *Social Networks, 32*, 345–357.

Rowe, J. W., & Kahn, R. L. (1998). *Successful aging.* New York, NY: Patheon.

Ruan, D. (1998). The content of the General Social Survey discussion networks: an exploration of General Social Survey discussion name generator in a Chinese context. *Social Networks, 20*(3), 247–264.

Sand, M., Fisher, W., Rosen, R., Heiman, J., & Eardley, I. (2008). Erectile dysfunction and constructs of masculinity and quality of life in the Multinational Men's Attitudes to Life Events and Sexuality (MALES) Study. *Journal of Sexual Medicine, 5*, 583–594.

Seeman, T., & Berkman, L. (1988). Structural characteristics of social networks and their relationship with social support in the elderly: Who provides support? *Social Science and Medicine, 26*, 737–749.

Seeman, T. E. (2000). Health promoting effects of friends and family on health outcomes in older adults. *American Journal of Health Promotion, 14*, 362–370.

Shaw, B. A., Krause, N., Liang, J., & Bennett, J. (2007). Tracking changes in social relations throughout late life. *Journals of Gerontology Series B: Psychological Sciences and Social Sciences, 62B*, S90–S99.

Shiovitz-Ezra, S., Leitsch, S., Graber, J., & Karraker, A. (2009). Quality of life and psychological health indicators in the National Social Life, Health, and Aging Project. *Journals of Gerontology Series B: Psychological Sciences and Social Sciences, 64B* (Suppl. 1), i30–i37.

Sorkin, D., Rook, K. S., & Lu, J. L. (2002). Loneliness, lack of emotional support, lack of companionship and the likelihood of having a heart condition in an elderly sample. *Annals of Behavioral Medicine, 24*, 290–298.

Steptoe, A., Owen, N., Kunz-Ebrect, S. R., & Brydon, L. (2004). Loneliness and neuroendocrine, cardiovascular and inflammatory stress responses in middle-aged men and women. *Psychoneuroendocrinology, 29*, 593–611.

Terhell, E. L., Broese van Groenou, M., & van Tilburg, T. (2007). Network contact changes in early and later postseparation years. *Social Networks, 29*, 11–24.

Thoits, P. A. (1992). Identity structures and psychological well-being: Gender and marital status comparisons? *Social Psychology Quarterly, 55*, 236–256.

Thoits, P. A. (2011). Mechanisms linking social ties and support to physical and mental health. *Journal of Health and Social Behavior, 52*, 145–161.

Utz, R. L., Carr, D., Nesse, R., & Wortman, C. B. (2002). The effect of widowhood on older adults' social participation: An evaluation of activity, disengagement and continuity theories. *Gerontologist, 42*, 522–533.

Waite, L., & Das, A. (2010). Families, social life, and well-being at older ages. *Demography, 47*, S87–S109.

Waite, L. J., & Gallagher, M. (2000). *The case for marriage.* New York, NY: Broadway Books.

Waite, L. J., & Hughes, M. E. (1999). At risk on the cusp of old age: Living arrangements and functional status among black, white and Hispanic adults. *Journal of Gerontology, 54B*, S136–S144.

Waite, L. J., & Joyner, K. (2001). Emotional and physical satisfaction with sex in married, cohabiting and dating sexual unions: Do men and women differ? In E. O. Laumann & R. T. Michael (Eds.), *Sex, love and health in America: Private choices and public policies* (pp. 239–269). Chicago, IL: University of Chicago Press.

Waite, L. J., Laumann, E. O., Das, A., & Schumm, L. P. (2009). Sexuality: Measures of partnerships, practices, attitudes, and problems in the National Social Life, Health, and Aging Study. *Journals of Gerontology Series B: Psychological Sciences and Social Sciences, 64B*(Suppl. 1), i56–i66.

Warren-Findlow, J., Seymour, R. B., & Shenk, D. (2010). Intergenerational transmission of chronic illness self-care: Results from the caring for hypertension in African-American families study. *Gerontologist, 51*, 64–75.

Weeks, D. G., Michela, J. L., Peplau, L. A., & Bragg, M. E. (1980). Relation between loneliness and depression: A structural equation analysis. *Journal of Personality and Social Psychology, 39*, 1238–1244.

Wellman, B., & Wortley, S. (1990). Different strokes from different folks: Community ties and social support. *American Journal of Sociology, 96*, 558–588.

York Cornwell, E., & Waite, L. J. (2009). Social disconnectedness, perceived isolation, and health among older adults. *Journal of Health and Social Behavior, 50*, 31–48.

York Cornwell, E., & Waite, L. J. (2012). Social network resources and management of hypertension: Evidence from a national sample of older adults. *Journal Health and Social Behavior, 52*, 215–231.

Zilbergeld, B. (1992). *The new male sexuality.* New York, NY: Bantam.

CHAPTER 10

Trajectories of Within-Relationship Relationship Quality, Relationship Satisfaction, and Sexual Satisfaction Among Young African American Women

J. DENNIS FORTENBERRY AND DEVON J. HENSEL

Experience and expression of sexuality in adolescence typically occurs in the context of relationships additionally characterized by attraction and affiliation, relative exclusivity, and duration over a period of time (Giordano, Manning, & Longmore, 2010). These relationships condition experiences in adulthood (Madsen & Collins, 2011) and challenge adolescents to manage the social and emotional aspects of relationships (e.g., sexual communication/negotiation, jealousy/love, or sexual desire; O'Sullivan & Brooks-Gunn, 2005). A range of dyadic behaviors, from sexual kissing to sexual intercourse, and the concomitant issues of satisfaction with those behaviors, are salient aspects of almost all adolescent romantic relationships (O'Sullivan, Cheng, Harris, & Brooks-Gunn, 2007). In fact, sexuality is an integral element of perceptions of romantic relationships, even among early adolescents (Royer, Keller, & Heidrich, 2009).

Among adults, sexual qualities of relationships change over time and contribute to overall relationship stability and duration (Ein-Dor & Hirschberger, 2012; La France, 2010). In fact, dissatisfaction with sexual aspects of relationships contributes to dissolution of marriages and long-term cohabitations (Byers, 2005; MacNeil & Byers, 2009). This intersection of romantic and sexual relationship elements among adolescents is infrequently addressed, especially as these elements evolve within the course of a single relationship and contribute to the relative stability and duration of the relationship. However, some research supports the importance of sexual aspects within the romantic relationships of adolescents (Auslander et al., 2007; O'Sullivan & Majerovich, 2008). This suggests that more detailed understanding of sexual satisfaction within adolescent relationships is warranted.

The focus of this chapter, then, is the within-relationship changes in three cognitive and emotional assessments of adolescent women's romantic/sexual relationships: relationship quality, relationship satisfaction, and sexual relationship satisfaction. The young women who participated in our research were African American, living in communities with prevalence of sexually transmitted infections that are among the highest in the United States. Thus, we purposefully focus attention on the subjective experiences of relationships among African American young women who are less visible in sexuality research and whose sexuality is typically problematized as "risky" for adverse outcomes such as sexually transmitted infections and unplanned pregnancy. Our focus on the young women's cognitive and emotional assessments of relatively long-lasting relationships (6–12 months) respects the importance of relationships in young women's lives in the context of our understanding that most relationships dissolve and are replaced over time by others. Our inquiry is also based on the assumption that a variety of sexual activities are integral to most adolescent relationships, and that the dimension of sexual satisfaction is as relevant for the relationships of young women as it is for adults.

PUBLIC HEALTH AND SEXUAL HEALTH IN YOUNG WOMEN

The inclusion of partnered sex in adolescent romantic relationships, with the attendant pregnancy and infection risks, gives these relationships public health relevance, as well as developmental importance. The threat of sexually transmitted infections accompanies much of the formal and informal sex education adolescents receive (Hogben, Chesson, & Aral, 2010; Robert & Sonenstein, 2010). Vaccination to prevent sexually transmitted human papillomavirus infections is recommended for 9- to 12-year-old girls, bringing additional emphasis on sexually transmitted infections as a consequence of sexual behavior (Mullins et al., 2012). Sexually transmitted infections themselves are an integral developmental experience for many contemporary American adolescent women, with up to 25% experiencing at least one sexually transmitted infection by age 20 (Forhan et al., 2009). Sexually transmitted infections may be an especially important experience for African American adolescent women, among whom rates of several types of infections are much higher than for women in other American racial-ethnic groups (Romero et al., 2007).

Serial relationships—often with expectations of exclusion of other romantic relationships—are characteristic patterns of heterosexual experience during contemporary adolescence and young adulthood (Seiffge-Krenke, 2003). Sexual exchange in romantic relationships is nearly universal, although sexual expressions may be as limited as subtle indications of attraction or include a complete repertoire of partnered sexual practices also associated with risk of unplanned pregnancy and sexually transmitted infection (Collins, Welsh, & Furman, 2009). The trajectories of adolescents' relationships may affect risk of sexually transmitted infection in at least three ways. First, prevention practices such as condom use decline over time, often in as little as 3 weeks after initiation of coitus, often accompanied by shift to hormonal forms of contraception (Fortenberry, Tu, Harezlak, Katz, & Orr, 2002). Second, sexual nonexclusivity is relatively common, but the occurrences are not uniformly distributed in the duration of a given relationship (Manning, Giordano, & Longmore, 2006). Rather, involvement with other partners is more common during the later weeks and months of a relationship, reflecting (perhaps causing) a deterioration in relationship quality (Matson, Adler, Millstein, Tschann, & Ellen, 2011). Adolescent women ending a relationship are more likely to have a sexually transmitted infection, especially when ending a relationship with the father of their baby (Kershaw et al., 2010). Finally, relationship trajectories are important because romantic relationships that end are typically replaced, often within days or weeks. In the parlance of epidemiology, these relationships are comprised of "new partners" (Ott, Katschke, Tu, & Fortenberry, 2011). A new partner, or the number of new partners, is consistently identified as a predictor of a number of different sexually transmitted infections (Jennings, Glass, Parham, Adler, & Ellen, 2004). However, perhaps as a reflection of the deterioration in relationships, many young women are already infected at the initiation of a relationship with a new partner (Ott, Harezlak, Ofner, & Fortenberry, 2012).

JUSTIFICATION FOR FOCUS ON AFRICAN AMERICAN WOMEN

This chapter focuses on African American adolescent women. This decision to base a scientific inquiry on a single racial category is contentious for a variety of reasons. Perhaps the most difficult issue is the recurrent tendency in epidemiologic, psychological, and social sciences to attribute differences between racial groups to differences assumed to be inherent in the racial categories. Many recognize the essentially social and political nature of racial categories but use race as a proxy for underlying causal factors that are unknown or unmeasured (Lorusso, 2011).

Racial group inferences are difficult to refute because, within an American context, centuries of conquest, colonization, slavery, immigration, economics, social policy, and cultural practice have created surprisingly enduring social commitment to race as a meaningful approach to population diversity. Racial categories have immense implications for almost all aspects of American life, especially sexually transmitted infections, where rates of some infections among African American adolescents are three times or more those of other groups (Centers for Disease Control & Prevention, 2012).

This suggests that our research should not be "color-blind." Rather, our responsibility is to translate the insights of research into better understanding of health disparities without depending on the inherent validity of the categories on which disparities are based (Duster, 2005). Although contemporary American racial group categories are defined to represent presumed continental (e.g., African, European, or Asian) genetic origins, these categories are unreliable for classification of human genomic diversity (Romualdi et al., 2002). However, these categories do reflect experiences of poverty, opportunity, social capital, discrimination, and environmental stress that likely condition ways in which adolescents develop and maintain romantic relationships (Cunningham et al., 2012; Seaton, Yip, Morgan-Lopez, & Sellers, 2012; Simons, Simons, Lei, & Landor, 2012). To best reflect these social origins of racial group differences, we have chosen to uniformly use the racial group term "African American" as defined by the US Office of Management and Budget, and in distinction to other groups: White, American Indian or Alaska Native, Asian, and Native Hawaiian or Other Pacific Islander (http://www.census.gov/population/race/).

Our final reason for exclusive focus on African American young women is as a subversion of much of existing sexuality and relationship research that addresses samples of European Americans, typically recruited from the rarified socioeconomic contexts of college classrooms. A relatively small research literature addresses the romantic relationships of African American adolescents (Eyre, Flythe, Hoffman, & Fraser, 2012; Giordano, Manning, & Longmore, 2005; Meier & Allen, 2009), and our description of the trajectories of African American women's relationship and sexual satisfaction additionally anchors these relationships in a sense of their normality and developmental importance.

TRAJECTORIES OF RELATIONSHIP CHARACTERISTICS

The epidemiologic importance of the dynamics of young women's romantic relationships highlights the importance of attention to the subjective relationship evaluations made as relationships begin, develop, and terminate. From a theoretical perspective, each relationship experience contributes to a higher order relationship knowledge that summarizes underlying processes such as attachment style, relational commitment, emotional experiences such as attraction, liking, and loving, and interpersonal relationship characteristics such as communication, conflict, and support (Jones & Furman, 2011; Manning, Giordano, Longmore, & Hocevar, 2011). Adolescents' subjective experience of romantic relationships suggests that relationship continuation or dissolution is based on cognitive and emotional assessments of the relationships qualities (Lee, Rogge, & Reis, 2010; Reis, Collins, & Berscheid, 2000). Factors such as relationship quality, relationship satisfaction, and sexual relationship satisfaction become relevant at this developmental point because of their association with relationship stability, which is associated with subsequent cohabitation among young African American women (Meier & Allen, 2009). Cohabitation is an important element of family formation among African

American adolescents and young adults, who have relatively low rates of family formation through marriage (Heuveline & Timberlake, 2004).

Relationship Quality

Relationship quality refers to a variously defined subjective evaluation of various dimensions of the relationship (Hassenbrauck & Fehr, 2002). For adolescents' romantic relationships, these dimensions include disclosure, enjoyment, conflict resolution, intimacy, and security (Collins, Welsh, & Furman, 2009). Relationship quality associated with relationship stability for a range of adult intimate relationships, including marriage (Cutrona, Russell, Burzette, Wesner, & Bryant, 2011; Hassenbrauck & Fehr, 2002). Relationship quality in adolescent romantic relationships is associated with less relationship conflict in young adulthood (Collins, Martino, Elliott, & Miu, 2011).

Less is known about the function of relationship quality among adolescent women. Relational scripts reflective of relationship quality—communication, mutual support, trust, emotional attachment—are often mentioned by young African American women (Eyre et al., 2012). In a sample of mostly African American adolescent women, higher relationship quality was associated with decreased likelihood of partner change over the succeeding month (Sayegh, Fortenberry, Anderson, & Orr, 2005). Relationship quality is associated with greater coital frequency and less condom use over time, although levels of average relationship quality remain relatively stable (Katz, Fortenberry, Zimet, Blythe, & Orr, 2000; Sayegh, Fortenberry, Shew, & Orr, 2006).

Relationship Satisfaction

Relationship satisfaction is a concept adopted from studies of adult romantic relationships, defined as "an affective response arising from one's subjective evaluation of the positive and negative dimensions associated with one's sexual relationship" (Lawrance & Byers, 1995, p. 268). The importance of relationship satisfaction in the stability of adult relationships is broadly accepted (Byers, 2001). An important element of relationship satisfaction is the idea that it is subject to revision in response to changes in individuals and accumulated experiences (Byers, 2005). Among adolescents, relationship satisfaction is associated with partner characteristics such as intelligence, sense of humor, and appearance (Andrinopoulos, Kerrigan, & Ellen, 2006; Regan, 1998). Relationship satisfaction has some developmental qualities, with higher satisfaction associated with greater shared activities, which increase from early into middle adolescence (Carlson & Rose, 2012). Shared activities and relational communality are important elements in relationship stability during middle and late adolescence (Peck, Shaffer, & Williamson, 2004; Sprecher,

2002). In general, relationship satisfaction in adolescent relationships is associated with sexual satisfaction, relationship quality, and relationship stability (Auslander et al., 2007). Likewise, relationship satisfaction is a correlate of greater perceived partner support, which is associated with increased coitus (Hensel, Fortenberry, & Orr, 2008).

Among African American adolescent women (compared to European American adolescent women), romantic relationships are described as less intimate, with less disclosure, lower frequency of contact (Giordano et al., 2005), and more sexual intimacy (Meier & Allen, 2009). Experiences such as family instability, discrimination, and poverty are associated with distrustful relational schemas that lead to less stable relationships during adolescence (Simons et al., 2012).

Sexual Relationship Satisfaction

Sexual relationship satisfaction can be thought of as a person's assessment of sexual interactions in a relationship as a function of expectations for sex within the relationship. Sex plays a complex role in the formation and maintenance of many adolescent relationships and serves different functions in relationships with different partners (Andrinopoulos et al., 2006; Giordano et al., 2010). Sexual interactions occur at many levels within a relationship, and the repertoire of interactions likely changes over time (O'Sullivan et al., 2007). Sexual relationship satisfaction also contributes to subsequent sexual and condom use events, with sexual satisfaction associated with higher relationship quality, decreased likelihood of partner change, and increased coital frequency (Sayegh et al., 2005). Within relationships, African American women see sex as an extension of emotional intimacy, especially when sex occurs later rather than earlier in the relationship (Eyre et al., 2012).

Young women's subjective assessments of relationship quality, relationship satisfaction, and sexual satisfaction clearly have relevance to the ways interpersonal behaviors (including sexual behaviors) are structured over time. These behaviors have implications for young women's health over time within a specific relationship, as well as influence health and well-being in the transition to subsequent relationships (Fortenberry et al., 2002). One challenge is design of research that captures romantic and sexual qualities of relationships and allows relatively precise measurement of the beginning and end of these relationships. We turn attention next to this topic.

STUDYING THE TRAJECTORIES OF YOUNG WOMEN'S RELATIONSHIPS

In considering various alternative designs for understanding the development of young women's relationships, we rejected potential methodologies such as a timeline follow-back method (Freedman, Thornton, & Camburn, 1988) as likely insensitive to emotional and cognitive assessments of relationships at a given time. Guided by earlier research experience with assembling and following cohorts of adolescents (Costa, Jessor, Donovan, & Fortenberry, 1995; Fortenberry, Costa, Jessor, & Donovan, 1997), and with frequently repeated interview and self-report methods of data collection (Fortenberry, Cecil, Zimet, & Orr, 1997), an inception cohort approach was chosen.

The cohort was assembled as part of a larger longitudinal cohort study locally called the Young Women's Project. Funding support was initially from the National Institute of Allergy & Infectious Diseases and subsequently from the National Institute of Child Health & Human Development. The project (started in 1999 and completed in 2009) was a study of sexual relationships, sexual behaviors, and sexually transmitted infections among young women in middle to late adolescence (Fortenberry et al., 2005). The 387 young women were between 14 and 17 years of age at enrollment. The young women were recruited from one of three primary care adolescent health clinics in Indianapolis, Indiana. These clinics serve primarily low- and middle-income families residing in areas with high rates of early childbearing and among the highest rates of sexually transmitted infections in the United States. As a result of this recruitment strategy, 90% of the young women reported their race as African American, and the average maternal education level was 12th grade. Neither relationship status nor partnered sexual experience was an eligibility criterion. Thus, the sample was homogeneous in terms of race and socioeconomic status but diverse in terms of experience with romantic and sexual relationships. However, all of the participants reported both relationship and partnered sexual experience over the course of the study.

Young women completed quarterly study visits for collection of interview and physical data related to the larger project. At enrollment and at each interview, participants identified up to five romantic partners, including friends, dating partners, boyfriends/girlfriends, and sexual partners. As a means of examining various types and stages of relationships, partners were not limited to those with whom a defined sexual behavior such as coitus had happened. This allowed us to capture nascent relationships, as well as those that were more advanced.

In each quarterly interview, young women provided partner-specific information related to relationship emotional, behavioral, and sexual content. At each quarterly interview, unique partner identifiers allowed longitudinal linkage of young women's relationship assessments with that partner. This research was approved by the institutional review board of the institution of the first author. Informed consent was obtained from each participant and permission obtained from a parent or legal guardian.

For the data presented in this chapter, we used a subset of African American young women (N = 284; 73.3% of participants in the larger study) who reported the same romantic partner in at least two consecutive quarters. This allows us to examine young women's relationship characteristics within relationships of at least 6 months duration.

MEASURING RELATIONSHIP QUALITY, RELATIONSHIP SATISFACTION, AND SEXUAL RELATIONSHIP SATISFACTION

At the time this study was conceived and designed (circa 1998), there were few validated measures of subjective assessments of relational and sexual qualities of relationships for adolescents. This was addressed by development of a new scale of Relationship Quality, and adaptation of measures of Relationship Satisfaction and Sexual Relationship Satisfaction used in studies of adults. *Relationship Quality* included six, 4-point Likert-type items (strongly disagree to strongly agree; $\alpha = 0.94$). Items consisted of statements of relationship characteristics (e.g., "We have a strong emotional relationship") that resemble those used in other measures of relationship quality (Hassenbrauck & Fehr, 2002). The scale range was 6–24, with higher scores indicating greater relationship quality. *Relationship Satisfaction* was five, 7-point semantic differential items ($\alpha = 0.95$) assessing a participant's feelings about the overall relationship with that partner (e.g., "very bad to very good") (Lawrance & Byers, 1995). This scale was developed for adults, based in social exchange theory (Sprecher, 1998). Pilot testing with adolescent women at study initiation showed high levels of comprehension, and the scale items were used without modification. Scale range was 5–35, with higher scores indicating greater relationship satisfaction. *Sexual Relationship Satisfaction* was five, 7-point semantic differential items ($\alpha = 0.95$) assessing a participant's feelings about the sexual relationship with that partner (e.g., "very bad to very good") (Lawrance & Byers, 1995). These scale items were developed in parallel to those for Relationship Satisfaction, and they also were used unchanged after pilot testing with adolescent women. Scale range was 5–35, with higher scores indicating greater sexual relationship satisfaction.

MODELING WITHIN-RELATIONSHIP TRAJECTORIES

Latent growth curve (LGC) analysis was used to model the parallel growth trajectories in Relationship Quality, Relationship Satisfaction, and Sexual Relationship Satisfaction (Bollen & Curran, 2006; Curran & Hussong, 2002). The LGC models include two simultaneously estimated components: the within-person model and the between-person model (Bollen & Curran, 2004). The basic linear form of these trajectories is characterized by a latent intercept factor, whose mean value represents the between-person initial value of the trajectory, and by a latent slope factor, whose mean value represents the between-person rate of change over time (Bollen & Curran, 2004). Significant variances in either factor denote meaningful between-person differences.

Relationships of the latent factors to the trajectory are nested within a restricted confirmatory factor analysis approach, as the measures of a given construct are used as multiple indicators on a given latent factor. Loadings are numerically defined relative not only to latent factor function but also to the passage of time. For the intercept, there is a static starting value, with up to four time points that are all fixed to a value of one. The slope factor's values are fixed from zero through three, respectively, to reflect a linear passage of time from the enrollment interview through Quarters 2, 3, and 4. A "freed loading" approach frees loadings from the slope factor to allow the model to accommodate "stretching" or "shrinking" in the trajectory shape (Bollen & Curran, 2006). This approach is typically used when a linear model provides suboptimal fit.

Because LGC methods alone account for time-lagged change within specific time frames, in certain circumstances, modifying the chosen LGC format to include autoregressive effects (e.g., between Quarter 1 and Quarter 3) provides a more comprehensive examination of change (Curran & Bollen, 2001). In contrast to LGC parameters, which use all available time points to gauge developmental change, autoregressive paths isolate time-specific effects, controlling for developmental effects (Bollen & Curran, 2006).

Analyses were carried out in three steps. First, an unconditional, two-factor (intercept and slope) LGC was estimated to model linear change over consecutive quarters for Relationship Quality, Relationship Satisfaction, and Sexual Relationship Satisfaction. Alternative unconditional models were evaluated that included freed loadings. Freed loadings allow estimation of the amount of variance between adjacent quarters (Bollen & Curran, 2006). The two-factor LGC model was retained when the change in chi-square between the freed loading and two-factor models was not significant (Table 10.3). Where differences of chi-square tests were marginally significant (e.g., $p > .05$ and $p < .10$), alternative measures of comparison were used to choose a model (e.g., improvement in global fit measures and significance of autoregressive paths). In all models, the latent intercept and slope factors were covaried. Next, the best fitting model of Relationship Quality, Relationship Satisfaction, and Sexual Relationship Satisfaction was retained and estimated together in a single triple-trajectory LGC. Our key interest here is the cross-domain covariance.

We employed a structural equation model (SEM) approach to simultaneously assess multiple developmental trajectories (Bollen & Curran, 2006; Curran & Hussong, 2002; Kim & Cicchetti, 2006). All analyses used AMOS, version 19.0 with a full information maximum likelihood (FIML) estimation method. FIML was used to adjust the analysis for respondents with differing numbers of annual visits and to produce the moment structure needed to estimate LGCs with an ordered categorical variable (Bollen & Curran, 2006).

Model fit was assessed through evaluation of several indices. In general, nonsignificant chi-square values, a comparative fit index (CFI) greater than 0.90, and root mean square error of approximation (RMSEA) less than 0.08 indicate acceptable model fit to the data (Browne & Cudeck, 1993).

OBTAINED TRAJECTORIES

Young women reported relationship quality, relationship satisfaction, and sexual relationship satisfaction for 508 individual partners. Of these, 165/508 (32.4%) reported on the same relationship for two consecutive quarters, 142/508 (27.9%) for three consecutive quarters, and 201/508 (40%) for at least four consecutive quarters (i.e., more than 1 year). For 179/201 (89%) of these longest lasting relationships, initiation of the consecutive reports was the first mention of that specific partner.

Average relationship quality, relationship satisfaction, and sexual relationship satisfaction were all in the high side of scale distribution. Quarter 1 and Quarter 2 scale means for relationships with only two consecutive quarters (i.e., relationships of shorter duration) were lower than those for relationships with three or four quarters (Table 10.1). Similarly, Quarter 3 scale means for relationships with four consecutive quarters were lower than those for relationships assessed at four consecutive quarters. Relationship Quality, Relationship Satisfaction, and Sexual Relationship Satisfaction declined from one quarter to the next (Table 10.1). The exception to this was in relationships with four quarters of assessments: Scale means for these relationships peaked at the second (rather than first) assessment and declined thereafter.

Correlations within relationship domains for relationships assessed at four consecutive quarters are shown in Table 10.2. Within all three domains, the size of correlation between Quarter 1 and Quarter 2 were smaller than correlations between Quarter 3 and Quarter 4. For example, the Quarter 1/Quarter 2 correlation for Relationship Quality was 0.43, compared to 0.49 for Quarter 3/Quarter 4. Similarly, the Quarter 1/Quarter 2 correlation for Relationship Satisfaction was 0.50 for Quarter 1/Quarter 2 compared to 0.63 for Quarter 3/Quarter 4. Sexual Relationship Satisfaction was 0.28 for Quarter 1/Quarter 2, compared to 0.76 for Quarter 3/Quarter 4.

Table 10.1. RELATIONSHIP QUALITY, RELATIONSHIP SATISFACTION, AND SEXUAL RELATIONSHIP SATISFACTION IN CONSECUTIVE QUARTERS OF RELATIONSHIPS OF AFRICAN AMERICAN, ADOLESCENT WOMEN

	Quarter 1 (mean, SD)	Quarter 2 (mean, SD)	Quarter 3 (mean, SD)	Quarter 4 (mean, SD)	Overall (mean, SD)
Relationship quality					
Two quarters	20.2 (3.5)	18.5 (4.1)	—	—	19.8 (3.7)
Three quarters	20.5 (3.3)	19.5 (3.5)	19.3 (3.9)	—	20.3 (3.8)
Four quarters	20.5 (3.2)	20.9 (2.6)	20.3 (4.1)	19.7 (3.9)	20.3 (3.6)
Relationship satisfaction					
Two quarters	28.7 (5.8)	27.9 (6.6)	—	—	28.3 (6.4)
Three quarters	29.5 (4.7)	28.2 (6.7)	26.2 (7.0)	—	28.7 (6.0)
Four quarters	29.9 (6.0)	30.1 (4.7)	29.9 (5.8)	28.0 (6.1)	29.4 (5.5)
Sexual relationship satisfaction					
Two quarters	28.9 (5.7)	29.5 (6.0)	—	—	29.3 (7.0)
Three quarters	30.6 (6.1)	29.2 (7.1)	28.5 (6.5)	—	30.3 (6.5)
Four quarters	31.3 (5.9)	32.1 (4.8)	31.8 (5.7)	30.9 (5.6)	31.0 (5.5)

Note. Two consecutive quarters, N = 165; three consecutive quarters, N = 142; four consecutive quarters, N = 201.

Table 10.2. CORRELATIONS OF RELATIONSHIP QUALITY, RELATIONSHIP SATISFACTION, AND SEXUAL RELATIONSHIP SATISFACTION IN CONSECUTIVE QUARTERS OF RELATIONSHIP DURATION

	RQ 2	RQ 3	RQ 4	RS 1	RS 2	RS 3	RS 4	SRS 1	SRS 2	SRS 3	SRS 4
Relationship quality, Quarter 1	0.43	0.34	0.08	0.32	0.39	0.10	−0.08	0.31	0.32	−0.003	−0.04
Relationship quality, Quarter 2	1.00	0.34	0.21	0.27	0.39	0.14	0.06	0.32	0.45	0.08	0.07
Relationship quality, Quarter 3		1.00	0.49	0.01	−0.03	0.37	0.32	0.02	0.16	0.38	0.30
Relationship quality, Quarter 4			1.00	0.15	−0.08	0.27	0.56	0.09	0.08	0.34	0.36
Relationship satisfaction, Quarter 1				1.00	0.50	0.34	0.33	0.84	0.27	0.17	0.16
Relationship satisfaction, Quarter 2					1.00	0.28	0.29	0.36	0.59	−0.01	0.09
Relationship satisfaction, Quarter 3						1.00	0.63	0.19	0.15	0.73	0.52
Relationship satisfaction, Quarter 4							1.00	0.20	0.18	0.48	0.61
Sexual relationship satisfaction, Quarter 1								1.00	0.28	0.14	0.12
Sexual relationship satisfaction, Quarter 2									1.00	0.19	0.22
Sexual relationship satisfaction, Quarter 3										1.00	0.76

Note. $p < 0.05$ for correlations of 0.25 and larger. Relationships reported for four consecutive quarters (12 months).

Correlations across relationship domains are also shown in Table 10.2. Across all three domains, cross-domain correlations in Quarter 1 were smaller than in subsequent quarters. The Quarter 1 correlation of Relationship Quality and Relationship Satisfaction was 0.32, while the Quarter 4 correlation was 0.56. The Quarter 1 correlation of Relationship Quality and Sexual Relationship Satisfaction was also lower than the Quarter 4 correlation ($r = 0.31$ and $r = 0.36$ for Quarter 1 and Quarter 4, respectively). However, a different pattern was seen for Relationship Satisfaction and Sexual Relationship Satisfaction, where the correlations were 0.84 and 0.61 for Quarter 1 and Quarter 4, respectively.

The unconditional covariance structure of intercepts and slopes of Relationship Quality, Relationship Satisfaction, and Sexual Relationship Satisfaction are shown in Table 10.3. Each covariance was significant at $p < 0.05$. Covariance was highest ($r = 0.86$) for the intercepts of Relationship Satisfaction and Sexual Relationship Satisfaction, possibly indicating the substantial theoretical overlap and common

Table 10.3. UNCONDITIONAL COVARIANCE OF INTERCEPT/SLOPE FOR
RELATIONSHIP QUALITY, RELATIONSHIP SATISFACTION, AND SEXUAL
RELATIONSHIP SATISFACTION

	Relationship Quality		Relationship Satisfaction		Sexual Relationship Satisfaction	
	Intercept	Slope	Intercept	Slope	Intercept	Slope
Relationship quality intercept	1.0	−0.34	—	−0.25	—	−0.34
Relationship satisfaction intercept	0.58	−0.21	1.0	−0.37	—	−0.63
Sexual relationship satisfaction intercept	0.61	−0.28	0.86	−0.38	1.0	−0.25

Note. All $p < 0.05$; dashes indicate redundant covariances omitted to reduce confusion.

method variance of these constructs. However, the substantially smaller covariance of Relationship Quality intercept with intercepts of Relationship Satisfaction and Sexual Relationship Satisfaction ($r = 0.58$ and $r = 0.61$, respectively) supports the independent contribution of the Relationship Quality domain from assessments of satisfaction.

The intercept of each construct (Relationship Quality, Relationship Satisfaction, and Sexual Relationship Satisfaction) covaried negatively with the slope of that construct (Table 10.3): The Relationship Quality intercept/slope covariance was −0.34; the Relationship Satisfaction intercept/slope covariance was −0.37; and the Sexual Relationship Satisfaction intercept/slope covariance was −0.25. These covariances indicate that relationships with higher initial Relationship Quality, Relationship Satisfaction, or Sexual Relationship Satisfaction declined more slowly than others.

The interrelationships of Relationship Quality, Relationship Satisfaction, and Sexual Relationship Satisfaction can be seen in the cross-domain intercept/slope covariances (Table 10.3). The Relationship Quality intercept/Relationship Satisfaction slope was −0.25. The Relationship Quality intercept/Sexual Relationship Satisfaction slope covariance was −0.34. The Relationship Satisfaction intercept/Sexual Relationship Satisfaction slope covariance was −0.63. These data suggest that initially positively evaluated relationships decline more slowly than less positively evaluated relationships.

The longitudinal associations of Relationship Quality, Relationship Satisfaction, and Sexual Relationship Satisfaction are shown in the triple LGC analysis shown in Table 10.4. Three observations about within-relationship trajectories of Relationship Quality, Relationship Satisfaction, and Sexual Relationship Satisfaction can be made. First, adjusted variance for the intercept mean indicates significant between-person differences in initial (Quarter 1) levels of Relationship Quality, Relationship Satisfaction, and Sexual Relationship Satisfaction. This is

Table 10.4. TRIPLE LATENT GROWTH CURVE OF RELATIONSHIP QUALITY, RELATIONSHIP SATISFACTION, AND SEXUAL RELATIONSHIP SATISFACTION

	Freed Loading, B	Intercept		Slope	
		Mean	Variance	Mean	Variance
Relationship quality	0.33*	19.9 (0.15)*	7.6 (0.88)*	–0.17 (0.12)	2.5 (0.58)*
Relationship satisfaction	NA	29.5 (0.27)*	19.8 (2.35)*	–0.51 (0.14)*	2.8 (0.62)*
Sexual relationship satisfaction	0.36*	30.3 (0.27)*	17.5 (3.29)*	–0.58 (0.26)*	7.9 (2.33)*

*$p < 0.05$.

consistent with selection of the sample based on relationship continuity of at least 6 months, as less satisfactory relationships were terminated and not included.

Second, the adjusted average slope for each of the domains was negative, although significantly so only for Relationship Satisfaction and Sexual Relationship Satisfaction. This shows a group-level decline over time in young women's assessments of these key indicators of relationship functioning. However, a caveat to this group-level change is the significant variance in the slopes of each domain. This demonstrates the marked between-person variation to be expected if some relationships continue over time and some cease.

Finally, the finding of significant freed loadings shows that declines for Relationship Quality and Sexual Relationship Quality are not smoothly linear over time. Rather, for these two relationship domains, most of the decline occurred between Quarter 2 and Quarter 3 (66% for Relationship Quality [B = 0.33]; 69% for Sexual Relationship Satisfaction [B = 0.36]) (Table 10.4). This is consistent with the finding in Table 10.1, where the highest mean scores in each relationship domain for relationships lasting four quarters were reported at Quarter 2. Thus, longer enduring relationships of adolescent women appear to undergo a period of improvement, subsequently followed by decline, especially in Relationship Quality and Sexual Relationship Satisfaction.

BUILDING MEANING FROM TRAJECTORIES

Adolescent romantic relationships are thought to be inherently short-lived and unstable. A relationship of 1-year duration seems short compared to adult standards for marriages and cohabitations with durations of decades. In this chapter, we focused on a single segment—one romantic/sexual partnership—in the larger relationship history of young, urban, African American women. All of the relationships lasted at least 6 months and many for at least 1 year. However, 1 year is about 7% of a 15-year-old's life, and an even larger proportion of her adolescence: These are not trivial interpersonal investments. The developmental salience of romantic/

sexual relationships in adolescence is increasingly recognized, with understanding of ways in which these relationships presage those of young adulthood (Furman & Wehner, 1997; Madsen & Collins, 2011; Montgomery & Sorell, 1998; Welsh, Haugen, Widman, Darling, & Grello, 2005; Zimmer-Gembeck, Siebenbruner, & Collins, 2001). These are relationships associated with experiences that reverberate through the emotional life course: the feelings of being in love, the feelings of strong sexual desire, the first coitus that for many signals the transition from adolescence to womanhood. These also are relationships that often have other enduring consequences such as pregnancy and sexually transmitted infections (Hensel & Fortenberry, 2011). Our perspective is that these issues all warrant detailed attention to these relatively short intervals of developmental time.

Within time-framed boundaries of a single relationship, three related cognitive and emotional relationship assessments—relationship quality, relationship satisfaction, and sexual relationship satisfaction—generally declined. Because the data were obtained from a larger longitudinal study, we know that in almost all instances, this decline was associated with relationship termination. Even in young women with relatively little relational experience, these three dimensions declined in concert, supporting the idea that adolescents bring relational schema to their assessments of relationships (Andersen & Cyranowski, 1994; Cyranowski & Andersen, 1998; Simons et al., 2012). These relational schema and self-schema may help explain how young adolescents assess somewhat ephemeral qualities such as satisfaction, especially with little actual experience in setting expectations for relationships (Tolman & McClelland, 2011). Some young women may include expectations for relationship dissolution in their understanding of relationship commitment, reflecting interest in obtaining a larger range of relationship experiences, or investment in a schooling or career trajectory thought to be in conflict with long-term romantic relationships (Halpern, Joyner, Udry, & Suchindran, 2000; Manning et al., 2011).

These data add to existing understanding of young women's romantic relationships. Focus on within-relationship evaluations of relationship characteristics shifts attention away from a perspective of adolescent relationships as largely empty of meaningful content (except violence, sexual coercion, unintended pregnancy, and sexually transmitted infection), largely animated by family or peer influences, and structured as dating and courtship processes (presumably oriented toward preparations for marriage). We also find it important that attention given to relationship experiences among African American youth be equal to that given to the study of health risk and adverse interpersonal consequences. The relationship experiences of these young women have been largely invisible in developmental literature on adolescent relationships (Ohye & Daniel, 1999). These are relationships that do not seem to have a clear social definition within an evolving adolescent relationship lexicon that includes terms like "hook-ups," "friends with benefits," "wifey," and "baby mama," as well as traditionally used words such as "girlfriend" (Bergdall et al., 2012; Manning et al., 2006).

The trajectories of relationship domains that condition relationship stability and dissolution achieve public health relevance when both past and new relationships involve dyadic sexual exchanges, especially when intervals between one relationship and the next are only a few days or weeks (Kraut-Becher & Aral, 2003). In economically disadvantaged communities (such as those in which our research was conducted) with high background prevalence of sexually transmitted infections, new partners are associated with substantial infection risk (Manning, Flanigan, Giordano, & Longmore, 2009). Our data demonstrate that more positive initial cognitive assessments of relationships are associated with slower rates of decline over time. Over the decade of highest sexually transmitted infection risk (approximately ages 15–25 years), longer relationship duration and fewer accumulated relationships could be associated with decreased experience with highly prevalent sexually transmitted infections such as chlamydia. One lesson that might be taken from these data is the importance of attention to relationship dynamics in the context of sexuality education in schools or in a variety of community-based organizations (Fisher et al., 2012; Hall, Moreau, & Trussell, 2012; Picot et al., 2012). These types of relationship dynamics are also important in the negotiation of some of the more enduring consequences of relationships such as school completion and children (Crockett & Beal, 2012; Kershaw et al., 2010).

Most important, our research experience with these young women demonstrated the unique value of lasting relationships. In this case, the relationships were between the young women participants (often including other members of their families) and our research team. We had the privilege of insight into intimate aspects of their daily lives. Hopefully, this chapter fulfills the obligation of that privilege by honoring all that our young women taught us about their lives.

REFERENCES

Andersen, B. L., & Cyranowski, J. M. (1994). Women's sexual self-schema. *Journal of Personality and Social Psychology, 67*, 1079–1100.

Andrinopoulos, K., Kerrigan, D., & Ellen, J. M. (2006). Understanding sex partner selection from the perspective of inner-city black adolescents. *Perspectives on Sexual and Reproductive Health, 38*, 132–138.

Auslander, B. A., Rosenthal, S. L., Fortenberry, J. D., Biro, F. M., Bernstein, D. I., & Zimet, G. D. (2007). Predictors of sexual satisfaction in an adolescent and college population. *Journal of Pediatric and Adolescent Gynecology, 20*, 25–28.

Bergdall, A. R., Kraft, J. M., Andes, K., Carter, M., Hatfield-Timajchy, K., & Hock-Long, L. (2012). Love and hooking up in the new millennium: Communication technology and relationships among urban African American and Puerto Rican young adults. *Journal of Sex Research, 49*, 570–582. doi: 10.1080/00224499.2011.604748.

Bollen, K. A., & Curran, P. J. (2004). Autoregressive latent trajectory (ALT) models: A synthesis of two traditions. *Sociological Methods and Research, 32*, 336–383.

Bollen, K. A., & Curran, P. J. (2006). *Latent curve models: A structural equation approach.* New York, NY: Wiley.

Browne, M. W., & Cudeck, R. (1993). Alternative ways of assessing model fit. In K. A. Bollen & J. S. Long (Eds.), *Testing structural equation models* (pp. 136–162). Newbury Park, CA: Sage.

Byers, E. S. (2001). Evidence for the importance of relationship satisfaction for women's sexual functioning. *Women and Therapy, 24*, 23–26.

Byers, E. S. (2005). Relationship satisfaction and sexual satisfaction: A longitudinal study of individuals in long-term relationships. *Journal of Sex Research, 42*, 113–118. doi: 10.1080/00224490509552264.

Carlson, W., & Rose, A. J. (2012). Brief report: Activities in heterosexual romantic relationships: Grade differences and associations with relationship satisfaction. *Journal of Adolescence, 35*, 219–224. doi: 10.1016/j.adolescence.2010.09.001.

Collins, R. L., Martino, S. C., Elliott, M. N., & Miu, A. (2011). Relationships between adolescent sexual outcomes and exposure to sex in media: Robustness to propensity-based analysis. *Developmental Psychology, 47*, 585–591. doi: 10.1037/a0022563.

Collins, W. A., Welsh, D. P., & Furman, W. (2009). Adolescent romantic relationships. *Annual Review of Psychology, 60*, 631–652.

Costa, F. M., Jessor, R., Donovan, J. E., & Fortenberry, J. D. (1995). Early initiation of sexual intercourse: The influence of psychosocial unconventionality. *Journal of Research on Adolescence, 5*, 93–121.

Crockett, L. J., & Beal, S. J. (2012). The life course in the making: Gender and the development of adolescents' expected timing of adult role transitions. *Developmental Psychology, 48*, 1727–1738. doi: 10.1037/a0027538.

Cunningham, T. J., Seeman, T. E., Kawachi, I., Gortmaker, S. L., Jacobs, D. R., Kiefe, C. I., & Berkman, L. F. (2012). Racial/ethnic and gender differences in the association between self-reported experiences of racial/ethnic discrimination and inflammation in the CARDIA cohort of 4 US communities. *Social Science and Medicine, 75*, 922–931.

Curran, P. J., & Bollen, K. A. (2001). The best of both worlds: Combining autoregressive and latent curve models. In L. M. Collins & A. G. Sayer (Eds.), *New methods for the analysis of change* (pp. 105–136). Washington, DC: American Psychological Association.

Curran, P. J., & Hussong, A. M. (2002). Structural equation modeling of repeated data: Latent curve analysis. In D. S. Moskowitz & S. L. Hershberger (Eds.), *Modeling intraindividual variability with repeated measures data: Methods and applications* (pp. 59–85). Mahwah, NJ: Erlbaum.

Cutrona, C. E., Russell, D. W., Burzette, R. G., Wesner, K. A., & Bryant, C. M. (2011). Predicting relationship stability among midlife African American couples. *Journal of Consulting and Clinical Psychology, 79*, 814–825.

Cyranowski, J. M., & Andersen, B. L. (1998). Schemas, sexuality, and romantic attachment. *Journal of Personality and Social Psychology, 74*, 1364–1379.

Duster, T. (2005). Medicine. Race and reification in science. *Science, 307*, 1050–1051.

Ein-Dor, T., & Hirschberger, G. (2012). Sexual healing: Daily diary evidence that sex relieves stress for men and women in satisfying relationships. *Journal of Social and Personal Relationships, 29*, 126–139. doi: 10.1177/0265407511431185.

Eyre, S. L., Flythe, M., Hoffman, V., & Fraser, A. E. (2012). Primary relationship scripts among lower-income, African American young adults. *Family Process, 51*, 234–249.

Fisher, C. M., Reece, M., Wright, E., Dodge, B., Sherwood-Laughlin, C., & Baldwin, K. (2012). The role of community-based organizations in adolescent sexual health promotion. *Health Promotion Practice, 13*, 544–552.

Forhan, S. E., Gottlieb, S. L., Sternberg, M. R., Xu, F., Datta, S. D., McQuillan, G. M., ... Markowitz, L. E. (2009). Prevalence of sexually transmitted infections among female adolescents aged 14 to 19 in the United States. *Pediatrics, 124*, 1505–1512.

Fortenberry, J. D., Cecil, H., Zimet, G. D., & Orr, D. P. (1997). Concordance between self-report questionnaires and coital diaries for sexual behaviors of adolescent women with sexually transmitted diseases. In J. Bancroft (Ed.), *Researching sexual behavior* (pp. 237–249). Bloomington: Indiana University Press.

Fortenberry, J. D., Costa, F. M., Jessor, R., & Donovan, J. E. (1997). Contraceptive behavior and adolescent lifestyles: A structural modeling approach. *Journal of Research on Adolescence, 7*, 307–329.

Fortenberry, J. D., Temkit, M., Tu, W., Katz, B. P., Graham, C. A., & Orr, D. P. (2005). Daily mood, partner support, sexual interest and sexual activity among adolescent women. *Health Psychology, 24*, 252–257.

Fortenberry, J. D., Tu, W., Harezlak, J., Katz, B. P., & Orr, D. P. (2002). Condom use as a function of time in new and established adolescent sexual relationships. *American Journal of Public Health, 92*, 211–213.

Freedman, D., Thornton, A., & Camburn, D. (1988). The life history calendar: A technique for collecting retrospective data. In C. C. Clogg (Ed.), *Sociological methodology* (pp. 37–68). Washington, DC: The American Sociological Association

Furman, W., & Wehner, E. A. (1997). Adolescent romantic relationships: A developmental perspective. *New Directions for Child Development, 78*, 21–36.

Giordano, P. C., Manning, W. D., & Longmore, M. A. (2005). The romantic relationships of African-American and white adolescents. *The Sociological Quarterly, 46*, 545–568. doi: 10.1111/j.1533-8525.2005.00026.x.

Giordano, P. C., Manning, W. D., & Longmore, M. A. (2010). Affairs of the heart: Qualities of adolescent romantic relationships and sexual behavior. *Journal of Research on Adolescence, 20*, 983–1013. doi: 10.1111/j.1532-7795.2010.00661.x.

Hall, K. S., Moreau, C., & Trussell, J. (2012). Associations between sexual and reproductive health communication and health service use among U.S. adolescent women. *Perspectives on Sexual and Reproductive Health, 44*, 6–12.

Halpern, C. T., Joyner, K., Udry, J. R., & Suchindran, C. (2000). Smart teens don't have sex (or kiss much either). *Journal of Adolescent Health, 26*, 213–225. doi: 10.1016/s1054-139x(99)00061-0.

Hassenbrauck, M., & Fehr, B. (2002). Dimensions of relationship quality. *Personal Relationships, 9*, 253–270.

Hensel, D. J., & Fortenberry, J. D. (2011). Adolescent mothers' sexual, contraceptive, and emotional relationship content with the fathers of their children following a first diagnosis of sexually transmitted infection. *Journal of Adolescent Health, 49*, 327–329.

Hensel, D. J., Fortenberry, J. D., & Orr, D. P. (2008). Variations in coital and noncoital sexual repertoire among adolescent women. *Journal of Adolescent Health, 42*, 170–176.

Heuveline, P., & Timberlake, J. M. (2004). The role of cohabitation in family formation: The United States in comparative perspective. *Journal of Marriage and Family, 66*, 1214–1230. doi: 10.1111/j.0022-2445.2004.00088.x.

Hogben, M., Chesson, H., & Aral, S. O. (2010). Sexuality education policies and sexually transmitted disease rates in the United States of America. *International Journal of STD and AIDS, 21*, 293–297.

Jennings, J., Glass, B., Parham, P., Adler, N., & Ellen, J. M. (2004). Sex partner concurrency, geographic context, and adolescent sexually transmitted infections. *Sexually Transmitted Diseases, 31*, 734–739.

Jones, M. C., & Furman, W. (2011). Representations of romantic relationships, romantic experience, and sexual behavior in adolescence. *Personal Relationships, 18*, 144–164. doi: 10.1111/j.1475-6811.2010.01291.x.

Katz, B. P., Fortenberry, J. D., Zimet, G. D., Blythe, M. J., & Orr, D. P. (2000). Partner-specific relationship characteristics and condom use among young people with sexually transmitted infections. *Journal of Sex Research, 37,* 69–75.

Kershaw, T. S., Ethier, K. A., Niccolai, L. M., Lewis, J. B., Milan, S., Meade, C., & Ickovics, J. R. (2010). Let's stay together: Relationship dissolution and sexually transmitted diseases among parenting and non-parenting adolescents. *Journal of Behavioral Medicine, 33,* 454–465. doi: 10.1007/s10865-010-9276-6.

Kim, J., & Cicchetti, D. (2006). Longitudinal trajectories of self-system processes and depressive symptoms among maltreated and nonmaltreated children. *Child Development, 77,* 624–639.

Kraut-Becher, J. R., & Aral, S. O. (2003). Gap length: An important factor in sexually transmitted disease transmission. *Sexually Transmitted Diseases, 30,* 221–225.

La France, B. H. (2010). Predicting sexual satisfaction in interpersonal relationships. *Southern Communication Journal, 75,* 195–214.

Lawrance, K-A., & Byers, E. S. (1995). Sexual satisfaction in long-term heterosexual relationships: The interpersonal exchange model of sexual satisfaction. *Personal Relationships, 2,* 267–285. doi: 10.1111/j.1475-6811.1995.tb00092.x.

Lee, S., Rogge, R. D., & Reis, H. T. (2010). Assessing the seeds of relationship decay. Using implicit evaluations to detect the early stages of disillusionment. *Psychological Science, 21,* 857–864.

Lorusso, L. (2011). The justification of race in biological explanation. *Journal of Medical Ethics, 37,* 535–539.

MacNeil, S., & Byers, E. S. (2009). Role of sexual self-disclosure in the sexual satisfaction of long-term heterosexual couples. *Journal of Sex Research, 46,* 3–14.

Madsen, S. D., & Collins, W. A. (2011). The salience of adolescent romantic experiences for romantic relationship qualities in young adulthood. *Journal of Research on Adolescence, 21,* 789–801. doi: 10.1111/j.1532-7795.2011.00737.x.

Manning, W. D., Flanigan, C. M., Giordano, P. C., & Longmore, M. A. (2009). Relationship dynamics and consistency of condom use among adolescents. *Perspectives on Sexual and Reproductive Health, 41,* 181–190.

Manning, W. D., Giordano, P. C., & Longmore, M. A. (2006). Hooking up: The relationship contexts of "nonrelationship" sex. *Journal of Adolescent Research, 21,* 459–483. doi: 10.1177/0743558406291692.

Manning, W. D., Giordano, P. C., Longmore, M. A., & Hocevar, A. (2011). Romantic relationships and academic/career trajectories in emerging adulthood. In F. D. Fincham & M. Cui (Eds.), *Romantic relationships in emerging adulthood* (pp. 317–333). New York, NY: Cambridge University Press.

Matson, P. A., Adler, N. E., Millstein, S. G., Tschann, J. M., & Ellen, J. M. (2011). Developmental changes in condom use among urban adolescent females: Influence of partner context. *Journal of Adolescent Health, 48,* 386–390.

Meier, A., & Allen, G. (2009). Romantic relationships from adolescence to young adulthood: Evidence from the National Longitudinal Study of Adolescent Health. *Sociological Quarterly, 50,* 308–335. doi: 10.1111/j.1533-8525.2009.01142.x.

Montgomery, M. J., & Sorell, G. T. (1998). Love and dating experience in early and middle adolescence: Grade and gender comparisons. *Journal of Adolescence, 21,* 677–689.

Mullins, T. L. K., Zimet, G. D., Rosenthal, S. L., Morrow, C., Ding, L., Shew, M., … Kahn, J. A. (2012). Adolescent perceptions of risk and need for safer sexual behaviors after first human papillomavirus vaccination. *Archives of Pediatrics and Adolescent Medicine, 166,* 82–88.

O'Sullivan, L. F., & Brooks-Gunn, J. (2005). The timing of changes in girls' sexual cognitions and behaviors in early adolescence: A prospective, cohort study. *Journal of Adolescent Health, 37*, 211–219.

O'Sullivan, L. F., Cheng, M. M., Harris, K. M., & Brooks-Gunn, J. (2007). I wanna hold your hand: The progression of social, romantic and sexual events in adolescent relationships. *Perspectives on Sexual and Reproductive Health, 39*, 100–107.

O'Sullivan, L. F., & Majerovich, J. (2008). Difficulties with sexual functioning in a sample of male and female late adolescent and young adult university students. *Canadian Journal of Human Sexuality, 17*, 109–121.

Ohye, B. Y., & Daniel, J. H. (1999). The "other" adolescent girls: Who are they? In N. G. Johnson, M. C. Roberts, & J. Worell (Eds.), *Beyond appeance: A new look at adolescent girls* (pp. 115–129). Washington DC: American Psychological Association.

Ott, M. A., Harezlak, J., Ofner, S., & Fortenberry, J. D. (2012). Timing of incident STI relative to sexual partner change in young women. *Sexually Transmitted Diseases, 39*, 747–749.

Ott, M. A., Katschke, A., Tu, W., & Fortenberry, J. D. (2011). Longitudinal associations among relationship factors, partner change, and sexually transmitted infection acquisition in adolescent women. *Sexually Transmitted Diseases, 38*, 153–157.

Peck, S. R., Shaffer, D. R., & Williamson, G. M. (2004). Sexual satisfaction and relationship satisfaction in dating couples: The contributions of relationship communality and favorability of sexual exchanges. *Journal of Psychology and Human Sexuality, 16*, 17–37. doi: 10.1300/J056v16n04_02.

Picot, J., Shepherd, J., Kavanagh, J., Cooper, K., Harden, A., Barnett-Page, E., . . . Frampton, G. K. (2012). Behavioural interventions for the prevention of sexually transmitted infections in young people aged 13-19 years: A systematic review. *Health Education Research, 27*, 495–512.

Centers for Disease Control and Prevention. (2012). *Sexually transmitted diseases surveillance 2011.* Atlanta, GA: US Department of Health and Human Services.

Regan, P. C. (1998). What if you can't get what you want? Willingness to compromise ideal mate selection standards as a function of sex, mate value, and relationship context. *Personality and Social Psychology Bulletin, 24*, 1294–1303.

Reis, H. T., Collins, W. A., & Berscheid, E. (2000). The relationship context of human behavior and development. *Psychological Bulletin, 126*, 844–872.

Robert, A. C., & Sonenstein, F. L. (2010). Adolescents' reports of communication with their parents about sexually transmitted diseases and birth control: 1988, 1995, and 2002. *Journal of Adolescent Health, 46*, 532–537.

Romero, E. G., Teplin, L. A., McClelland, G. M., Abram, K. M., Welty, L. J., & Washburn, J. J. (2007). A longitudinal study of the prevalence, development, and persistence of HIV/ sexually transmitted infection risk behaviors in delinquent youth: Implications for health care in the community. *Pediatrics, 119*, e1126–e1141.

Romualdi, C., Balding, D., Nasidze, I. S., Risch, G., Robichaux, M., Sherry, S. T., . . . Barbujani, G. (2002). Patterns of human diversity, within and among continents, inferred from biallelic DNA polymorphisms. *Genome Research, 12*, 602–612.

Royer, H. R., Keller, M. L., & Heidrich, S. M. (2009). Young adolescents' perceptions of romantic relationships and sexual activity. *Sex Education, 9*, 395–408. doi: 10.1080/14681810903265329.

Sayegh, M. A., Fortenberry, J. D., Anderson, J. G., & Orr, D. P. (2005). Effects of relationship quality on chlamydia infection among adolescent women. *Journal of Adolescent Health, 37*, 163.

Sayegh, M. A., Fortenberry, J. D., Shew, M., & Orr, D. P. (2006). The developmental association of relationship quality, hormonal contraceptive choice and condom non-use among adolescent women. *Journal of Adolescent Health, 39*, 388–395.

Seaton, E. K., Yip, T., Morgan-Lopez, A., & Sellers, R. M. (2012). Racial discrimination and racial socialization as predictors of African American adolescents' racial identity development using latent transition analysis. *Developmental Psychology, 48,* 448–458. doi: 10.1037/a0025328.

Seiffge-Krenke, I. (2003). Testing theories of romantic development from adolescence to young adulthood: Evidence of a developmental sequence. *International Journal of Behavioral Development, 27*(6), 519–531. doi: 10.1080/01650250344000145.

Simons, R. L., Simons, L. G., Lei, M. K., & Landor, A. M. (2012). Relational schemas, hostile romantic relationships, and beliefs about marriage among young African American adults. *Journal of Social and Personal Relationships, 29,* 77–101. doi: 10.1177/0265407511406897.

Sprecher, S. (1998). Social exchange theories and sexuality. *Journal of Sex Research, 35,* 32–43.

Sprecher, S. (2002). Sexual satisfaction in premarital relationships: Associations with satisfaction, love, commitment, and stability. *Journal of Sex Research, 39,* 190–196. doi: 10.1080/00224490209552141.

Tolman, D. L., & McClelland, S. I. (2011). Normative sexuality development in adolescence: A decade in review, 2000–2009. *Journal of Research on Adolescence, 21,* 242–255. doi: 10.1111/j.1532-7795.2010.00726.x.

Welsh, D. P., Haugen, P. T., Widman, L., Darling, N., & Grello, C. M. (2005). Kissing is good: A developmental investigation of sexuality in adolescent romantic couples. *Sexuality Research and Social Policy, 2,* 32–41. doi: 10.1525/srsp.2005.2.4.32.

Zimmer-Gembeck, M. J., Siebenbruner, J., & Collins, W. A. (2001). Diverse aspects of dating: Associations with psychosocial functioning from early to middle adolescence. *Journal of Adolescence, 24,* 313–336.

CHAPTER 11

Personality Effects on Risky Sexual Behavior

The Importance of Dynamic Situational

Processes and Relational Contexts

M. LYNNE COOPER AND RUIXUE ZHAOYANG

The overwhelming majority of past research on sexual behavior, especially risky sexual behavior, has focused on interindividual differences in background and demographic factors, and health-specific knowledge, attitudes, and beliefs. With few exceptions, however, such factors are only modestly related to risky sexual behaviors. In one particularly comprehensive meta-analytic review, for example, an average meta-analytic r of .08 (range = .02 to .18) was found across 24 effects linking condom use to such factors as gender, race, age, education, religiosity, sexual and sexually transmitted disease history, perceived threat of HIV, HIV knowledge, and prior sex education (Sheerhan, Abraham, & Orbell, 1999). More recent meta-analytic reviews yield similar results (e.g., Albarracin, Johnson, Fishbein, & Muellerleile, 2001; Albarracin, Kumkale, & Johnson, 2004; Casey, Timmermann, Allen, Krahn, & Turkiewicz, 2009; Newcomb & Mustanski, 2011), with most effects in the .05 to .15 range. Indeed, the largest meta-analytic associations with factors of this sort observed in any of the aforementioned reviews fell in the .25 to .35 range and involved associations between condom use and narrowly targeted beliefs or attitudes specific to condom use, such as self-efficacy for use (Casey et al., 2009) or perceived control over use (Albarracin et al., 2001, 2004).

Research examining personality in relation to sexual behaviors indicates that trait effects are also of modest magnitude. The most consistent patterns of effects have been found for two dimensions of personality: conscientiousness (marked by responsibility, orderliness, and self-control) and agreeableness (marked by humility, trust, cooperation, and sympathy). Using data from 52 nations representing 10 regions of the world, Schmitt (2004) obtained an average r of .14 between (low) conscientiousness and sexual promiscuity. In a meta-analysis of 53 studies, Hoyle, Fejfar, and Miller (2000) reported overall effect sizes ranging from .14 (sex without a condom) to .21 (number of sex partners) for impulsivity or low constraint (a core feature of [low] conscientiousness). Similarly, Bogg and Roberts (2004) reported meta-analytic r's ranging from .09 to .15 for specific facets of (low) conscientiousness and risky sex behaviors, with the largest association found for impulsivity. For agreeableness and (low) trait aggression, Hoyle and colleagues (2000) reported meta-analytic rs ranging from −.20 (number of partners) to −.23 (high-risk encounters), whereas Schmitt obtained an r of −.14 between agreeableness and sexual promiscuity in the 52-nation study.

Results appear weaker or more inconsistent for differences in other personality traits. For example, openness to experience (marked by curiosity, imagination, and sophistication) was unrelated or weakly related to diverse forms of risky sexual behavior in both the Hoyle et al. meta-analysis and the Schmitt cross-cultural study. Neuroticism (marked by negative affect, moodiness, reactivity, and low self-esteem) was also unrelated to sexual promiscuity in the 52-nation study ($r = .01$) but was inconsistently related (r's ranged from −.05 to .27) across different measures of neuroticism and sexual behaviors in the Hoyle et al. meta-analysis. Weak results (average meta-analytic $r = .05$) were also reported by Crepaz and Marks (2001), who meta-analyzed associations between trait-like measures of depression, anxiety, and hostility and risky sexual behaviors. Finally, extraversion (marked by sociability, assertiveness, excitement seeking, and positive emotionality) exhibited similar inconsistencies. Hoyle et al. (2000) reported meta-analytic r's ranging from −.09 to .15 depending on sexual behavior and extraversion measure, whereas Schmitt obtained an r of .13 between extroversion and sexual promiscuity in the 52-nation study. In sum, even the most consistently linked personality traits—conscientiousness and agreeableness—reveal only modest associations with most measures of sexual behavior, including risky ones.

Although situational and relationship factors exhibit stronger associations, on average, than most intraindividual difference factors, the absolute magnitude of these associations is in most instances surprisingly modest. For example, situational factors such as arousal (Sheerhan et al., 1999) and alcohol use (Cooper, 2002; Graves & Leigh, 1995) are only modestly related to condom use, with effect sizes typically smaller than .10. Indeed, the only situational factor to show a stronger relationship in the Sheerhan et al. meta-analysis was condom availability ($r = .41$), a behavior so closely tied to actual condom use that one might wonder why the association was only .41.

Finally, relationship factors yield, on average, the most robust associations, though they tend to be modest in size. For example, using self-report data on six different sexual events (e.g., the most recent occasion of sexual intercourse) collected from a randomly selected community sample of approximately 1,800 adolescents (aged 13 to 19 years at baseline) followed over a 12-year period, Cooper (2010) found that having a new or casual partner accounted for 3% of the variance in risk discussion and about 7% of the variance (i.e., r's ~ in the .25–.30 range) in both alcohol use in connection with sex and condom use. Meta-analyses of the effects of partner characteristics on condom use also reveal small to moderate effects, with r's ranging from .11–.30, for having a nonmonogamous partner, partner attitudes about condoms, and communication with the partner about safe sex (Noar, Carlyle, & Cole, 2006; Sheerhan et al., 1999). Indeed, the single strongest meta-analytic r reported in these two meta-analyses was found between condom use and communication with the partner specifically about using a condom ($r = .46$ in the Sheerhan et al. analysis, but only .25 in the Noar et al. analysis).

In sum, the effects of most intraindividual factors, including personality, are small, frequently accounting for no more than 1% to 2% of the variance in a range of sexual behaviors. Moreover, although situational and relationship factors tend to show larger effects, the absolute value of these effects is also relatively modest, typically accounting for no more than 2% to 3% of the variance in the case of situational factors and 5%–10% of the variance in the case of relationship factors. The relatively modest magnitude of these effects raises serious questions about the value or appropriateness of theoretical and empirical approaches taken in past research. In the following section, we outline what we see as some of the key issues contributing to the limited explanatory power of past research.

LIMITATIONS OF PAST RESEARCH

Historically, efforts to understand sexual behavior came out of a public health tradition and were motivated by concerns for preventing negative consequences of sexual behavior, such as unplanned pregnancies and sexually transmitted infections. This led to a focus on rational models such as the Health Belief Model (Janz & Becker, 1984) and on factors such as knowledge and beliefs that could be easily changed, to the relative neglect of more psychologically sophisticated conceptualizations, particularly those emphasizing the motivational and emotional bases of health behavior (see Rodin & Salovey, 1989, for a review). Second and relatedly, the vast majority of research also focused on sexual behavior at the level of the individual, with little attention to the intrinsically interpersonal nature of sex (Kelly & Kalichman, 1995; Misovich, Fisher, & Fisher, 1997). Third, past research tended to view sexual behavior as a stable and enduring property of the person, rather than something that is dynamic and changes across partners, sexual situations, and time. Indeed, the overwhelming majority of past studies (92% in one meta-analysis; Sheerhan et al., 1999) used global measures of risky sexual behavior (e.g., "How often in the past year did you use a condom?") that require respondents to aggregate their behavior across partners, occasions, and time to arrive at a single overall estimate. Such a strategy is not only more error prone (Loftus, Smith, Klinger, &

Fiedler, 1992; Lucas & Baird, 2006) but also precludes the examination of potentially important qualitative differences across partners, situations, or time.

Finally, as Gullone and Moore (2000) pointed out, the majority of past studies examined only one or a few factors in isolation. This is true not only of studies focused on personality as predictors, the target of Gullone and Moore's comment, but also of research on sexual behaviors in general. As a result, we know little about the unique or nonoverlapping predictive validity of individual factors, be they at the level of the person, the situation, or the relationship. Perhaps more important, this narrow focus has prevented the testing of integrated theoretical models that distinguish more proximal and distal influences, and specify plausible mediating mechanisms. Finally, by focusing on factors individually, few studies have even considered the possibility that intraindividual, relational, and situational factors combine or interact to shape sexual behavior.

In the following sections, we draw on data from several different studies to illustrate some of the most important downsides of the predominant approaches taken in past research.

Treating Sexual Behavior as a Stable, Enduring Property of the Person

As previously discussed, past research has relied almost exclusively on global or aggregate measures of sexual behavior. Because global measurement strategies require aggregating behaviors, they are capable of modeling interindividual differences (i.e., differences between people) in behavior, but not within-person variation across situations, partners, and time. Of course, the extent to which this is problematic depends on how much of the total variability in sexual behavior lies at the between- versus within-person levels. If most of the variation in these behaviors exists between people, then global measurement strategies may indeed provide an easy and economical way to model sexual behaviors and the factors that cause them. However, if substantial portions of the variation exist within a person across occasions, partners, and time, then global measurement strategies are inadequate to the task.

To examine this issue, we decomposed the variance in five risky sexual behaviors (viz., drinking proximal to intercourse, having sex with a risky partner, discussing risk factors with the partner before sex, not using a condom, and not using a form of noncoital birth control) using event-level data from the first three waves of the previously described longitudinal study in which respondents reported on two sexual experiences at each wave—the last time they had sex and the first time they had sex with that partner. In this way, descriptive information was obtained for each person on up to six different sexual occasions (7,653 events in total; see Cooper, 2010, for details). To decompose the variance, events were nested under the person and an unconditional model (i.e., a model which has no predictors; Nezlek, 2001) was estimated for each behavior. Results of these analyses revealed that, on average, 25%

of the variance in the five risk behaviors was due to between-person differences, whereas 75% was due to variability within the person across situations, partners, and time. Partner risk showed the smallest proportion of within-person variability (66%), whereas condom use (81%), alcohol use (81%), and level of commitment to one's sexual partner (86%) showed the largest proportions.

One might argue, however, that the design of this study overestimates, perhaps even substantially, the amount of within-person variability. After all, analyses were based on reports of sexual events that took place over roughly 12 years, during a developmental period (adolescence into young adulthood) that encompasses nearly unparalleled growth and change. Moreover, the sample of events included qualitatively different types of sexual experiences (e.g., with both new and established partners) as well as, in most cases, events with three different sexual partners. Thus, it is perhaps not surprising that such a large percentage of the variance was due to variability within the person across occasions, partners, and time.

To provide an alternate and more conservative estimate of the amount of within-person variability in sexual experience, we analyzed data from 1,598 sexual events provided by 144 young adult couples who completed an event report each time they had sexual intercourse over an approximately 3-week period (see Zhaoyang & Cooper, 2013, for details on the study design and method). Because couples in this study had been together on average more than 2 years, these sexual events can be seen as capturing a sample of everyday sexual experiences, experiences that on the whole should not differ that dramatically from one another. These data also permit a more refined decomposition of variance in sexual feelings and behaviors. Not only can we estimate variance due to between- and within-person sources, as before, but we can also estimate variance due to the couple.

Accordingly, we nested sex event reports under individuals and individuals under couples and once again estimated a series of unconditional models (Nezlek, 2001). This time, however, we decomposed the total variance in reports of seven different feelings and behaviors (i.e., feelings of arousal, love, negative mood, and satisfaction, as well as the number of different sexual activities, drinking proximal to intercourse, and condom use) into their between-couple, between-person, and within-person components. Results of these analyses are summarized in Figure 11.1.

As shown in Figure 11.1, feelings of arousal, satisfaction, and negative mood varied substantially more at the within-person level, perhaps not so surprisingly, than at the between-person or between-couple levels. Interestingly, feelings of love—commonly seen as the emotional glue that holds relationships together—also varied nearly as much as the more traditional feeling states.

The last three sets of bars illustrate results for the three behaviors. As shown, the number of actual behaviors (e.g., kissing, oral sex, vaginal sex, etc.) engaged in across these sexual occasions was highly variable at the within-person level, exhibiting on average seven times more within-person variance, and three times more between-couple variance, than between-person variance. In contrast, the lion's share of the variance in both alcohol use and condom use occurred at the between-couple level.

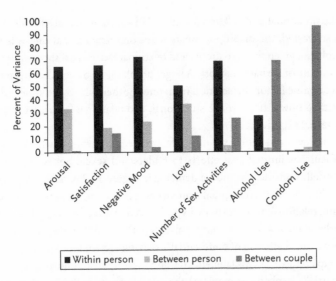

Figure 11.1: Decomposition of variance in sexual feelings and behaviors into between-couple, between-person, and within-person components.

Such a pattern indicates that whereas couples differed markedly from one another in their average levels of both behaviors, differences within a couple were comparatively small (i.e., perhaps not surprisingly, couple members reported highly similar behaviors). Indeed, couple-level differences accounted for nearly all of the variance in condom use (96%), whereas significant variability in alcohol use existed at the between-couple and within-person levels.

In sum, these data indicate that most sexual behaviors and all sexual feelings, including love, vary more within a person across sexual occasions than between-persons. Moreover, for those behaviors that did not conform to this pattern, most of the variance occurred between couples rather than between persons. Thus, across both studies and for all behaviors examined, only a relatively small portion of the variance occurred at the between-person level, which ironically is the only type of variance that the predominant methodological approaches used in the field (e.g., analyses of cross-sectional, individual-level data) are suited to capture. Although it is true that some unknown portion of the within-person variance is due to error (Raudenbush & Bryk, 2002), these results nevertheless underscore the limitations of predominant approaches that are insensitive to within-person sources of variation in sexual behavior, as well as to interpersonal and couple-level causes of these behaviors.

Focusing on Individual-Level Factors and Treating Causes in Isolation

As just discussed, past research has focused disproportionately on stable, intrapersonal causes of sexual behavior such as personality, while neglecting potentially important situational and relational causes. However, as our brief review of past research suggested, the disproportionate focus on intrapersonal causes is not the whole problem, given that situational and relational factors also show modest associations with most sexual behaviors. A larger problem, we believe, has been the tendency to examine factors in isolation from one another, which has impeded efforts to understand how intrapersonal, situational, and relational factors work together to shape sexual experience.

In the following sections, we illustrate two primary ways in which this overly narrow focus has limited past efforts to understand sexual behavior. First, however, we briefly consider the model depicted in Figure 11.2 as a way to place these processes in a broader conceptual framework. As shown, personality, situational factors, and relationship contexts are hypothesized to directly predict sexual experience (paths labeled "a"). Personality is also hypothesized to indirectly shape sexual behavior via the likelihood of preferentially seeking certain types of situational and relationship contexts (paths labeled "b"), and in turn these contexts are thought to at least partially explain (or mediate) the effects of intraindividual differences on sexual behavior (paths "a" × "b"). In addition, situational and relationship contexts are hypothesized to moderate the strength or nature of personality effects on sexual behavior (paths labeled "c"). Importantly, because interactions are symmetrical, this also means that personality can be seen as moderating the effects of situational and relational contexts on behavior. Finally, background and demographic characteristics are viewed as more distal factors that directly (paths labeled "d") and indirectly (via their influence on personality and the likelihood of selecting into or creating different types of environments) predict sexual behavior. As previously indicated, the present chapter focuses on two of these mechanisms: (1) the indirect effects of personality on sexual behavior as mediated by the tendency to seek different types of situational and relationship contexts, and (2) the moderating effects of these contexts on personality.

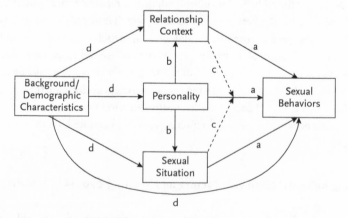

Figure 11.2: Person-in-context model of sexual behavior. (Adapted from Cooper, 2010, *Journal of Personality and Social Psychology*.)

Situational and Relational Contexts as Mediators of Intraindividual (Personality) Effects

According to Snyder and Ickes (1985), this first mechanism reflects a dynamic transaction between person and environment in which individuals with certain traits or predispositions actively select or construct (through evoking characteristic responses or by active manipulation) the social contexts in which they feel most comfortable (i.e., are most ego syntonic), and these contexts in turn selectively reinforce certain behaviors and response patterns. In other words, personality *indirectly* shapes sexual behavior by selectively directing people toward compatible sexual situations and relationship contexts.

Evidence for this mechanism (path "b" in Fig. 11.2), a mechanism we refer to as niche seeking, comes from several different lines of research. For example, data from the previously described longitudinal study of adolescents showed that individuals who were dispositionally high in avoidant attachment were significantly less likely than either secure or anxiously attached adolescents to be in a serious, committed relationship as long as 15 years later (Cooper, Albino, Michaes, Levitt, & Collins, 2004). Using data from this same study, we also found that individuals who strongly endorsed enhancement motives for sex (e.g., reported having sex because it was exciting or fun) in their late teens and early twenties were significantly more likely to report having recently had sex with a stranger (defined as someone they met that same day or evening) nearly 10 years later (Cooper, Barber, Zhaoyang, & Talley, 2011). Similarly, in a diary study of college students who had recently experienced a break-up (Barber & Cooper, 2014), we found that students high (vs. low) in enhancement motives were significantly more likely to have sex with someone other than their ex-partner, as well as to have significantly more sex partners in the semester following the break-up (see Cooper et al., 2011). Together these data suggest that some individuals, by virtue of their discomfort with intimacy or their dispositional preferences for excitement, selectively avoid committed, intimate contexts, deliberately seek out more casual ones, or both.

Conversely, we have also shown that individuals who value intimacy preferentially seek out specific relational contexts in which their needs for emotional closeness can be most easily satisfied. For example, in the previously described longitudinal study, we found that intimacy motives interacted with the number of sex partners in the past 6 months to predict change in partners over a 1.4-year period (Cooper, Shapiro, & Powers, 1998, Study 4). As shown in Figure 11.3, plotting the interaction showed that intimacy motives predicted a significant *positive* change in the number of partners among individuals who initially had no sex partners, a significant *negative* change among those who had more than one sex partner, and *no* change among those who had one sex partner, thus suggesting that over time high intimacy-motive individuals preferentially sought out a relational context in which their intimacy needs were likely to be met—that is, a context involving a single sexual partner.

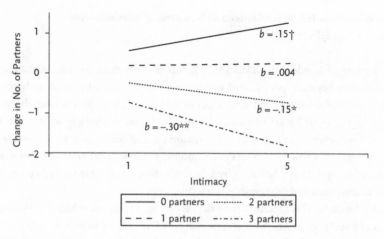

Figure 11.3: Interaction of intimacy motive × number of partners at baseline predicting change in partners. $^\dagger p < .10$. $^* p < .05$. $^{**} p < .01$. (From Cooper, Shapiro, & Powers, 1998, *Journal of Personality and Social Psychology*.)

In this same study, we also found that high-intimacy-motive individuals were more likely to move into or stay in an exclusive relationship over time, and importantly that these relationship contexts in turn explained significant variance in the individual's subsequent sexual behavior. For example, individuals high in intimacy motives at baseline were more likely to be in an exclusive relationship 1.4 years later, and as a result of being in an exclusive relationship had both less frequent intercourse and less risky sex. Interestingly, the opposite pattern of mediated effects was found for enhancement motives—that is, individuals who were initially high in enhancement motives were more likely to be single or unattached at follow-up, and consequently had both more frequent intercourse and riskier sex.

In one final example, we examined the effects of attachment styles assessed in adolescence on the nature and quality of relationships established during emerging adulthood (i.e., in the early to mid-twenties; Collins, Cooper, Albino, & Allard, 2002). As shown in Figure 11.4, our results revealed that individuals who had an avoidant attachment style in adolescence chose partners some 6 years later who, by the partner's own report, had less healthy personalities: They reported higher levels of negative emotionality, a diminished sense of personal competence, and low warmth. Not surprisingly, these partners—again by their own admission—behaved in less relationship supportive ways, and these relationship-undermining behaviors in turn adversely affected both the partner's and the individual's own relationship quality, including the quality of their intimate and sexual experiences.

In short, we have presented evidence from several different studies, using both self- and partner reports, showing that individuals by virtue of their personal preferences and needs selectively seek out certain types of relational and sexual niches, and that these niches in turn shape the individual's subsequent sexual experiences. Clearly, studies that focus predominantly on a single cause or category of causes

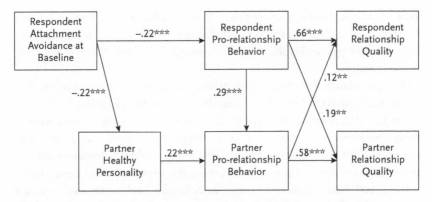

Figure 11.4: Model linking attachment avoidance at baseline to own and partner relationship quality 6 years later. ** $p < .01$. *** $p < .001$. (Reprinted with permission from Collins, Cooper, Albino & Allard, 2002, *Journal of Personality.*)

cannot model the types of transactional processes we have observed between persons and the relational and situational contexts they seek, or the influences that these contexts in turn exert on the nature and quality of the individual's sexual experience.

Situational and Relational Contexts as Moderators of Intraindividual Characteristics

Thus far we have focused on what Snyder and Ickes (1985) called transactional mechanisms, mechanisms in which individuals seek out or create certain relational contexts, and these contexts in turn shape behavior. However, contexts matter in another, entirely different way. Individuals with different preferred styles of behaving or with different needs, values, and goals routinely adjust their behavior to exploit the unique opportunities or accommodate the particular constraints imposed by the environments they inhabit. To the extent that this is true, different relational contexts may trigger different responses depending on the opportunities and constraints they present, and how these fit (or fail to fit) with the individual's preferred styles of behaving, needs, goals, and so on. Such mechanisms should manifest in the form of person × context or person × situation interactions (effects labeled "c" in Fig. 11.2).

In the following section, we present data from several past studies in which we tested interactions between situational or relationship contexts and intraindividual characteristics, including both personality traits and dispositional motives. Although such interactions can take on a range of theoretically meaningful forms (see Cooper, Talley, Sheldon, Levitt, & Barber, 2008, for a discussion), in the present chapter, we examine a particular form of person × environment interaction involving what Mischel (1977) referred to as strong versus weak situations. According to Mischel, strong situations have clear injunctive and descriptive norms, are more likely to be scripted, and afford the individuals in them little choice in how they behave. In contrast, weak situations have less clear norms, are less likely to be scripted, and allow people to behave in many different ways. Thus, individuals have far greater latitude to express their individuality in weak than strong situations, suggesting that personality should be more strongly linked to behavior in weak than strong situations.

In close relationship contexts, we believe that a key determinant of situation strength is the degree of interdependence between partners, such that highly interdependent situations or relationship contexts act as strong situations, whereas those characterized by low levels of interdependence act as weak situations. Interdependent situations are those in which an individual's outcomes are intimately bound up with, or contingent on, those of his or her partner (Kenny, Kashy, & Cook, 2006), such that an individual, by definition, has less autonomy and control over his or her own behavior. Accordingly, the more highly interdependent a situation, the less an individual can behave autonomously, and consequently the less strongly his or her own personality, preferences, and needs should predict his or her sexual experiences. Evidence in support of this premise comes from several different studies (described below).

Using data from the previously described longitudinal study of adolescents, we tested the hypothesis that individual differences in motives for sex would more strongly predict sexual experience among single or unattached individuals compared with their coupled counterparts (Cooper et al., 1998, Studies 3 and 4). Consistent with expectation, we found a reliable pattern of relationship status × motive interactions predicting sexual experience in both cross-sectional and longitudinal analyses. For example, we found that a dispositional preference to have sex for fun or excitement (i.e., enhancement motives) significantly positively predicted risky sexual behaviors and intercourse frequency in cross-sectional analyses, as well as increases over time in the number of partners among those who were single. In contrast, enhancement motives were unrelated or more weakly related to each of these outcomes among those who were in a relationship. Likewise, as shown in Figure 11.5, the dispositional preference to use sex as a way to minimize or escape

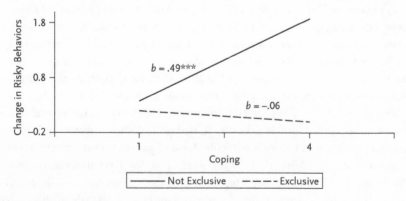

Figure 11.5: Sex motive × relationship status interaction predicting risky sexual behaviors. *** $p < .001$. (From Cooper, Shapiro, & Powers, 1998, *Journal of Personality and Social Psychology*.)

negative mood states (i.e., coping motives for sex) significantly positively predicted risky sexual behaviors in cross-sectional analyses, as well as increases over time in the number of risky behaviors among those who were unattached. However, no such association was found among those who were in a relationship.

In another study (Cooper, 2010), we tested the possibility that individual differences in personality would be more strongly linked to sexual experience among those whose relationships were new (vs. established) or more casual (vs. more committed). We reasoned that new relationships would be less interdependent, as interdependence develops over time with shared experience and partner interactions (see Rusbult & Van Lange, 2003 for a review), and likewise that casual relationships would be less interdependent as interdependence is a hallmark of committed relationships (Agnew, Van Lange, Rusbult, & Langston, 1998).

To test these ideas, we used the previously described data from the first three waves of the longitudinal study in which respondents reported on two recent sexual experiences, one involving a first-time sex partner and the other involving the most recent sexual experience with that same partner (7,653 events in total; see Cooper, 2010). Ratings of relationship commitment and a variety of sexual behaviors were collected for each sexual event. Because people vary substantially in the extent to which first-sex occasions occur with more casual versus serious partners (Christopher & Roosa, 1991), ratings of relationship commitment were only moderately correlated ($r = .45$) with the first versus subsequent distinction ($0 =$ first, $1 =$ subsequent). Thus, we were able to use these data to analyze each effect controlling for the other, to determine whether similar patterns were observed across these alternative instantiations of the interdependence construct.

Results of these analyses revealed, as expected, that more than half (13 of 25) of all trait–risk behavior associations examined were moderated by situation type, commitment level, or both. Moreover, the overwhelming majority of these effects, when plotted, showed that personality traits were more strongly associated with sexual experience on occasions with new versus established partners, as well as on occasions with casual versus serious ones. For example, communal orientation (marked by warmth, a concern for others, and a preference for close, intimate relationships) significantly, positively predicted the degree of prior risk discussion with the partner on first but not subsequent sex occasions, and on occasions with casual but not serious partners. Similarly, agency (marked by social skill and dominance, along with a positive focus on the self) significantly, positively predicted the amount of prior risk discussion on first sex occasions, but not on later ones.

Particularly striking was the consistent pattern of moderation observed for sexual venturesomeness (a preference for novel, risky, and exciting sexual activities) and impulsivity (the tendency to act hastily and without forethought), widely regarded as two of the most reliable and robust predictors of risky sexual behaviors (Bogg & Roberts, 2004; Devieux et al., 2002; Hoyle et al., 2000). Not only were eight out of the ten tested associations involving these two traits moderated by situation type, relationship context, or both, but the majority of these cases (five of eight) distinguished contexts in which a significant, positive association existed between the trait (i.e., venturesomeness or impulsivity) and risk behavior versus no association whatsoever. Two of these effects are illustrated in Figure 11.6.

Finally, we examined the possibility that individual differences in the need for or concern with partner approval serve as a marker of interdependence to the extent that the outcomes of those who are high in partner approval motives should depend more on the partner and less on one's own needs and preferences. Accordingly, we speculated that partner approval motives would moderate the link between intraindividual differences and sexual behavior, such that the behavior of individuals who are higher (vs. lower) on partner approval motives would be less strongly determined by their own, and more strongly determined by their partner's, needs and preferences. We tested this idea using data from a subset of participants in the previously described longitudinal study who were interviewed with their sexual partners (see Cooper et al., 2008).

As expected, results revealed a consistent pattern of interactions indicating that partner needs and preferences more strongly determined sexual experience among

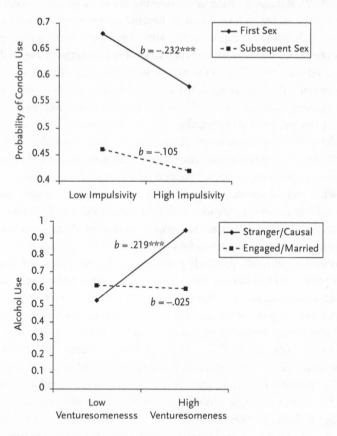

Figure 11.6: Representative person × situation and person × relationship interactions predicting risky sexual behavior. *** $p < .001$. (From Cooper, 2010, *Journal of Personality and Social Psychology*.)

women who were high (vs. low) in partner approval motives. Figure 11.7 provides an illustrative example of the form of the interaction. As shown, the male partner's desire to have sex for enhancement reasons significantly positively predicted female partner reports of the frequency of sexual intercourse (top panel) and of sexual satisfaction (bottom panel), but only among women who were high in partner approval motives. Although interactions of this form were also observed among men, the pattern was less consistent across predictors and sexual outcomes. Finally, we found little support for the idea that one's own needs and preferences less strongly determined behavior among individuals who high in partner approval motives.

In sum, we have presented evidence from several different studies indicating that the effects of personality and motives vary significantly across relational and situational contexts: They are substantially more predictive in contexts and situations that are less interdependent, and indeed they are often completely unrelated to the nature or quality of sexual experiences in highly interdependent contexts. Moreover, the predictive utility of partner needs and preferences was also found to be greater for individuals whose outcomes were presumably highly dependent on their partner's approval. Such findings clearly illustrate the limitations of examining predictors in isolation, and they also help to explain why the main effect of many traits may be only weakly related to sexual behavior outcomes.

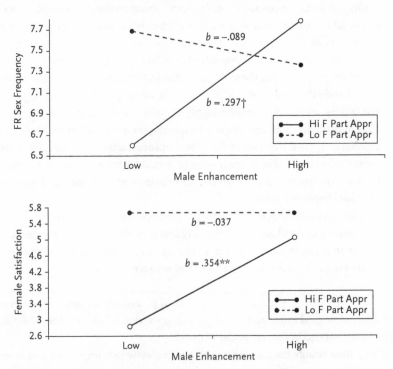

Figure 11.7: Representative approval motive × partner motive interactions predicting sexual behavior. FR, female report; Hi(Lo) F Part Appr, high(low) female partner approval. $+ p < .10$. $** p < .01$. (From Cooper et al. 2008.)

SUMMARY AND IMPLICATIONS FOR FUTURE RESEARCH

The data presented in the present chapter support four main conclusions about the nature of sexual experience:

1. Most sexual behaviors and all sexual feelings, including love, varied more within a person across sexual occasions than between persons, and this was true even in the context of a single, established partnership. Moreover, for those behaviors that did not conform to this pattern, more variance was found between couples than between persons. Thus, across both data sets and for all behaviors examined, only a relatively small portion of the variance occurred at the between-person level, which ironically is the only type of variance that the predominant methodological approaches used in the field are suited to capture.

2. People choose relational and situational contexts that are compatible with their needs, goals, and preferred styles of behaving, and these contexts in turn shape their sexual experience. Such findings suggest that the effects of intraindividual differences are at least in part mediated or explained by the interpersonal environments people choose or create by virtue of their personalities.

3. The effects of intraindividual characteristics on sexual behavior vary consistently, and in many cases substantially, across situational and relational contexts. In particular, we showed that many trait–behavior associations are stronger in contexts or situations characterized by low levels of interdependence, and weaker or nonexistent in highly interdependent contexts. Because interaction effects are symmetrical, these findings also indicate that the strength of situational and relational contexts likewise varies across levels of traits (e.g., context effects are stronger among highly impulsive individuals; see Fig. 11.6). Thus, most traits do not predispose to specific sexual behaviors and feelings in a global or typical way, just as the effects of sexual situations and relationship contexts do not invariably predispose to particular types of sexual outcomes. Rather, in most cases, it is the unique combination of the person and the situation that shapes behavior.

4. And finally, depending on one's partner for approval increases partner control over one's sexual outcomes, particularly among women. It does not, however, appear to result in a corresponding decrease in the importance of one's own needs and preferences as a determinant of sexual outcomes.

Taken together, these data have a number of potentially important theoretical and methodological implications for research on sexual behaviors. These implications are elaborated in the remainder of the chapter.

First, these results lend strong support to the view that important and meaningful within-person differences in sexual behavior exist. Indeed, the fact that sexual behaviors varied substantially more within-person than they did, on average, between persons underscores the limitations of predominant strategies used in past research, which have focused on relatively static properties of the person and used global measures of risk and protective behaviors aggregated across situations and partners. Such strategies are not only incapable of explaining the majority of variance in sexual behaviors but also obscure the most informative aspect of these behaviors: their variability. As Mischel and Shoda (1995) have argued, identifying and understanding reliable patterns of cross-situational variability in behavior must lie at the core of any successful effort to explain human behavior. According to Mischel (1999), it is through the study of this variability—of the unique patterns of behavior exhibited across situations or contexts—that the true meaning of interindividual (or trait) differences is most likely to be revealed. Thus, it is this level of analysis that has the greatest potential to illuminate the psychological dynamics that underlie sexual behavior and ultimately to yield findings that can be translated into meaningful social policy and change efforts. For example, gaining a more nuanced understanding of how individuals with different motive or personality profiles behave with more casual versus intimate sexual partners, or how their behavior changes over time as a relationship develops, could provide the basis for interventions tailored to the behavioral tendencies of particular individuals in specific relational contexts.

Together these considerations indicate that strategies seeking to understand within-person variability in sexual behaviors across situations, partners, and time must play a more prominent role in future research. Toward that end, studies using diary methods should prove particularly informative. However, simply using designs that faithfully model within-person variability will not be enough. Future research will also need to develop more complex, contextualized theoretical models that explain the variability in behavior within a person across situations and relationship partners, as well as assessment tools that more faithfully capture this variability.

Second, although past research has focused disproportionately on the individual as the locus of explanation for sexual behaviors, our review of past research as well as the analyses presented herein indicate that, relative to individual-level factors, situational and relational factors are equally if not more important determinants of sexual behavior. Indeed, as we have shown, failure to take situational and relationship contexts into account risks seriously underestimating the predictability of sexual behavior. Thus, we believe that all studies—including studies of single or unattached individuals—must take explicit account of the situational and relational contexts in which sexual behaviors occur.

However, the optimal way to accomplish this remains an open question. In our past research, we have used several approaches for assessing sexual experience that we believe capture much of the meaningful variance due to contextual factors without being unduly burdensome and, as such, may provide useful models for others. Cooper and Orcutt (2000), for example, used cross-sectional data from a single wave of interviews from the previously described longitudinal study to examine the within-person effects of relationship commitment on condom use and drinking proximal to intercourse. Individuals with one or two sexual partners in the past 6 months were asked a set of seven questions about the nature of the relationship with each partner, as well as his or her sexual experiences with that partner. Due to concerns about fatigue effects, those with three or more partners answered a parallel set of seven questions for up to two partners or partner types. For example, an individual who had three partners (one primary and two secondary) would answer the same set of questions, first, for his or her primary partner and then for the two secondary partners together (see Cooper & Orcutt, 2000, for details). Thus, although some aggregation of experience was still required, respondents were at least aggregating across partners that were relatively similar on the key dimension of commitment.

Event-level assessments focused on recent sexual experiences represent another way to generate within-person data in the context of a cross-sectional survey. Cooper, Peirce, and Huselid (1994), for example, examined sexual experiences on two occasions of intercourse, the most recent occasion (occurring, on average, within the last 2 days) and the first time the individual had sex with their most recent partner (occurring, on average, about 1 year ago). Although Cooper and colleagues used these data to examine the within-person effects of drinking alcohol on risky sexual behavior, as well as the generalizability of these effects across new and established sexual partners, they could have been used to examine the within-person effects of relationship stage or commitment on the nature and quality of sexual experience (and, in fact, were used this way in a subsequent publication as part of a larger, event-level data set; see Cooper, 2010).

Although we have not used timeline follow-back procedures in our own research, this approach provides yet another option that can be used to generate within-person data on sexual experiences in the context of a cross-sectional study. For example, Weihardt and colleagues (Weinhardt, Carey, Carey, Maisto, & Gordon, 2001) used this procedure to collect data from 123 sexually active participants on 3,026 sexual events experienced over a 3-month period. A structured interview was used in which participants first provided the initials of their sexual partners over the last 3 months along with basic information needed to categorize the nature of the relationship with each partner. (In this particular study, they used three categories—new, casual, and frequent/regular.) With the aid of a calendar, participants filled in special (e.g., birthdays, holidays, vacations) and recurring events, and then around these events, filled in all occasions on which they had a sexual encounter. Sexual encounters were linked with specific partners such that the nature and quality of those experiences could be examined within a person across individual partners or partner types.

Of course, event-level assessments of specific sexual events can also be used as part of a diary study (see Zhaoyang & Cooper, 2013, for an example). While this approach provides perhaps the richest and most accurate within-person data, it also poses a substantially greater burden on both the researcher and the participants. For this reason, we believe that these other approaches provide an excellent trade-off. They can be implemented in the context of a cross-sectional study and, with the possible exception of the timeline follow-back procedure, require the addition of only a few more questions than traditional global assessments. Yet they enable the researcher to use powerful analytic tools (such as multilevel modeling) to examine sexual experiences and how they differ within a person across relational contexts that differ in the degree of interdependence.

Third, although measurement approaches such as this are promising, they are not designed to yield a nuanced or multifaceted description of situational and relational contexts. For that purpose, more refined models that identify the specific parameters or dimensions that underpin these contexts and shape sexual experience within them will need to be developed. Interdependence theory may provide one useful framework for thinking about these issues. According to Rusbult and Van Lange (2003), interdependence theory provides a functional analysis of the structure of social situations that interacting people encounter, and relates classes of situations to the particular types of goals and motives that are relevant to dealing with them. As such, it seems particularly well suited to the task of identifying the key dimensions that underlie and control sexual experiences with novel or casual partners as well as with established and committed ones.

Fourth, the data presented herein suggest that understanding sexual behavior in highly interdependent contexts poses a particularly difficult challenge. Indeed, the limited ability of one's own personality to predict sexual behavior in committed relationship contexts, along with the fact that the majority of variance in some sexual behaviors was shown to reside at the couple rather than individual level, underscores the need for a careful and systematic consideration of the specific individual- and couple-level factors that account for sexual behavior in interdependent contexts such as these. Indeed, the profound psychological differences that exist between highly interdependent versus minimally interdependent relational contexts suggest that qualitatively different dynamics and wholly different factors may shape sexual behaviors within the two contexts. Accordingly, future research will need to move away from the idea of a single, overarching theoretical model for understanding sexual behavior and instead embrace the notion of at least two distinct models to account for sexual experiences that occur within minimally interdependent versus highly interdependent contexts.

Fifth, the diminished predictability of intraindividual traits and characteristics in committed relationship contexts also highlights the need to include both couple members whenever studying sexual behavior among interdependent dyads. As Kenny and Cook (1999) point out, designs that include individuals rather than couples assume that one's behavior is caused by his or her own standing on important predictors—an assumption we have shown to be false in many instances. The fact that, in at least some instances, partner needs and preferences may be more predictive of an individual's sexual experiences than his or her own needs and preferences lends additional weight to this recommendation. Thus, moving away from the predominant focus on individuals to the inclusion of both couple members appears to be key.

Finally, the evidence presented in this chapter illustrates the fundamental impossibility of developing a truly adequate explanatory model of sexual behavior by focusing on any set of factors in isolation, be they at the individual, situational, or relational level. Moreover, simply assessing these factors and examining them as main effects is not enough. Building an adequate explanatory model will instead require careful and systematic attention to the myriad ways in which these factors interact both within and across levels to shape sexual behavior. Although the model depicted in Figure 11.2 provides a useful starting point, it is overly general and needs to be systematically elaborated to include specific factors within the general categories identified and, more important, to reflect the unique dynamics that are likely to underpin sexual behaviors in minimally versus highly interdependent contexts.

In closing, the present chapter has attempted to illustrate some of the key ways in which the predominant approaches used to study human sexual experience in the past are incapable of adequately modeling sexual behaviors and the factors that cause them. By so doing, we hope to point the way toward approaches that will ultimately yield a deeper and richer understanding of sexual behavior, one that by necessity embraces both its dynamic and relational nature.

REFERENCES

Agnew, C. R., Van Lange, P. A. M., Rusbult, C. E., & Langston, C. A. (1998). Cognitive interdependence: Commitment and the cognitive representation of close relationships. *Journal of Personality and Social Psychology, 74*, 939–954.

Albarracín, D., Johnson, B. T., Fishbein, M., & Muellerleile, P. (2001). Theories of reasoned action and planned behavior as models of condom use: A meta-analysis. *Psychological Bulletin, 127*, 142–161.

Albarracin, D., Kumkale, G. T., & Johnson, B. T. (2004). Influences of social power and normative support on condom use decisions: A research synthesis. *AIDS Care, 16*, 700–723.

Barber, L. L., & Cooper, M. L. (2014). Sex on the rebound: Factors influencing sexual behavior following a relationship breakup. *Archives of Sexual Behavior, 43*, 251–265.

Bogg, T., & Roberts, R. W. (2004). Conscientiousness and health related behaviors: A meta-analysis of the leading behavioral contributors to mortality. *Psychological Bulletin, 130*, 887–917.

Casey, M. K., Timmerman, L., Allen, M., Krahn, S., & Turkiewicz, K. L. (2009). Response and self-efficacy of condom use: A meta-analysis of this important element of AIDS education and prevention. *Southern Communication Journal, 74*, 57–78.

Christopher, F. S., & Roosa, M. W. (1991). Factors affecting sexual decisions in the premarital relationships of adolescents and young adults. In K. McKinney & S. Sprecher (Eds.), *Sexuality in close relationships* (pp. 111–134). Hillsdale, NJ: Erlbaum.

Collins, N. L., Cooper, M. L., Albino, A., & Allard, L. (2002). Psychosocial vulnerability from adolescence to adulthood: A prospective study of attachment style differences in relationship functioning and partner choice. *Journal of Personality, 70*, 965–1008.

Cooper, M. L. (2002). Alcohol use and risky sexual behavior among college students and youth: Evaluating the evidence. *Journal of Studies on Alcohol/Supplement, 14*, 101–117.

Cooper, M. L. (2010). Toward a person X situation model of sexual risk-taking behaviors: Illuminating the conditional effects of traits across sexual situations and relationship contexts. *Journal of Personality and Social Psychology, 98*, 319–341.

Cooper, M. L., Albino, A., Micheas, L., Pioli, M., Levitt, A., & Collins, N. (2004). *Attachment style differences in sexual motivation and experience: Developmental, dyadic, and daily perspectives.* Invited talk given at the 60th Birthday Celebration in Honor of Phillip R. Shaver, Distinguished Professor, University of California at Davis.

Cooper, M. L., Barber, L., Zhaoyang, R., & Talley, A. E. (2011). Motivational pursuits in the context of human sexual relationships. *Journal of Personality, 79*, 1333–1368.

Cooper, M. L., & Orcutt, H. K. (2000). Alcohol use, condom use, and partner type among heterosexual adolescents and young adults. *Journal of Studies on Alcohol, 3*, 413–419.

Cooper, M. L., Peirce, R. S., & Huselid, R. F. (1994). Substance use and sexual risk taking among black adolescents and white adolescents. *Health Psychology, 13*, 251–262.

Cooper, M. L., Shapiro, C. M., & Powers, A. M. (1998). Motivations for sex and sexual behavior among adolescents and young adults: A functional perspective. *Journal of Personality and Social Psychology, 75*, 1528–1558.

Cooper, M. L., Talley, A., Sheldon, M. S., Levitt, A., & Barber, L. (2008). A dyadic perspective on approach and avoidance motives for sex. In A. J. Elliot (Ed.), *Handbook of approach and avoidance motivation* (pp. 615–631). New York, NY: Psychology Press.

Crepaz, N., & Marks, G. (2001). Are negative affective states associated with HIV sexual risk behavior? A meta-analytic review. *Health Psychology, 20*, 291–299.

Devieux, J., Malow, R., Stein, J., Jennings, T., Lucenko, B., Averhart, C., & Kalichman, S. (2002). Impulsivity and HIV risk among adjudicated alcohol-and other drug-abusing adolescent offenders. *AIDS Education and Prevention, 14*, 24–35.

Graves, K., & Leigh, B. (1995). The relationship of substance use to sexual activity among young adults in the United States. *Family Planning Perspectives, 30*, 18–23.

Gullone, E., & Moore, S. (2000). Adolescent risk-taking and the five-factor model of personality. *Journal of Adolescence, 23*, 393–407.

Hoyle, R. H., Fejfar, M. C., & Miller, J. D. (2000). Personality and sexual risk taking: A quantitative review. *Journal of Personality, 66*, 1203–1231.

Janz, N. K., & Becker, M. H. (1984). The health belief model: A decade later. *Health Education Quarterly, 11*, 1–47.

Kelly, J. A., & Kalichman, S. C. (1995). Increased attention to human sexuality can improve HIV-AIDS prevention efforts: Key research issues and directions. *Journal of Consulting and Clinical Psychology, 63*, 907–918.

Kenny, D. A., & Cook, W. L. (1999). Partner effects in relationship research: Conceptual issues, analytic difficulties, and illustrations. *Personal Relationships, 6*, 433–448.

Kenny, D. A., Kashy, D. A., & Cook, W. L. (2006). *Dyadic data analysis.* New York, NY: Guilford Press.

Loftus, E. F., Smith, K., Klinger, M., & Fiedler, J. (1992) Memory and mismemory for health events. In J. M. Tanur (Ed.), *Questions about questions: Inquiries into the cognitive bases of surveys* (pp. 102–137). New York, NY: Russell Sage.

Lucas, R. E., & Baird, B. M. (2006). Global self-assessment. In M. Eid & E. Diener (Eds.), *Handbook of psychological measurement: A multimethod perspective* (pp. 29–42). Washington, DC: American Psychological Association.

Mischel, W. (1977). The interaction of person and situation. In D. Magnusson & N. S. Endler (Eds.), *Personality at the crossroads: Current issues in interactional psychology* (pp. 333–352). Hillsdale, NJ: Erlbaum.

Mischel, W. (1999). Personality coherence and disposition in a cognitive affective personality system (CAPS) approach. In D. Cervone & Y. Shoda (Eds.), *The coherence of* personality: Social-cognitive bases of consistency, variability, and organization (pp. 37–60). New York, NY: Guilford Press.

Mischel, W., & Shoda, Y. (1995). A cognitive-affective system theory of personality: Re-conceptualizing situations, dispositions, dynamics, and invariance in personality structure. *Psychological Review, 102,* 246–268.

Misovich, S. J., Fisher, J. D., & Fisher, W. A. (1997). Close relationships and elevated HTV risk behavior: Evidence and possible underlying psychological processes. *Review of General Psychology, 1,* 72–107.

Newcomb, M. E., & Mustanski, B. (2011). Moderators of the relationship between internalized homophobia and risky sexual behavior in men who have sex with men: A meta-analysis. *Archive of Sexual Behavior, 40,* 189–199.

Nezlek, J. B. (2001). Multilevel random coefficient analyses of event and interval contingent data in social and personality psychology research. *Personality and Social Psychology Bulletin, 27,* 771–785.

Noar, S. M., Carlyle, K., & Cole, C. (2006). Why communication is crucial: Meta-analysis of the relationship between safer sexual communication and condom use. *Journal of Health Communication, 11,* 365–390.

Raudenbush, S. W., & Bryk, A. S. (2002). *Hierarchical linear models: Applications and data analysis methods* (2nd ed.). Thousand Oaks, CA: Sage.

Rodin, J., & Salovey, P. (1989). Health psychology. *Annual Review of Psychology, 40,* 533–579.

Rusbult, C. E., & Van Lange, P. A. M. (2003). Interdependence, interaction, and relationships. *Annual Review of Psychology, 54,* 351–375.

Schmitt, D. P. (2004). The big five related to risky sexual behavior across 10 world regions: Differential personality association of sexual promiscuity and relationship infidelity. *European Journal of Personality, 18,* 301–319.

Sheeran, P., Abraham, C., & Orbell, S. (1999). Psychosocial correlates of heterosexual condom use: A meta-analysis. *Psychological Bulletin, 125,* 90–132.

Snyder, M., & Ickes, W. (1985). Personality and social behavior. In E. Aronson & G. Lindzey (Eds.), *Handbook of social psychology* (pp. 248–305). New York, NY: Random House.

Weinhardt, L. S., Carey, M. P., Carey, K. B., Maisto, S. A., & Gordon, C. M. (2001). The relation of alcohol use to HIV-risk sexual behavior among adults with a severe and persistent mental illness. *Journal of Consulting and Clinical Psychology, 69,* 77–84.

Zhaoyang, R., & Cooper, M. L. (2013). Body satisfaction and couple's daily sexual experience: A dyadic perspective. *Archives of Sexual Behavior, 42*(6), 985–998.

PART FOUR

Summary: Putting It All Together

CHAPTER 12

Synthesizing Social and Clinical Approaches to Relationships and Health

SUSAN C. SOUTH

The contributions to this edited volume bring together different theories, methods, approaches, and findings from social and clinical psychological explorations of interpersonal relationships and health. While certainly there are other scientific fields that concern themselves with the links between relationships and health, we focused in this book on social and clinical psychological mechanisms for several reasons: (1) psychologists are uniquely suited to understand how socially constructed groups, including intimate pair bonds and families, impact individual functioning; (2) social and clinical are the branches of psychology that have historically had the most interest in relationships; and (3) the editors of this volume are, respectively, a social and clinical psychologist who felt that bringing together these two research worlds would offer rich potentials for cross-talk among disciplines. Of course, the final collection of contributors to this volume included not only social and clinical psychology researchers but developmental psychologists, sociologists, and a physician working in an adolescent medicine unit. What unites the authors is that they are all using social or clinical mechanisms to understand relationships and their impact on health.

That being said, it is interesting that even the lines between social and clinical psychology begin to blur as we read through these chapters. Classically, clinical psychologists are interested in individual differences in what goes wrong with people and, when applied to relationships, this generally translate into how mental illness impacts relationships (and vice versa), what causes disturbed relationships, and prevention and intervention efforts for unhappy, conflicted, or violent couples and families. Social psychologists are also interested in distressed relationships, but they tend to focus on broader normative processes (e.g., commitment) rather than individual differences. Across the various authors and chapters in this volume, we find researchers crossing traditional boundaries to use the theories, methods, and approaches of not only social and clinical psychology but also from genetics, immunology, endocrinology, and other fields. This final synthesizing chapter presents five cross-cutting themes that emerge across the chapters.

THE IMPORTANCE OF QUANTITY AND QUALITY
OF SOCIAL RELATIONSHIPS

One of the strongest themes to emerge from the various chapters in this volume was the importance of not only relationships per se, but the right type of relationships. For example, greater social connections are related to reduced risk for cardiovascular disease (Chapter 2), and the experience of divorce, the loss of perhaps the most important adult relationship, predicts greater mortality (Chapter 4). Many of the chapters in this volume, however, make the point that those in our social network, whether spouses, friends, or others, must be involved in our lives in the right way (e.g., Chapters 2, 5, and 9). There are times in which a close relationship can become a burden and negatively impact health behaviors or health outcomes.

Several of the chapters describe research examining how the quality of one's marital relationship impacts behavioral and physiological health variables. Loving and Keneski (Chapter 1) provide a thorough and lively introduction to the field of psychoneuroimmunology. In particular, they focus on the groundbreaking work by Kiecolt-Glaser and colleagues, who were among the first researchers to document the importance of social relationships for health outcomes (Kiecolt-Glaser & Newton, 2001). Since these original studies documented how quality of social relationships, particularly marital conflict, can have a direct effect on immune functioning, researchers have broadened the scope of inquiry to examine other types of health outcomes. Smith and colleagues (Chapter 2), for example, review a program of research aimed at examining when and how marital functioning, not just marital status per se, impacts cardiovascular disease.

Another important advance in this area of research is the investigation of partner effects—or how aspects of one's partner can affect one's own health and well-being. For instance, Cooper and Zhaoyang (Chapter 11) describe how type of sexual partner (i.e., new or committed) affects the impact of personality on risky sexual behavior. Stephens and colleagues (Chapter 5) also suggest that both spouses are negatively, emotionally affected by the chronic illness suffered by only one partner. There is now substantial research suggesting that a partner's mental health can impact his or her spouse's well-being (Chapter 6, this volume; South, Krueger, & Iacono, 2011; Whisman & Baucom, 2012). These lines of evidence suggest a continued need for examining relationships and health from the perspective of all members of the dyad/family.

THE CHANGING DEMOGRAPHICS OF
INTERPERSONAL RELATIONSHIPS

One implicit theme that ran through many of the chapters was the changing look of relationships, particularly in the United States in 2014. It is well known that approximately half of all first marriages will end in divorce (see Chapter 4). Add to this the increasing age at first marriage and the number of couples who choose to cohabit (before or instead of marrying; Kreider, 2005), as well as the growing number of gay and lesbian couples who choose to enter into civil unions or marriages (in the 17 states and the District of Columba where such marriage is legal as of this writing); as a whole, these changes mean that the modal intimate pair bond is quite different than it was just 30 years ago. Even the Centers for Disease Control and Prevention list 11 different types of intimate partners for purposes of surveying intimate partner violence rates (Chapter 7). Most research on "relationships" and health, however, focuses on the marital relationships of middle- or upper-class heterosexual community participants. We know much less about the quality, communication, interactions, and other aspects of relationship functioning of nonmarried, non-White, homosexual individuals from a diverse range of socioeconomic status. This is slowly, but surely, starting to change. Beach, for instance, explicitly states in Chapter 6 that the couple and family discord model of depression is an expansion of the marital discord model that specifically allows for "a range of romantic couple relationships" (p. 133).

Societal and cultural changes apply not only to intimate romantic relationship pair bonds but also to the makeup and composition of families today. The combination of divorce and remarriage, childbirth during cohabitation, single mothers who are not with committed romantic partners, and both domestic and international adoption (including adoption by homosexual parents) means that today's family is more diverse than ever before. As just one example, more than 40% of births in the United States in 2010 (Martin et al., 2012) were to unwed mothers. No longer is there a "norm" for what families in the United States, and elsewhere, look like. And as with intimate romantic relationships, research on families has only begun to scratch the surface of these various combinations of family members. Future research will need to expand to cover all of these possible family units, to see how they differ (or not) from two-parent, married mother and father units that have dominated Western psychological research on intimate relationships and health. As just one example, research by South and colleagues (2013) found that marital satisfaction of mothers who had recently adopted a child was predicted by partner support, fatigue, and socioeconomic status, not by factors unique to the adoption process, suggesting more similarities than differences between adoptive and biological parents' relationship functioning.

As we move forward, research will also need to expand to cover other aspects of relationships and health that have been traditionally understudied. This volume is fortunate to include chapters from three noted research groups studying, one way or another, aspects of sexual relationships. Two of our contributors focus on sexual relationships of adolescents; obviously this is an important cohort because of the increased risk of sexually transmitted diseases among teenagers and young adults. But our contributors tackle unique and interesting questions not often studied with regard to teenage sexuality—the importance of the interplay between personality and environment on sexual decision-making (Chapter 11) and sexual relationship satisfaction of African American adolescent women (Chapter 10).

THE CENTRALITY OF METHODS

The title of this volume very deliberately includes the word *mechanisms*, and inherent in the study of mechanisms is the importance of using good method. The chapters in this volume include a diverse and exciting use of methods that are starting to uncover some of the mechanisms that explain the observed associations between relationships and health. Several authors emphasize the importance of physiological measures. Sbarra and colleagues (Chapter 4) note that much of the work in the area of relationships and stress-related health outcomes focuses on autonomic nervous system activity, with a particular emphasis on cardiovascular reactivity (see also Chapter 2). Another widely studied physiological variable is cortisol, a stress hormone that is the ultimate end product of the HPA axis. It has been examined in relation to couple interactions (e.g., Kiecolt-Glaser et al., 1996) and coregulation of mood states in couples (Saxbe & Repetti, 2010). Slatcher and colleagues (Chapter 3) give an excellent overview of work examining cortisol in family relationships, including children. They also describe an exciting new program of research using naturalistic measures (the EAR technique) to understand how family conflict impacts cortisol levels and, ultimately, aspects of physical functioning (i.e., asthma). Cummings and colleagues (Chapter 8) also review research that has linked altered cortisol responses in children to marital conflict. In their recent work, they have begun examining the interplay between cortisol and autonomic nervous system activity, an illustrative example of how researchers can attend to multiple physiological systems at once. While genetic techniques have not been as widely utilized as these other measures, it is likely that this will change as the technology becomes cheaper and researchers begin to hypothesize logical connections between potential genetic mechanisms, relationships, and health outcomes. Beach (Chapter 6) for example, details a fascinating program of research looking at measured gene × environment interactions.

Other authors in this volume stress the importance of collecting behavioral measures that may explain links between relationships and health. Murphy and his colleagues (Chapter 7) review the use of the ATSS paradigm, in which participants are asked to respond as naturally as possible to a simulated scenario involving their partner, as a way of eliciting cognitive variables that form part of the biopsychosocial model of interpersonal violence. Smith and colleagues (Chapter 2) have also used behavioral interactions between married couples; of note, they often go behind standard conflict discussion tasks, using supportive tasks designed to elicit positive dimensions of couple behavior or even collaborative problem-solving tasks. These authors also advocate for the use of daily diary methods with couples, to examine the transactional nature of interactions between individual- and couple-level variables (see also Chapter 5). Cooper and Zhaoyang (Chapter 11) use event-level data to examine variance in risky sexual behaviors. Using hierarchical linear modeling, they determined that most of the variability in risky behaviors (e.g., condom use) could be attributed to within-person variation across time, partner, and situation, not between-person differences. This was vitally important in showing that it is not simply characteristics of the person (e.g., personality traits, demographic variables) but an interplay between personality and immediate context of the environment that impacts decisions about sexual behavior.

It is worth emphasizing in this discussion of methods the critical need to explicitly define the variables of interest, whether it is the assessment of social support, health outcome, or some type of mediating mechanism. Stephens and colleagues (Chapter 5) assessed two aspects of social control—encouragement and warning—which were associated with treatment adherence in *opposite* directions. As another group of authors in this volume noted, marital quality may not be a unidimensional concept, and researchers should attempt to assess both negative and positive aspects (Chapter 2). Indeed, there may be a discrete "cut point" beyond which distressed couples are particularly at risk for a host of associated negative outcomes (Chapter 6). Marital conflict can also be understood as an umbrella term for different, maladaptive types of strategies, each of which may have different relationships to outcome variables (Chapter 8). Finally, Loving and Keneski (Chapter 1) note that psychoneuroimmunology studies often have nuanced and methodologically advanced measures of physiological functioning but gross and generalized measures of *stress*.

There is one caveat to our generally positive endorsement of these myriad methodologies. As Smith and colleagues note, "in most studies individual-level risk factors (e.g., personality, emotional adjustment) and social-environmental factors (e.g., social support, isolation, relationship quality) are examined separately" (Chapter 2, p. 45). We advocate for a systematic, multilevel, and longitudinal investigation of giinterpersonal relationships and health, with incorporation of individual-, family-, and environmental-level contextual factors. Sbarra and colleagues (Chapter 4) recommend that research into interpersonal relationships and health should focus on both macro- and micro-level processes. Further, research should focus on long-term longitudinal investigations of relationships and health (Chapter 8), as the impact of relationship changes (e.g., divorce), relationship functioning (e.g., parent–child relations), or exposure to conflict or violence may exert the most important or deleterious effects much later in development. This type of longitudinal, multimethod design will necessitate more complicated analyses, including multilevel modeling and/or longitudinal modeling, which our contributors, like many in the field, are already utilizing. Fortenberry and Hensel (Chapter 10) provide an elegant example of latent growth curve modeling with regard to relationship trajectories and relationship and sexual satisfaction. Following these suggestions may necessitate greater collaborations across disciplines and researchers, which of course can carry additional burdens. However, the cost is likely to be outweighed by the benefits in knowledge gained.

MY KINGDOM FOR A THEORY

Again and again, the contributions to this volume emphasize the importance of theory as a guide for explorations of mechanisms linking interpersonal relationships and well-being. These theories differ as to the ultimate outcome variables, predictors, and mediating/moderating variables, but at a minimum they offer testable hypotheses about biological, environmental, and social pathways from relationships to health. Slatcher (Chapter 3) points to the glucocorticoid resistance theory of why stress is linked to cortisol and poor health. Beach's (Chapter 6) couple and family discord model of depression leads to testable hypotheses about effects of interventions. Cumming's (Chapter 8) emotional security theory sets a framework for examining the effect of interparental conflict on children's health and well-being. Fitting with other authors' calls for multiple levels of analysis, emotional security theory specifically aims to describe the mechanisms and the environmental contexts that explain how family conflict affects child adjustment. Murphy and colleagues (Chapter 7) advocate for the use of a biopsychosocial model of intimate partner violence that includes variables at multiple levels of analysis, including neurobiological, trauma, alcohol, and cultural beliefs, with a particular focus on social information processing as a key mediator between distal and proximal risk factors and perpetration of partner violence. Certainly, these theories are not etched in stone and may, in fact, change as more research is conducted; for example, Murphy and colleagues note that earlier theories of intimate partner violence have not been able to account for subsequent contradictory research (e.g., feminist theories of intimate partner violence and findings that suggest bidirectional aggression between men and women in violent couples).

A WORTHY GOAL: INTERVENTION AND PREVENTION

One particularly worthy goal of understanding social and clinical mechanisms between interpersonal relationships and health, beyond purely scientific advancement, is to ultimately find ways to alleviate problems at this nexus. Some of the effects of relationships on health outcomes described by the contributors to this volume may take years, if not decades, to unfold (e.g., early parental relationships and later adolescent outcomes, see Chapters 6 and 8; marital relationships and atherosclerosis leading to cardiovascular disease, see Chapter 2), while others are more proximal and immediate, including risky sexual behavior leading to sexually transmitted diseases (Chapters 10 and 11) or intimate partner violence and associated legal, mental, and physical health costs (Chapter 7). Thus, the types of intervention or prevention efforts with families, couples, or other important social support figures in a person's life may differ markedly depending on outcome timelines.

Several of our contributors are either currently incorporating their work into intervention and prevention efforts or detail findings that could be implemented into current strategies. Beach (Chapter 6) points to couples treatments that are effective in ameliorating depressive symptoms in the context of distressed and conflicted intimate relationships. He also describes fascinating research which suggests that parents' response to treatment may depend in part on genetic characteristics of their children. Work by Stephens and colleagues (Chapter 5) suggests that certain strategies, including providing encouragement, support, and understanding rather than criticism and irritation, could be implemented right away in couples dealing with chronic disease management. It is our hope that as research into relationships and health continues to progress, the work from our excellent contributors and others will continue to inform strategies that can buffer the negative effects and augment the positive effects of interpersonal relationships on health and well-being.

REFERENCES

Kiecolt-Glaser, J. K., & Newton, T. L. (2001). Marriage and health: His and hers. *Psychological Bulletin, 127*, 472–503.

Kiecolt-Glaser, J. K., Newton, T. L., Cacioppo, J. T., MacCallum, R. C., Glaser, R., & Malarkey, W. B. (1996). Marital conflict and endocrine function: Are men really more physiologically affected than women? *Journal of Consulting and Clinical Psychology, 64*, 324–332.

Kreider, R. M. (2005). *Number, timing, and duration of marriages and divorces: 2001. Current Population Reports, P70-97*. Washington, DC: US Census Bureau.

Martin, J. A., Hamilton, B. E., Ventura, S. J., Osterman, M. J. K., Wilson, E. C., & Matthews, T. J. (2012). *Births: Final data for 2010. National Vital Statistics Reports, 61*. Hyattsville, MD: National Center for Health Statistics.

Saxbe, D., & Repetti, R. L. (2010). For better or for worse? Coregulation of couples' cortisol levels and mood states. *Joural of Personality and Social Psychology, 98*, 92–103.

South, S. C., Foli, K. J., & Lim, E. (2013). Predictors of relationship satisfaction in adoptive mothers. *Journal of Social and Personal Relationships, 30*, 545–563.

South, S. C., Krueger, R. F., & Iacono, W. G. (2011). Understanding general and specific connections between psychopathology and marital distress: A model based approach. *Journal of Abnormal Psychology, 120*, 935–947.

Whisman, M. A., & Baucom, D. H. (2012). Intimate relationships and psychopathology. *Clinical Child and Family Psychology Review, 15*, 4–13.

INDEX

attachment anxiety (*Cont.*)
   separation threat, 95
   stress responses and, 23
attachment avoidance
   conflict behaviors and interleukin-6, 26
   long-term sexual relationships, 259, 260, 261
   stress responses and, 23
attachment theory, 4. *See also* adult attachment
   downstream health effects, 26
   emotional security theory (EST), 9, 181
   PNI approaches, 6
   social defense of children, 182
autonomic nervous system (ANS), 187

Baron, C., 6
Beach, S. R. H., 8, 133, 138, 140, 149, 195, 277,
   278, 280, 281
Behavioral Family Intervention (BFI), 141
behavioral genetics, 56
behavioral marital therapy (BMT), 138–139
Benjamin, M., 162
biological intermediaries, 95
   divorce, social psychophysiology of, 100–101
biological perspectives, 5. *See also* genetic factors
   mortality and social relationships, 18–19
biomeasures, 206
biopsychosocial model, major assumptions, 9–10
blood pressure reactivity, 49
   ambivalent others, 97–98
   divorce-related emotional intrusion, 95
   gender differences over divorce distress, 99
   poor sleep, 53
Bodenmann, G., 139
Bogg, T., 253
borderline personality disorder (BPD), 53–54
Bowlby, J., 23–24
Bradbury, T. N., 135
Brockmann, H., 94
Brody, G. H., 149
Brooks, K. P., 25
Bugyi, P., 93

Cairns, E., 194
"calm and connect" model, 49–50
cancer, 219
cardiovascular disease (CVD)
   behavioral risk factors, 35
   childhood and adolescence, 35, 57
   divorce impact, 100
   lifestyle behaviors, 110
   marital status and quality, 36–37
   modifiable risk factors, 35–36
   posttraumatic stress disorder (PTSD), 53
   psychosocial characteristics, 35
   significance, 34

stress management approaches, 59
stress-related mechanisms, 54
transactional trajectory model, 57–58
cardiovascular reactivity (CVR), 48
cardiovascular responses, 47–49
   men's divorce experience, 99
   social support and, 97–98
cardiovascular system
   allostatic load, 72
   attachment security and insecurity, 24
   overview, 6–7
caregivers of infants, 77–78
Caska, C., 6
Centers for Disease Control and Prevention
   (CDC), 157
chemotherapy, 18
Chen, E., 22
Cheung, R. Y. M., 9
child abuse
   child cortisol levels, 79
   genetic changes, 149
   physical, 171
child adjustment, 180
   emotional security theory and, 183–184
   parental depressive symptoms related,
     188–191
child adversity, 149–150
child cortisol levels, 77–81
   child abuse, 79
   infancy and early childhood, 77–78
   middle childhood, 78–79
   prenatal, 77
children. *See also* emotional security theory
   (EST); marital conflict
   asthma, 81–82
   genetic factors, 147
   impact of parental destructive conflict, 179
   intergenerational patterns of conflict,
     171, 173
   psychopathology and parents' depressive
     symptoms, 136
   social competence model, 164
China, 192
chronic illness
   as couple problem, 7–8, 109, 281
   diabetes management, 111–112
   incidence, 109–110
   intimate partner violence (IPV), 158
   mid to late life, 109–111
   persuasion research, 127
   risk factors, 110
   self-care treatment, 110
   self-regulation and social regulation, 112–114
   spouse's role in management, 112
   type 2 diabetes, 111